Sexually Transmitted Diseases

SOURCEBOOK

Sixth Edition

Health Reference Series

Sixth Edition

Sexually Transmitted Diseases

SOURCEBOOK

Basic Consumer Health Information about Sexual Health and the Screening, Diagnosis, Treatment, and Prevention of Common Sexually Transmitted Diseases (STDs), including Chancroid, Chlamydia, Gonorrhea, Herpes, Hepatitis, Human Immunodeficiency Virus/Acquired Immunodeficiency Syndrome (HIV/AIDS), Human Papillomavirus (HPV), Syphilis, and Trichomoniasis

Along with Facts about Risk Factors and Complications, Trends and Disparities in Infection Rates, Tips for Discussing STDs with Sexual Partners, a Glossary of Related Terms, and Resources for Additional Help and Information

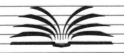

OMNIGRAPHICS

615 Griswold, Ste. 901, Detroit, MI 48226

Bibliographic Note

Because this page cannot legibly accommodate all the copyright notices, the Bibliographic Note portion of the Preface constitutes an extension of the copyright notice.

* * *

Omnigraphics, Inc.

Editorial Services provided by Omnigraphics, Inc.,
a division of Relevant Information, LLC

Keith Jones, *Managing Editor*

* * *

Copyright © 2016 Relevant Information, LLC
ISBN 978-0-7808-1518-6
E-ISBN 978-0-7808-1519-3

Library of Congress Cataloging-in-Publication Data

Names: Omnigraphics, Inc.

Title: Sexually transmitted diseases sourcebook: basic consumer health information about sexual health and the screening, diagnosis, treatment, and prevention of common sexually transmitted diseases (STDs), including chancroid, chlamydia, gonorrhea, herpes, hepatitis, human immunodeficiency virus/acquired immunodeficiency syndrome (HIV/AIDS), human papillomavirus (HPV), syphilis, and trichomoniasis; along with facts about risk factors and complications, trends and disparities in infection rates, tips for discussing stds with sexual partners, a glossary of related terms, and resources for additional help and information.

Description: Sixth edition. | Detroit, MI: Omnigraphics, [2016] | Series: Health reference series | Includes bibliographical references and index.

Identifiers: LCCN 2016011521 (print) | LCCN 2016014568 (ebook) | ISBN 9780780815186 (hardcover: alk. paper) | ISBN 9780780815193 (ebook) | ISBN 9780780815193 (eBook)

Subjects: LCSH: Sexually transmitted diseases--Popular works.

Classification: LCC RC200.2.S387 2016 (print) | LCC RC200.2 (ebook) | DDC 616.95/1--dc23

LC record available at http://lccn.loc.gov/2016011521

Table of Contents

Part III: Complications That May Accompany STD Infection

Part IV: STD Testing and Treatment Concerns

Part V: STD Risks and Prevention

Part VI: Healthy Living with HIV

Part VII: Additional Help and Information

Preface

About This Book

Every year, more than 20 million people in the United States are diagnosed with sexually transmitted diseases (STDs), costing the American healthcare system nearly $16 billion in direct medical costs alone. The Centers for Disease Control and Prevention (CDC) reports that diagnosing, treating, and preventing these potentially life-threatening STDs is one of the greatest public health challenges today. For some STDs, such as the easily treatable chlamydia, the rates of reported cases are on the rise, especially among adolescent girls and young women. The diagnosis rates of other STDs, such as HIV (human immunodeficiency virus), have decreased in recent years due to increased education and prevention efforts. Regardless of prevalence or severity, all STDs have significant health consequences if they are not diagnosed and treated.

Sexually Transmitted Diseases Sourcebook, Sixth Edition, offers basic information about sexual health and the screening, diagnosis, treatment, and prevention of common sexually transmitted diseases, including chancroid, chlamydia, gonorrhea, herpes, hepatitis, human immunodeficiency virus (HIV/AIDS), human papillomavirus (HPV), syphilis, and trichomoniasis. It discusses trends in STD rates, developments in STD vaccine research, tips on talking to doctors and sexual partners, a glossary of related terms, and resources for additional help and information.

How to Use This Book

This book is divided into parts and chapters. Parts focus on broad areas of interest. Chapters are devoted to single topics within a part.

Part I: Introduction to Sexually Transmitted Diseases (STDs) identifies the parts of the male and female reproductive system and discusses STD trends in the United States and worldwide. It also examines the impact of these diseases on women, men, children and teens, and older adults. The part concludes with statistical information on racial and ethnic minorities disproportionately affected by STDs.

Part II: Types of STDs identifies the symptoms, diagnoses, and treatments of common types of STDs, including chancroid, chlamydia, donovanosis, gonorrhea, herpes, hepatitis, HPV, lymphogranuloma venereum, syphilis, and trichomoniasis. The part also includes information on how HIV causes AIDS and the disease's transmission, testing, and treatment, as well as strategies for living with HIV and paying for medical care.

Part III: Complications That May Accompany STD Infection provides information about infections and syndromes that may develop after sexual contact, such as bacterial vaginosis, cytomegalovirus, yeast infection, intestinal parasites, molluscum contagiosum, sexually transmitted gastrointestinal syndromes, pubic lice, and scabies. The part also provides information about conditions related to STDs that can cause long-term health complications for men and women, including cervicitis, congenital syphilis, epididymitis, infertility and pregnancy complications, pelvic inflammatory disease, and vaginitis.

Part IV: STD Testing and Treatment Concerns offers information on HIV testing, screening recommendations for STDs and addresses common issues associated with STD testing, such as maintaining confidentiality and discussing STDs with healthcare providers. Information about the fake and unproven STD treatment products is also included.

Part V: STD Risks and Prevention discusses sexual behaviors that increase the likelihood of STD transmission, such as choosing high-risk partners and using illegal substances. The part also offers tips on talking to sexual partners and adolescents about STDs and addresses the effectiveness of sexual and abstinence education as forms of STD prevention. The part concludes with information about preventing STDs by using safer sex, by using medication after a known exposure to STDs, by preventing the transmission of these diseases from a pregnant woman to her child, and by using STD vaccines and microbicides.

Part VI: Healthy Living with HIV discusses the various aspects involved in living with HIV. It also discusses medical care related to HIV, and how family planning, dieting, and smoking and substance abuse can have an impact on an individual living with HIV. The part concludes with information on traveling abroad with HIV.

Part VII: Additional Help and Information provides a glossary of important terms related to sexually transmitted diseases and a directory of organizations that offer information to people with STDs or their sexual partners.

Bibliographic Note

This volume contains documents and excerpts from publications issued by the following U.S. government agencies: Agency for Heathcare Research and Quality (AHRQ); Centers for Disease Control and Prevention (CDC); National Cancer Institute (NCI); National Institute of Allergy and Infectious Diseases (NIAID); National Institute of Neurological Disorders and Stroke (NINDS); National Institutes of Health (NIH); National Institute on Deafness and Other Communication Disorders (NIDCD); National Institute on Drug Abuse (NIDA); Office of Disease Prevention and Health Promotion (ODPHP); Office on Women's Health (OWH); U.S. Department of Health and Human Services (HHS); U.S. Department of Veterans Affairs (VA); U.S. Equal Employment Opportunity Commission (EEOC); and U.S. Food and Drug Administration (FDA).

In addition, this volume contains copyrighted documents from the following organization: The Nemours Foundation.

It may also contain original material produced by Omnigraphics, Inc. and reviewed by medical consultants.

About the Health Reference Series

The *Health Reference Series* is designed to provide basic medical information for patients, families, caregivers, and the general public. Each volume takes a particular topic and provides comprehensive coverage. This is especially important for people who may be dealing with a newly diagnosed disease or a chronic disorder in themselves or in a family member. People looking for preventive guidance, information about disease warning signs, medical statistics, and risk factors for health problems will also find answers to their questions in the *Health Reference Series*. The *Series*, however, is not intended to serve as a tool for diagnosing illness, in prescribing treatments, or as a substitute for the physician/patient relationship. All people concerned about medical symptoms or the possibility of disease are encouraged to seek professional care from an appropriate health care provider.

A Note about Spelling and Style

Health Reference Series editors use *Stedman's Medical Dictionary* as an authority for questions related to the spelling of medical terms and the *Chicago Manual of Style* for questions related to grammatical structures, punctuation, and other editorial concerns. Consistent adherence is not always possible, however, because the individual volumes within the *Series* include many documents from a wide variety of different producers, and the editor's primary goal is to present material from each source as accurately as is possible. This sometimes means that information in different chapters or sections may follow other guidelines and alternate spelling authorities.

Medical Review

Omnigraphics contracts with a team of qualified, senior medical professionals who serve as medical consultants for the *Health Reference Series*. As necessary, medical consultants review reprinted and originally written material for currency and accuracy. Citations including the phrase, "Reviewed (month, year)" indicate material reviewed by this team. Medical consultation services are provided to the *Health Reference Series* editors by:

Dr. Vijayalakshmi, MBBS, DGO, MD
Dr. Senthil Selvan, MBBS, DCH, MD
Dr. K. Sivanandham, MBBS, DCH, MS (Research), PhD

Our Advisory Board

We would like to thank the following board members for providing initial guidance on the development of this series:

- Dr. Lynda Baker, Associate Professor of Library and Information Science, Wayne State University, Detroit, MI

- Nancy Bulgarelli, William Beaumont Hospital Library, Royal Oak, MI

- Karen Imarisio, Bloomfield Township Public Library, Bloomfield Township, MI

- Karen Morgan, Mardigian Library, University of Michigan-Dearborn, Dearborn, MI

- Rosemary Orlando, St. Clair Shores Public Library, St. Clair Shores, MI

Health Reference Series *Update Policy*

The inaugural book in the *Health Reference Series* was the first edition of *Cancer Sourcebook* published in 1989. Since then, the *Series* has been enthusiastically received by librarians and in the medical community. In order to maintain the standard of providing high-quality health information for the layperson the editorial staff at Omnigraphics felt it was necessary to implement a policy of updating volumes when warranted.

Medical researchers have been making tremendous strides, and it is the purpose of the *Health Reference Series* to stay current with the most recent advances. Each decision to update a volume is made on an individual basis. Some of the considerations include how much new information is available and the feedback we receive from people who use the books. If there is a topic you would like to see added to the update list, or an area of medical concern you feel has not been adequately addressed, please write to:

Managing Editor
Health Reference Series
Omnigraphics, Inc.
615 Griswold, Ste. 901
Detroit, MI 48226

Part One

Introduction to Sexually Transmitted Diseases (STDs)

Chapter 1

Overview of Sexual Health and the Reproductive System

Chapter Contents

3

Section 1.1

Female Reproductive System

This section includes text excerpted from "Female Reproductive System," © 2016 The Nemours Foundation/KidsHealth®. For more information, visit www.kidshealth.org. Reprinted with permission.

About Human Reproduction

All living things reproduce. Reproduction—the process by which organisms make more organisms like themselves—is one of the things that sets living things apart from nonliving matter. But even though the reproductive system is essential to keeping a species alive, unlike other body systems, it's not essential to keeping an individual alive.

In the human reproductive process, two kinds of sex cells, or gametes, are involved. The male gamete, or sperm, and the female gamete, the egg or ovum, meet in the female's reproductive system. When the sperm fertilizes, or meets, the egg, this fertilized egg is called the zygote. The zygote goes through a process of becoming an embryo and developing into a fetus.

Both the male and female reproductive systems are essential for reproduction. The female needs a male to fertilize her egg, even though it is she who carries offspring through pregnancy and childbirth.

Humans, like other organisms, pass certain characteristics of themselves to the next generation through their genes, the special carriers of human traits. The genes that parents pass along are what make their children similar to others in their family, but also what make each child unique. These genes come from the male's sperm and the female's egg.

Most species have two sexes: male and female. Each sex has its own unique reproductive system. They are different in shape and structure, but both are specifically designed to produce, nourish, and transport either the egg or sperm.

Components of the Female Reproductive System

Unlike the male, the human female has a reproductive system located entirely in the pelvis. The external part of the female reproductive organs is called the vulva, which means covering. Located between the legs, the vulva covers the opening to the vagina and other reproductive organs located inside the body.

The fleshy area located just above the top of the vaginal opening is called the mons pubis. Two pairs of skin flaps called the labia (which means lips) surround the vaginal opening. The clitoris, a small sensory organ, is located toward the front of the vulva where the folds of the labia join. Between the labia are openings to the urethra (the canal that carries urine from the bladder to the outside of the body) and vagina. Once girls become sexually mature, the outer labia and the mons pubis are covered by pubic hair.

A female's internal reproductive organs are the vagina, uterus, fallopian tubes, and ovaries.

The vagina is a muscular, hollow tube that extends from the vaginal opening to the uterus. The vagina is about 3 to 5 inches (8 to 12 centimeters) long in a grown woman. Because it has muscular walls, it can expand and contract. This ability to become wider or narrower allows the vagina to accommodate something as slim as a tampon and as wide as a baby. The vagina's muscular walls are lined with mucous membranes, which keep it protected and moist.

The vagina serves three purposes:

1. It's where the penis is inserted during sexual intercourse.

2. It's the pathway that a baby takes out of a woman's body during childbirth, called the birth canal.

3. It provides the route for the menstrual blood (the period) to leave the body from the uterus.

A thin sheet of tissue with one or more holes in it called the hymen partially covers the opening of the vagina. Hymens are often different from female to female. Most women find their hymens have stretched or torn after their first sexual experience, and the hymen may bleed a little (this usually causes little, if any, pain). Some women who have had sex don't have much of a change in their hymens, though.

The vagina connects with the uterus, or womb, at the cervix (which means neck). The cervix has strong, thick walls. The opening of the cervix is very small (no wider than a straw), which is why a tampon can never get lost inside a girl's body. During childbirth, the cervix can expand to allow a baby to pass.

The uterus is shaped like an upside-down pear, with a thick lining and muscular walls—in fact, the uterus contains some of the strongest muscles in the female body. These muscles are able to expand and contract to accommodate a growing fetus and then help push the baby out during labor. When a woman isn't pregnant, the uterus is only about 3 inches (7.5 centimeters) long and 2 inches (5 centimeters) wide.

At the upper corners of the uterus, the fallopian tubes connect the uterus to the ovaries. The ovaries are two oval-shaped organs that lie to the upper right and left of the uterus. They produce, store, and release eggs into the fallopian tubes in the process called ovulation. Each ovary measures about 1½ to 2 inches (4 to 5 centimeters) in a grown woman.

There are two fallopian tubes, each attached to a side of the uterus. The fallopian tubes are about 4 inches (10 centimeters) long and about as wide as a piece of spaghetti. Within each tube is a tiny passageway no wider than a sewing needle. At the other end of each fallopian tube is a fringed area that looks like a funnel. This fringed area wraps around the ovary but doesn't completely attach to it. When an egg pops out of an ovary, it enters the fallopian tube. Once the egg is in the fallopian tube, tiny hairs in the tube's lining help push it down the narrow passageway toward the uterus.

The ovaries are also part of the endocrine system because they produce female sex hormones such as estrogen and progesterone.

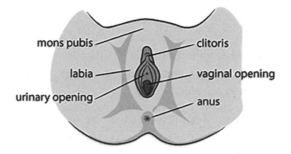

Figure 1.1. *Female Reproductive System*

What the Female Reproductive System Does

The female reproductive system enables a woman to:

- produce eggs (ova)

- have sexual intercourse

- protect and nourish the fertilized egg until it is fully developed

- give birth

Sexual reproduction couldn't happen without the sexual organs called the gonads. Although most people think of the gonads as the male testicles, both sexes actually have gonads: In females the gonads are the ovaries. The female gonads produce female gametes (eggs); the male gonads produce male gametes (sperm). After an egg is fertilized by the sperm, the fertilized egg is called the zygote.

When a baby girl is born, her ovaries contain hundreds of thousands of eggs, which remain inactive until puberty begins. At puberty, the pituitary gland, located in the central part of the brain, starts making hormones that stimulate the ovaries to produce female sex hormones, including estrogen. The secretion of these hormones causes a girl to develop into a sexually mature woman.

Toward the end of puberty, girls begin to release eggs as part of a monthly period called the menstrual cycle. Approximately once a month, during ovulation, an ovary sends a tiny egg into one of the fallopian tubes.

Unless the egg is fertilized by a sperm while in the fallopian tube, the egg dries up and leaves the body about 2 weeks later through the uterus—this is menstruation. Blood and tissues from the inner lining of the uterus combine to form the menstrual flow, which in most girls lasts from 3 to 5 days. A girl's first period is called menarche.

It's common for women and girls to experience some discomfort in the days leading to their periods. Premenstrual syndrome (PMS) includes both physical and emotional symptoms that many girls and women get right before their periods, such as acne, bloating, fatigue, backaches, sore breasts, headaches, constipation, diarrhea, food cravings, depression, irritability, or difficulty concentrating or handling stress. PMS is usually at its worst during the 7 days before a girl's period starts and disappears once it begins.

Many girls also experience abdominal cramps during the first few days of their periods caused by prostaglandins, chemicals in the body that make the smooth muscle in the uterus contract. These involuntary contractions can be either dull or sharp and intense.

It can take up to 2 years from menarche for a girl's body to develop a regular menstrual cycle. During that time, her body is adjusting to the hormones puberty brings. On average, the monthly cycle for an adult woman is 28 days, but the range is from 23 to 35 days.

Fertilization

If a female and male have sex within several days of the female's ovulation, fertilization can occur. When the male ejaculates (when semen leaves a male's penis), between 0.05 and 0.2 fluid ounces (1.5 to 6.0 milliliters) of semen is deposited into the vagina. Between 75 and 900 million sperm are in this small amount of semen, and they "swim" up from the vagina through the cervix and uterus to meet the egg in the fallopian tube. It takes only one sperm to fertilize the egg.

About a week after the sperm fertilizes the egg, the fertilized egg (zygote) has become a multicelled blastocyst. A blastocyst is about the size of a pinhead, and it's a hollow ball of cells with fluid inside. The blastocyst burrows itself into the lining of the uterus, called the endometrium. The hormone estrogen causes the endometrium to become thick and rich with blood. Progesterone, another hormone released by the ovaries, keeps the endometrium thick with blood so that the blastocyst can attach to the uterus and absorb nutrients from it. This process is called implantation.

As cells from the blastocyst take in nourishment, another stage of development, the embryonic stage, begins. The inner cells form a flattened circular shape called the embryonic disk, which will develop into a baby. The outer cells become thin membranes that form around the baby. The cells multiply thousands of times and move to new positions to eventually become the embryo.

After approximately 8 weeks, the embryo is about the size of an adult's thumb, but almost all of its parts—the brain and nerves, the heart and blood, the stomach and intestines, and the muscles and skin—have formed.

During the fetal stage, which lasts from 9 weeks after fertilization to birth, development continues as cells multiply, move, and change. The fetus floats in amniotic fluid inside the amniotic sac. The fetus receives oxygen and nourishment from the mother's blood via the placenta, a disk-like structure that sticks to the inner lining of the uterus and connects to the fetus via the umbilical cord. The amniotic fluid and membrane cushion the fetus against bumps and jolts to the mother's body.

Pregnancy lasts an average of 280 days—about 9 months. When the baby is ready for birth, its head presses on the cervix, which begins to relax and widen to get ready for the baby to pass into and through the vagina. The mucus that has formed a plug in the cervix loosens, and with amniotic fluid, comes out through the vagina when the mother's water breaks.

When the contractions of labor begin, the walls of the uterus contract as they are stimulated by the pituitary hormone oxytocin. The contractions cause the cervix to widen and begin to open. After several hours of this widening, the cervix is dilated (opened) enough for the baby to come through. The baby is pushed out of the uterus, through the cervix, and along the birth canal. The baby's head usually comes first; the umbilical cord comes out with the baby and is cut after the baby is delivered.

The last stage of the birth process involves the delivery of the placenta, which at that point is called the afterbirth. After it has separated from the inner lining of the uterus, contractions of the uterus push it out, along with its membranes and fluids.

Problems of the Female Reproductive System

Some girls might experience reproductive system problems, such as:

Problems of the Vulva and Vagina

- **Vulvovaginitis** is an inflammation of the vulva and vagina. It may be caused by irritating substances (such as laundry soaps or bubble baths) or poor personal hygiene (such as wiping from back to front after a bowel movement). Symptoms include redness and itching in the vaginal and vulvar areas and sometimes vaginal discharge. Vulvovaginitis also can be caused by an overgrowth of Candida, a fungus normally present in the vagina.

- **Nonmenstrual vaginal bleeding** is most commonly due to the presence of a vaginal foreign body, often wadded-up toilet paper. It may also be due to urethral prolapse, in which the mucous membranes of the urethra protrude into the vagina and form a tiny, doughnut-shaped mass of tissue that bleeds easily. It also can be due to a straddle injury (such as when falling onto a gymnastics beam or bicycle frame) or vaginal trauma from sexual abuse.

- **Labial adhesions**, the sticking together or adherence of the labia in the midline, usually appear in infants and young girls. Although there are usually no symptoms associated with this condition, labial adhesions can lead to an increased risk of urinary tract infection. Sometimes topical estrogen cream is used to help separate the labia.

Problems of the Ovaries and Fallopian Tubes

- **Ectopic pregnancy** occurs when a fertilized egg, or zygote, doesn't travel into the uterus, but instead grows rapidly in the fallopian tube. A woman with this condition can develop severe abdominal pain and should see a doctor because surgery may be necessary.

- **Endometriosis** occurs when tissue normally found only in the uterus starts to grow outside the uterus—in the ovaries, fallopian tubes, or other parts of the pelvic cavity. It can cause abnormal bleeding, painful periods, and general pelvic pain.

- **Ovarian tumors**, although they're rare, can occur. Girls with ovarian tumors may have abdominal pain and masses that can be felt in the abdomen. Surgery may be needed to remove the tumor.

- **Ovarian cysts** are noncancerous sacs filled with fluid or semi-solid material. Although they are common and generally harmless, they can become a problem if they grow very large. Large cysts may push on surrounding organs, causing abdominal pain. In most cases, cysts will disappear on their own and treatment is unnecessary. If the cysts are painful, a doctor may prescribe birth control pills to alter their growth or they may be removed by a surgeon.

- **Polycystic ovary syndrome** is a hormone disorder in which too many male hormones (androgens) are produced by the ovaries. This condition causes the ovaries to become enlarged and develop many fluid-filled sacs, or cysts. It often first appears during the teen years. Depending on the type and severity of the condition, it may be treated with drugs to regulate hormone balance and menstruation.

- **Ovarian torsion**, or the twisting of the ovary, can occur when an ovary becomes twisted because of a disease or a developmental abnormality. The torsion blocks blood from flowing through the blood vessels that supply and nourish the ovaries. The most common symptom is lower abdominal pain. Surgery is usually necessary to correct it.

Menstrual Problems

A variety of menstrual problems can affect girls, including:

- **Dysmenorrhea** is when a girl has painful periods.

- **Menorrhagia** is when a girl has a very heavy periods with excess bleeding.

- **Oligomenorrhea** is when a girl misses or has infrequent periods, even though she's been menstruating for a while and isn't pregnant.

- **Amenorrhea** is when a girl has not started her period by the time she is 16 years old or 3 years after starting puberty, has not developed signs of puberty by age 14, or has had normal periods but has stopped menstruating for some reason other than pregnancy.

Infections of the Female Reproductive System

- **Sexually transmitted diseases (STDs)**. Also called sexually transmitted infections (STIs), these include pelvic inflammatory disease (PID), human immunodeficiency virus/acquired immunodeficiency syndrome (HIV/AIDS), human papillomavirus (HPV, or genital warts), syphilis, chlamydia, gonorrhea, and genital herpes (HSV). Most are spread from one person to another by sexual contact.

- **Toxic shock syndrome**. This uncommon but life-threatening illness is caused by toxins released into the body during a type of bacterial infection that is more likely to develop if a tampon is left in too long. It can produce high fever, diarrhea, vomiting, and shock.

If you think your daughter may have symptoms of a problem with her reproductive system or if you have questions about her growth and development, talk to your doctor—many problems with the female reproductive system can be treated.

Section 1.2

Male Reproductive System

"The Male Reproductive System,"
© 2016 Omnigraphics, Inc.
Reviewed December 2015.

The Male Reproductive System

Like all living things, human beings reproduce. Reproduction is essential for the survival of a species. Most species have males and females for that purpose, with each sex having its own reproductive system.

What Are the Differences between the Male and Female Reproductive Systems?

There are many differences between male and female reproductive systems. Unlike the human female reproductive system, most of the parts of the male reproductive system are situated outside the body. Where the female reproductive system releases only one egg every month during the menstrual process, the male reproductive system can produces millions of sperm cells in a day. Each system also has a primary function which is unique to the reproduction process. The main function of the male reproductive system is to produce and deliver sperm as well as produce hormones such as testosterone, which is responsible for many of the important physical changes the male goes through during puberty. In addition to being critical for the natural development of a boy, testosterone is essential to the male reproductive system because it stimulates the ongoing production of sperm.

Function of Male Reproductive System

The external parts of the male reproductive system consist of the penis, scrotum, and testicles.

The internal organs, or accessory glands, include the epididymis, vas deferens, seminal vesicles, urethra, prostate gland, bulbourethral glands and the ejaculatory duct.

External Organs

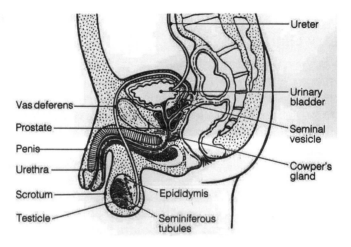

Figure 1.2. *Male Reproductive System*

Penis

The penis is the male organ used during intercourse. It consists of two main parts, the shaft and the glans. The glans is a cone-shaped structure situated at the end of the penis and is covered by foreskin, which is a thin, loose layer of skin, which is sometimes removed by a medical procedure called circumcision. Circumcision is done for many reasons; for hygiene; social, religious or cultural reasons. The tip of the penis contains the opening of the urethra, a tube that transports urine and semen. Inside, the penis consists of sponge-like tissues which absorb blood and makes the penis become erect for intercourse.

Scrotum

The scrotum is a bag-like structure that can be found behind the penis. It contains the testicles, which produce sperm, the male gamete, and sex hormones. Scrotum protects the testicles and adjusts the body temperature to ensure the survival of sperm. Scrotum contains special muscles in its wall which helps it to contract and relax according to the body temperature necessary for the proper functioning of the sperm.

Testicles

Also called testes, the testicles are two oval organs inside the scrotum. Testicles produce hormones including testosterone, and create sperm. The sperm are produced by seminiferous tubules inside the testes.

Accessory Glands

Urethra

The urethra is a long tube that carries urine from the urinary bladder. In boys, it also brings semen out of the body, during ejaculation. During sexual intercourse, when the penis becomes erect, urine is blocked and only the semen is allowed to come out of the urethra.

Epididymis

One of the accessory organs of the male reproductive system, the epididymis is found inside the body. Before transporting the sperm to vas deferens, epididymis matures the sperm cells.

Vas Deferens

The vas deferens is a long muscular tube connecting the epididymis and the pelvic area. The vas deferens is the duct system that carries semen—the sperm nourishing fluid—to the urethra.

Other accessory glands of the male reproductive system include the **ejaculatory ducts** which empty semen into the urethra; the **seminal vesicles** responsible for producing the majority of the fluid found in semen; the **prostate gland** which produces fluids that nourish and protect the sperm, and the **bulbourethral or Cowper's glands** which produce pre-ejaculate to provide lubrication for semen to pass through the urethra.

What Does the Male Reproductive System Do?

All of the organs that make up the male reproductive system are designed to work in harmony to generate and release sperm into the female's vagina during sexual intercourse. Once released into the vagina if a healthy sperm meets a mature egg conception can begin. In addition, the male reproductive system produces hormones that play a vital role in ensuring that a boy will develop into a sexually mature man who is capable of reproducing.

Chapter 2

Understanding Sexually Transmitted Diseases (STDs)

Chapter Contents

Section 2.1

What Is an STD?

This section includes text excerpted from "Sexually Transmitted Diseases (STDs): Overview," National Institute of Child Health and Human Development (NICHD), May 28, 2013.

Sexually Transmitted Diseases (STDs): Overview

Sexually transmitted diseases (STDs), also known as sexually transmitted infections (STIs), are typically caused by bacteria or viruses and passed from person to person during sexual contact with the penis, vagina, rectum, or mouth. The symptoms of STDs/STIs vary between individuals, depending on the cause, and many people may not experience symptoms at all. Many STDs/STIs have significant health consequences. Together with other scientists' investigations at the NIH, the NICHD's research focuses on understanding sexual risk-taking behaviors that increase the likelihood of individuals contracting STDs/STIs, on developing more effective educational interventions to prevent STDs/STIs, and on defining the consequences and optimal treatments for STIs, especially in pregnant women.

What Are STDs and Sexually Transmitted Infections (STIs)?

STDs are a group of illnesses that are passed from person to person during sexual intercourse, oral sex, or sex play. These diseases can be caused by bacteria, viruses, yeasts, or parasites and are spread through intimate sexual contact involving the penis, vagina, mouth, or anus. STDs are also called venereal diseases or STIs. Health care professionals prefer the term "infection" rather than "disease," because it is possible for a person to have no symptoms but still carry the bacterium or virus and require treatment. Scientists have identified more than 20 different STDs/STIs.

How Many People Are Affected by or at Risk for a Sexually Transmitted Disease or Sexually Transmitted Infection (STD/STI)?

Anyone who has had or is having sexual intercourse or oral sex, or who has participated or is participating in sex play, is at risk for acquiring an STD/STI. Fortunately, it is possible for a person to decrease his or her risk by having protected sex and knowing his or her STD/STI status and that of his or her partner. Still, the Centers for Disease Control and Prevention (CDC) estimates nearly 20 million new cases of these reportable STDs/STIs (gonorrhea, chlamydia, syphilis) occur each year in the United States—almost half of them among young people 15 to 24 years of age.

While not the most common STD/STI, HIV/AIDS is one of the most devastating and most well known. Recent data from the CDC indicate that 1.1 million Americans have HIV:

- One in five is unaware that they have the virus.

- Approximately 50,000 Americans become infected with HIV each year.

- 15,529 people with AIDS died in 2010.

What Are the Symptoms of a Sexually Transmitted Disease or Sexually Transmitted Infection (STD/STI)?

People with STDs/STIs may feel ill and notice some of the following signs and symptoms:

- Unusual discharge from the penis or vagina

- Sores or warts on the genital area

- Painful or frequent urination

- Itching and redness in the genital area

- Blisters or sores in or around the mouth

- Abnormal vaginal odor

- Anal itching, soreness, or bleeding

- Abdominal pain

- Fever

In some cases, people with STDs/STIs have no symptoms, and over time the symptoms, if present, can improve on their own. However, it is common for individuals to have an STD/STI and pass it on to others without knowing it.

If you are concerned that you or your sexual partner may have an STD/STI, talk to your health care provider. Even if you do not have symptoms, it is possible you may have an STD/STI that needs to be treated to ensure your and your partner's sexual health.

What Causes a Sexually Transmitted Disease or Sexually Transmitted Infection (STD/STI)?

There are two major causes of STDs/STIs:

1. Bacteria, including chlamydia, gonorrhea, and syphilis

2. Viruses, including HIV/AIDS, herpes simplex virus, human papillomavirus (HPV), hepatitis B virus, and cytomegalovirus, yeasts and protozoan parasites, such as Trichomonas vaginalis, or insects such as crab lice or scabies mites, cause STDs/STIs.

Any STD/STI can be spread through sexual intercourse, and some STDs/STIs also are spread through oral sex and sex play. Ejaculation does not have to occur for an STD/STI to be passed from person to person. Sharing contaminated needles used to inject drugs or using contaminated body piercing and tattooing equipment also can transmit some infections, such as HIV or hepatitis B and C.

A few diseases (such as CMV and molluscum contagiosum) can be sexually transmitted but are also spread through nonsexual, close contact. Regardless of how a person is exposed, once a person is infected by an STD/STI, he or she can spread the infection to other people through oral, vaginal, or anal sex, even if he or she has no symptoms.

STDs/STIs are of particular concern in pregnant women, because some infections can be passed on to the infant before birth or during delivery. However, the risk of transmission from mother to infant can be lowered, and it is important for every expectant mother to be screened.

For example, HIV can be passed from mother to infant during pregnancy before birth, at the time of delivery, or after birth during breastfeeding. This transmission can be prevented through treatment with certain medications during pregnancy and near delivery. After birth, women who have HIV should refrain from breastfeeding their infants if safe alternatives, such as infant formula, are available, further reducing the infant's risk.

In other cases, if the mother has an infection such as gonorrhea or herpes, in which risks of transmission are high during delivery, other steps can be taken to reduce the likelihood that the infant will be infected. In these instances, health care providers can treat the pregnant woman for the STD/STI before birth, or the infant can be delivered by cesarean section (also referred to as C section).

CMV affects about 1% of all births. A pregnant woman infected with CMV can transmit the infection to the fetus in the womb, or it can be passed to the infant during delivery or by breastfeeding. She could also pass it to her newborn after birth if the child comes into contact with her body fluids (for example, saliva or urine) carrying the virus. If a health care provider suspects that a woman has a CMV infection during pregnancy, an ultrasound examination, blood tests, and other tests are done to assess the health of the fetus. Most infants who were infected with the virus during pregnancy do not have any detectable problems after birth. But, 10% or 20% will have serious problems, including deafness and intellectual disabilities. If fetal testing shows increased risk of serious problems, some women opt to end the pregnancy. Researchers are studying antiviral drugs, immune treatments, and other medical approaches to control the infection during pregnancy. Some research is focusing on vaccines to prevent CMV infection.

What Are Some Types of Sexually Transmitted Diseases or Sexually Transmitted Infections (STDs/STIs)?

Approximately 20 different infections are known to be transmitted through sexual contact. Here are descriptions of some of the most common and well known:

- Chlamydia

- Gonorrhea

- Genital Herpes

- HIV/AIDS

- Human Papillomavirus (HPV)

- Syphilis

- Bacterial Vaginosis

- Trichomoniasis
- Viral Hepatitis

How Do Health Care Providers Diagnose a Sexually Transmitted Disease or Sexually Transmitted Infection (STD/STI)?

Any person who is sexually active should discuss his or her risk factors for STDs/STIs with a health care provider and ask about getting tested. If you are sexually active, it is important to remember that you may have an STD/STI and not know it because many STDs/STIs do not cause symptoms. You should get tested and have regular checkups with a health care provider who can help assess and manage your risk, answer your questions, and diagnose and treat an STD/STI if needed.

Starting treatment quickly is important to prevent transmission of infections to other people and to minimize the long-term complications of STDs/STIs. Recent sexual partners should also be treated to prevent re-infection and further transmission.

Some STDs/STIs may be diagnosed during a physical exam or through microscopic examination of a sore or fluid swabbed from the vagina, penis, or anus. This fluid can also be cultured over a few days to see whether infectious bacteria or yeast can be detected. The effects of human papilloma virus (HPV), which causes genital warts and cervical cancer, can be detected in a woman when her health care provider performs a pap smear test and takes samples of cells from the cervix to be checked microscopically for abnormal changes. Blood tests are used to detect infections such as hepatitis A, B, and C or HIV/AIDS.

Because sexually transmitted diseases are passed from person to person and can have serious health consequences, the health department notifies people if they have been exposed to certain STDs/STIs. Not all STDs/STIs are reported, though. If you receive a notice, it is important to see a health care provider, be tested, and start treatment right away.

Screening is especially important for pregnant women, because many STDs/STIs can be passed on to the fetus during pregnancy or delivery. During an early prenatal visit, with the help of her health care provider, an expectant mother should be screened for these infections, including HIV and syphilis. Some of these STDs/STIs can be cured with drug treatment, but not all of them. However, even if the infection is not curable, a pregnant woman can usually take measures to protect her infant from infection.

Is There a Cure for Sexually Transmitted Diseases and Sexually Transmitted Infections (STDs/STIs)?

Viruses such as HIV, genital herpes, human papillomavirus, hepatitis, and cytomegalovirus cause STDs/STIs that cannot be cured. People with an STD/STI caused by a virus will be infected for life and will always be at risk of infecting their sexual partners, although for many viruses treatment significantly reduces this risk. Treatments are available to cure STDs/STIs caused by bacteria, yeast, or parasites.

What Are the Treatments for Sexually Transmitted Diseases and Sexually Transmitted Infections (STDs/STIs)?

STDs/STIs caused by bacteria, yeast, or parasites can be treated with antibiotics. These antibiotics are most often given by mouth (orally). However, sometimes they are injected or applied directly to the affected area. Whatever the infection, and regardless of how quickly the symptoms resolve after beginning treatment, the infected person must take all of the medicine prescribed by the health care provider to ensure that the STD/STI is completely treated.

Although treatments, complications, and outcomes vary among viral STDs/STIs depending on the particular virus (HIV, genital herpes, human papillomavirus, hepatitis, or cytomegalovirus), health care providers can provide treatments to reduce the symptoms and the progression of most of these illnesses. For example, medications are available to limit the frequency and severity of genital herpes outbreaks while reducing the risk that the virus will be passed on to other people.

Individuals with HIV need to take special antiretroviral drugs that control the amount of virus they carry. These drugs, called highly active antiretroviral therapy, or HAART, can help people live longer, healthier lives. If a woman with HIV becomes pregnant, these medicines also can reduce the chance that her fetus or infant will get the infection.

Being tested and treated for STDs/STIs is especially important for pregnant women because some STDs/STIs may be passed on to their infants during pregnancy or delivery. Testing women for these STDs/STIs early in their pregnancy is important, so that steps can be taken to help ensure delivery of a healthy infant. The necessary treatment will depend on the type of STD/STI involved.

Section 2.2

Factors Contributing to the Spread of STDs

This section includes text excerpted from "Sexually
Transmitted Diseases," U.S. Department of Health and
Human Services (HHS), February 15, 2016.

Biological Factors

STDs are acquired during unprotected sex with an infected partner.
Biological factors that affect the spread of STDs include:

- **Asymptomatic nature of STDs**. The majority of STDs
  either do not produce any symptoms or signs, or they produce
  symptoms so mild that they are unnoticed; consequently,
  many infected persons do not know that they need medical
  care.

- **Gender disparities.** Women suffer more frequent and more
  serious STD complications than men do. Among the most serious
  STD complications are pelvic inflammatory disease, ectopic pregnancy (pregnancy outside of the uterus), infertility, and chronic
  pelvic pain.

- **Age disparities.** Compared to older adults, sexually active
  adolescents ages 15 to 19 and young adults ages 20 to 24 are at
  higher risk for getting STDs.

- **Lag time between infection and complications**. Often, a
  long interval, sometimes years, occurs between acquiring an
  STD and recognizing a clinically significant health problem.

Social, Economic, and Behavioral Factors

The spread of STDs is directly affected by social, economic, and
behavioral factors. Such factors may cause serious obstacles to STD
prevention due to their influence on social and sexual networks, access
to and provision of care, willingness to seek care, and social norms
regarding sex and sexuality. Among certain vulnerable populations,

historical experience with segregation and discrimination exacerbates the influence of these factors.

Social, economic, and behavioral factors that affect the spread of STDs include:

- **Racial and ethnic disparities.** Certain racial and ethnic groups (mainly African American, Hispanic, and American Indian/Alaska Native populations) have high rates of STDs, compared with rates for whites. Race and ethnicity in the United States are correlated with other determinants of health status, such as poverty, limited access to health care, fewer attempts to get medical treatment, and living in communities with high rates of STDs.

- **Poverty and marginalization.** STDs disproportionately affect disenfranchised people and people in social networks where high-risk sexual behavior is common, and either access to care or health-seeking behavior is compromised.

- **Access to health care.** Access to high-quality health care is essential for early detection, treatment, and behavior-change counseling for STDs. Groups with the highest rates of STDs are often the same groups for whom access to or use of health services is most limited.

- **Substance abuse.** Many studies document the association of substance abuse with STDs. The introduction of new illicit substances into communities often can alter sexual behavior drastically in high-risk sexual networks, leading to the epidemic spread of STDs.

- **Sexuality and secrecy.** Perhaps the most important social factors contributing to the spread of STDs in the United States are the stigma associated with STDs and the general discomfort of discussing intimate aspects of life, especially those related to sex. These social factors separate the United States from industrialized countries with low rates of STDs.

- **Sexual networks.** Sexual networks refer to groups of people who can be considered "linked" by sequential or concurrent sexual partners. A person may have only 1 sex partner, but if that partner is a member of a risky sexual network, then the person is at higher risk for STDs than a similar individual from a non-risky network.

Emerging Issues in Sexually Transmitted Diseases

There are several emerging issues in STD prevention:

- Each State needs to address system-level barriers to the implementation of expedited partner therapy for the treatment of chlamydia and gonorrheal infections.

- Enhanced data collection on demographic and behavioral variables, such as the sex of an infected person's sex partner(s), is essential to understanding the epidemiology of STDs and to guiding prevention efforts.

- Innovative communication strategies are critical for addressing issues of disparities, facilitating HPV vaccine uptake, and normalizing perceptions of sexual health and STD prevention, particularly as they help reduce health disparities.

- It is necessary to coordinate STD prevention efforts with the health care delivery system to leverage new developments provided by health reform legislation.

Chapter 3

The Global HIV/AIDs Epidemic

Global Statistics

HIV, the virus that causes AIDS, is one of the world's most serious health and development challenges:

- According to the World Health Organization (WHO) Exit Disclaimer, there were approximately 36.9 million people worldwide living with HIV/AIDS at the end of 2014. Of these, 2.6 million were children (<15 years old).

- According to WHO, Exit Disclaimer an estimated 2.0 million individuals worldwide became newly infected with HIV in 2014. This includes over 220,000 children (<15 years). Most of these children live in sub-Saharan Africa and were infected by their HIV-positive mothers during pregnancy, childbirth or breastfeeding.

- A UNAIDS report Exit Disclaimer shows that of the 36.9 million people living with HIV globally, 17.1 do not know they have the virus and need to be reached with HIV testing services, and around 22 million do not have access to HIV treatment, including 1.8 million children.

This chapter includes text excerpted from "The Global HIV/AIDS Epidemic," U.S. Department of Health and Human Services (HHS), November 25, 2015.

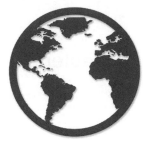

36.9 MILLION

people worldwide are currently living
with HIV/AIDS.

Figure 3.1. *AIDS/HIV Facts*

- The vast majority of people living with HIV are in low- and middle-income countries. According to WHO, Exit Disclaimer sub-Saharan Africa is the most affected region, with 25.8 million people living with HIV in 2014. Sub-Saharan Africa accounts for almost 70 percent of the global total of new HIV infections.

- According to WHO, Exit Disclaimer an estimated 34 million people have died from AIDS-related causes so far, including 1.2 million in 2014.

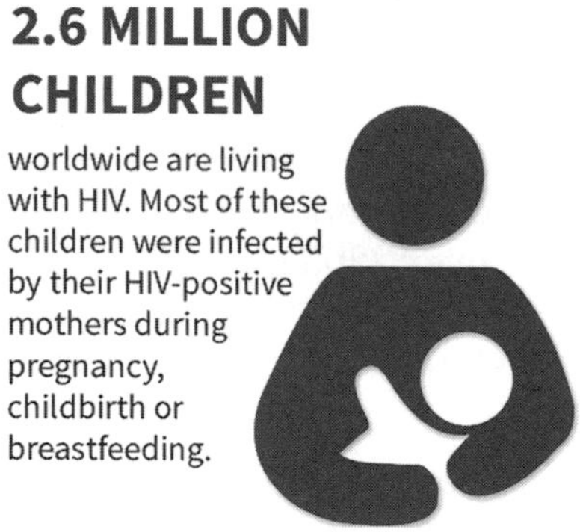

2.6 MILLION CHILDREN

worldwide are living
with HIV. Most of these
children were infected
by their HIV-positive
mothers during
pregnancy,
childbirth or
breastfeeding.

Figure 3.2. *HIV Stats*

- Despite advances in our scientific understanding of HIV and its prevention and treatment as well as years of significant effort by the global health community and leading government and civil society organizations, most people living with HIV or at risk for

The vast majority of people living
with HIV are in low- to middle-income
countries, particularly in
Sub-Saharan Africa.

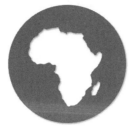

Figure 3.3. *HIV and AIDS in Africa*

IIIV do not have access to prevention, care, and treatment, and there is still no cure. However, effective treatment with antiretroviral drugs can control the virus so that people with HIV can enjoy healthy lives and reduce the risk of transmitting the virus to others.

- The HIV epidemic not only affects the health of individuals, it impacts households, communities, and the development and economic growth of nations. Many of the countries hardest hit by HIV also suffer from other infectious diseases, food insecurity, and other serious problems.

- Despite these challenges, there have been successes and promising signs. New global efforts have been mounted to address the epidemic, particularly in the last decade. Prevention has helped to reduce HIV prevalence rates in a small but growing number of countries and new HIV infections are believed to be on the decline. In addition, the number of people with HIV receiving treatment in resource-poor countries has dramatically increased in the past decade. According to UNAIDS, Exit Disclaimer in June 2015, 15.8 million people living with HIV were accessing antiretroviral therapy (ART) globally, up from 13.6 million in June 2014.

- Progress has been made in preventing mother-to-child transmission of HIV and keeping mothers alive. According to UNAIDS, Exit Disclaimer in 2014, 73% of the estimated 1.5 million pregnant women living with HIV globally were accessing antiretroviral therapy to avoid transmission of HIV to their children; new HIV infections among children were reduced by 58% from 2000 to 2014.

Chapter 4

Trends in STD Infection in the United States

National Overview of Sexually Transmitted Diseases (STDs)

All Americans should have the opportunity to make choices that lead to health and wellness. Working together, interested, committed public and private organizations, communities, and individuals can take action to prevent sexually transmitted diseases (STDs) and their related health consequences. In addition to federal, state, and local public support for STD prevention activities, local community leaders can promote STD prevention education. Health care providers can assess their patients' risks and talk to them about testing. Parents can better educate their children about STDs and sexual health. Individuals can use condoms consistently and correctly, and openly discuss ways to protect their health with partners and providers. As noted in the Institute of Medicine report, The Hidden Epidemic: Confronting Sexually Transmitted Diseases, surveillance is a key component of all our efforts to prevent and control these diseases.

This chapter summarizes national surveillance data for 2014 on the three notifiable diseases for which there are federally funded control programs: chlamydia, gonorrhea, and syphilis.

This chapter includes text excerpted from "Sexually Transmitted Disease Surveillance 2014," Centers for Disease Control and Prevention (CDC), November 2015.

Chlamydia

In 2014, a total of 1,441,789 cases of *Chlamydia trachomatis* infection were reported to the CDC. This case count corresponds to a rate of 456.1 cases per 100,000 population, an increase of 2.8% compared with the rate in 2013. This overall increase follows the first time since nationwide reporting for chlamydia began that the overall rate of reported cases of chlamydia decreased from 2011 to 2013. While the rate in women from 2013–2014 increased 1.3% and the rate in men increased 6.8%, the rate among women aged 15–19 years decreased 4.2%, continuing a decline in that group since 2011.

In 2014, the overall rate of chlamydial infection in the United States among women (627.2 cases per 100,000 females) based on reported cases was over two times the rate among men (278.4 cases per 100,000 males), reflecting the larger number of women screened for this infection. However, with the increased availability of urine testing, men are increasingly being tested for chlamydial infection. During 2010–2014, the chlamydia rate in men increased 22%, compared with a 6% increase in women during this period. Rates varied among different racial and ethnic minority populations. In 2014, the chlamydia rate in blacks was 6 times the rate in whites, and the rate among American Indians/Alaska Natives was almost 4 times the rate among whites.

Gonorrhea

In 2009, the national rate of reported gonorrhea cases reached an historic low of 98.1 cases per 100,000 population. However, during 2009–2012, the rate increased slightly each year, to 106.7 cases per 100,000 population in 2012. In 2013, the rate decreased to 105.3 cases per 100,000 population. But in 2014, a total of 350,062 gonorrhea cases were reported, and the national gonorrhea rate increased to 110.7 cases per 100,000 population.

The increase in gonorrhea rate during 2013–2014 was observed primarily among men. Gonorrhea rates among men increased in every region of the United States, while gonorrhea rates among women increased in the South and West but decreased in the Northeast and Midwest.

In 2014, the rate of reported gonorrhea cases remained highest among blacks (405.4 cases per 100,000 population). The rate among blacks was 10.6 times the rate among whites (38.3 cases per 100,000 population). The gonorrhea rate among American Indians/Alaska Natives (159.4 cases per 100,000 population) was 4.2 times that of whites. While rates of gonorrhea during 2010–2014 have been declining among blacks, they have increased in all other racial/ethnic groups. In American Indian/Alaska Natives, they have increased 104% during this time period.

Antimicrobial resistance remains an important consideration in the treatment of gonorrhea. With increased resistance to the fluoroquinolones and declining susceptibility to cefixime, dual therapy with ceftriaxone and azithromycin is now the only CDC recommended treatment for gonorrhea. In 2014, increases in minimum inhibitory concentrations (MICs) of cephalosporins (cefixime and ceftriaxone) were observed after decreases in 2012 and 2013. While the percentage of isolates with reduced azithromycin susceptibility has remained stable (between 0.3% and 0.6% of all isolates tested) in previous years, between 2013 and 2014, this percentage jumped up to 2.5%. Continued monitoring of susceptibility patterns to these antibiotics is critical.

Syphilis

In 2000 and 2001, the national rate of reported primary and secondary (P&S) syphilis cases was 2.1 cases per 100,000 population, the lowest rate since reporting began in 1941. However, the P&S syphilis rate has increased almost every year since 2000–2001. In 2014, a total of 19,999 P&S syphilis cases were reported, and the national P&S syphilis rate increased to 6.3 cases per 100,000 population, the highest rate since 1994. During 2000–2014, the rise in the P&S syphilis rate was primarily attributable to increased cases among men and, specifically, among gay, bisexual, and other men who have sex with men (collectively referred to as MSM). However, during 2013–2014, the rate increased both among men (14.4%) and among women (22.7%) This increase among women is of particular concern because congenital syphilis cases tend to increase as the rate of P&S syphilis among women increases.

During 2013–2014, the overall male and female P&S syphilis rates increased in every region of the country. Nationally, P&S syphilis rates increased in every 5-year age group of those 15–44 years of age and in every race/ethnicity group except for Native Hawaiians/Other Pacific Islanders during 2013–2014.

In 2014, men accounted for 91% of all cases of P&S syphilis. And, of those male cases for whom sex of sex partner was known, 83% were MSM. Reported cases of P&S syphilis continued to be characterized by a high rate of HIV co-infection, particularly among MSM. In 2014, 26 states reported both sex of sex partner and HIV status (HIV-positive or HIV-negative) for at least 70% of P&S syphilis cases. Among P&S

syphilis cases with known HIV-status in these states, 51% of cases among MSM were HIV-positive, compared with 11% of cases among MSW, and 6% of cases among women.

Rates in women remained unchanged between 2011 and 2013 but increased 22% between 2013 and 2014. In 2014, 1,840 cases of P&S syphilis were reported in women compared with 1,500 in 2013. The 2013 rate of congenital syphilis (9.1 cases per 100,000 live births) marked the first increase in congenital syphilis since 2008. During 2013–2014, the rate increased 27.5%. There were 458 cases of congenital syphilis reported in 2014 compared with 359 in 2013.

Significant racial and ethnic disparities in STD rates persist. In 2014, the P&S syphilis rate among blacks was 5.4 times the rate among whites. In some subgroups, however, disparities were even higher. The 2014 P&S syphilis rates among black and American Indian/Alaska Native women were between 9–10 times the rates for whites. While rates of congenital syphilis increased in most race/ethnicity groups during 2013–2014, they were 10 times higher in blacks than in whites and over 3 times higher in Hispanics and in American Indian/Alaska Natives than in whites.

Chapter 5

Women and STDs

Chapter Contents

Section 5.1

STDs in Women

This section includes text excerpted from "STDs in Women and Infants," Centers for Disease Control and Prevention (CDC), November 17, 2015.

Public Health Impact

Women and infants are at significant risk for long-term consequences of STDs. A woman's relationship status with her male partner, in particular, has been identified as an important predictor of her sexual health. In addition to social factors such as poverty and lack of access to quality STD services, a woman may be unable to negotiate safer sexual practices, such as condom use, which can significantly affect her sexual and reproductive health, as well as the health of her unborn baby.

As an example of how social factors can impact women's health, a perceived shortage of available men in a community can cause women to be more accepting of their partners' concurrent sexual relationships, and partner concurrency is a factor associated with increased risk for STDs. Because it may be her male partner's risk, rather than the woman's that increases a woman's risk for STDs, even a woman who has only one partner may be obliged to practice safer sex such as using condoms. A number of studies have found significant associations between condom use and socio-demographic characteristics, including age, income, education, and acculturation.

Women infected with *C. trachomatis* or N. gonorrhoeae can develop pelvic inflammatory disease (PID), which, in turn, can lead to reproductive morbidity such as ectopic pregnancy and tubal factor infertility. An estimated 10%–20% of women with chlamydia or gonorrhea may develop PID if they do not receive adequate treatment. Among women with PID, tubal scarring can cause infertility in 8% of women, ectopic pregnancy in 9%, and chronic pelvic pain in 18%.

About 80%–90% of chlamydial infections10 and up to 80% of gonococcal infections in women are asymptomatic. These infections are detected primarily through screening. Because the symptoms associated with PID can be nonspecific, up to 85% of women with PID delay seeking medical care, thereby increasing the risk for infertility and ectopic pregnancy. Data from two randomized controlled trials of chlamydia screening suggest that such screening programs reduce PID incidence.

Human papillomavirus (HPV) infections are highly prevalent in the United States, especially among young sexually active women. Although most HPV infections in women resolve within 2 years, they are a major concern because persistent infection with specific types of the virus can cause abnormal cervical cells to be noted on a Papanicolaou (Pap) smear. These abnormal cells can progress to cervical cancer. Other types cause genital warts, low-grade Pap smear abnormalities, and, rarely, recurrent respiratory papillomatosis in infants born to infected mothers.

Impact on Pregnancy Outcomes

Chlamydia and gonorrhea can result in adverse outcomes of pregnancy, including neonatal ophthalmia and, in the case of chlamydia, neonatal pneumonia. Although topical prophylaxis of infants at delivery is effective for prevention of gonococcal ophthalmia neonatorum, prevention of neonatal pneumonia requires prenatal detection and treatment.

Genital infections with herpes simplex virus (HSV) are extremely common, can cause painful outbreaks, and can have serious consequences for pregnant women and their infants.

When a woman has a syphilis infection during pregnancy, she can transmit the infection to the fetus in utero. Transmission can result in fetal death or an infant born with physical and mental developmental disabilities. Most cases of congenital syphilis are easily preventable if women are screened for syphilis and treated early during prenatal care.

Observations

Chlamydia—United States

Chlamydial infections in women are usually asymptomatic and screening is necessary to identify most infections. Routine chlamydia screening of sexually-active young women has been recommended by CDC since 1993. Rates of reported cases among women increased steadily from the early 1990s likely reflecting expanded screening coverage and use of more sensitive diagnostic tests. During 2011–2013, rates decreased from 643.4 to 619.0 cases per 100,000 females and then increased 1.3% to 627.2 per 100,000 in 2014.

Chlamydia rates are highest among young women, the population targeted for screening. During 2013–2014, rates of reported chlamydia decreased 4.2% among females aged 15–19 years and increased 1.6% among females aged 20–24 years. Regionally, chlamydia case rates are highest among women in the South, with a rate of 694.4 per 100,000 females in 2014. Rates of reported chlamydia exceeded gonorrhea rates among women in all regions.

Gonorrhea—United States

Like chlamydia, gonorrhea is often asymptomatic in women. Thus, gonorrhea screening is an important strategy for the identification of gonorrhea among women. Large-scale screening programs for gonorrhea in women began in the 1970s. After an initial increase in cases detected through screening, rates of reported gonorrhea cases for both women and men declined steadily throughout the 1980s and early 1990s and then declined more gradually in the late 1990s and the 2000s. After reaching a 40-year low in 2009 (104.5 cases per 100,000 females), the gonorrhea rate for women increased slightly each year during 2009–2011, but then decreased each year during 2012–2014. In 2014, the gonorrhea rate among women decreased to 101.3 cases per 100,000 females.

The gonorrhea rate among women was slightly higher than the rate among men during 2001–2012, but the rate among men was higher than the rate among women in 2013 and 2014. Gonorrhea rates are highest among young women. Among young women and adolescents, rates were highest in 2014 among 19-year old females (643.9 per 100,000 females).

Congenital Syphilis

Trends in congenital syphilis usually follow trends in primary and secondary syphilis (P&S) among women, with a lag of 1–2 years. The rate of reported P&S syphilis cases among women declined 95.4% (from 17.3 to 0.8 cases per 100,000 females) during 1990–2004. Since 2004, the rate has fluctuated. It increased during 2005–2008 to 1.5 cases per 100,000 females in 2008, decreased during 2009–2011 to 0.9 cases per 100,000 females in 2011, and plateaued at 0.9 cases per 100,000 females during 2012–2013. In 2014, the P&S syphilis rate among women increased to 1.1 cases per 100,000 females. This represents a 22.2% increase relative to 2013.

Similarly, the reported rate of congenital syphilis cases declined by 92.4% during 1991–2005, from a peak of 107.6 cases per 100,000 live births in 1991 to 8.2 cases per 100,000 live births in 2005, but has fluctuated since 2005. The congenital syphilis rate increased during 2006–2008 to 10.5 cases per 100,000 live births in 2008, decreased during 2009–2012 to 8.4 cases per 100,000 live births in 2012, and subsequently increased each year in 2013 and 2014, to 11.6 cases per 100,000 live births in 2014. This increase in 2014 represents a 27.5% increase relative to 2013 and a 19.6% increase relative to 2010.

As in previous years, the highest rates of P&S syphilis among women and the highest rates of congenital syphilis were observed in the South. However, all regions experienced an increase in the rate of P&S syphilis among women and the rate of congenital syphilis during 2013–2014. The largest increases in the rate of P&S syphilis among women were seen in the West (50.0%), followed by the Midwest (28.5%), Northeast (25%), and South (7.1%). The largest increases in the rate of congenital syphilis were seen in the Northeast (74.1%), followed by the West (63.6%), the Midwest (32.8%), and the South (9.2%).

Although most cases of congenital syphilis occur among infants whose mothers have had some prenatal care, late or limited prenatal care has been associated with congenital syphilis. Failure of health care providers to adhere to maternal syphilis screening recommendations also contributes to the occurrence of congenital syphilis.

Pelvic Inflammatory Disease (PID)

Accurate estimates of pelvic inflammatory disease (PID) and tubal factor infertility resulting from chlamydial and gonococcal infections are difficult to obtain, in part because definitive diagnoses of these conditions can be complex. Published data suggest overall declining rates of women diagnosed with PID in the United States in both hospital and ambulatory settings. The National Disease and Therapeutic Index (NDTI) provides estimates of initial visits to office-based, private physicians for PID. NDTI estimated that from 2004–2013 the number of visits to such physicians for PID among women aged 15–44 decreased (39.8%) from 123,000 to 88,000 visits. The 2014 NDTI data were not obtained in time to include them in this report. Several suggestions have been put forth as factors that could influence PID rates, including increases in chlamydia and gonorrhea screening coverage, more sensitive diagnostic technologies, and availability of single-dose therapies that increase adherence to treatment. While PID is declining nationally, it still causes an enormous amount of unnecessary and expensive morbidity.

Section 5.2

How Do STDs Impact Women Differently Than Men?

This section includes text excerpted from "10 Ways STDs Impact Women Differently from Men," Centers for Disease Control and Prevention (CDC), April 2011. Reviewed April 2016.

STDs in Women

Sexually transmitted diseases (STDs) remain a major public health challenge in the U.S., especially among women, who disproportionately bear the long-term consequences of STDs. For example, each year untreated STDs cause infertility in at least 24,000 women in the U.S., and untreated syphilis in pregnant women results in infant death in up to 40 percent of cases. Testing and treatment are keys to reducing disease and infertility associated with undiagnosed STDs. Why are women so severely affected by STDs?

Below are 10 ways STDs impact women differently from men.

1. A Woman's Anatomy Can Place Her at a Unique Risk for STD Infection, Compared to a Man.

- The lining of the vagina is thinner and more delicate than the skin on a penis, so it's easier for bacteria and viruses to penetrate.

- The vagina is a good environment (moist) for bacteria to grow.

2. Women Are Less Likely to Have Symptoms of Common STDs—Such as Chlamydia and Gonorrhea—Compared to Men.

- If symptoms do occur, they can go away even though the infection may remain.

38

3. Women Are More Likely to Confuse Symptoms of an STD for Something Else.

- Women often have normal discharge or think that burning/itching is related to a yeast infection.

- Men usually notice symptoms like discharge because it is unusual.

4. Women May Not See Symptoms as Easily as Men.

- Genital ulcers (like from herpes or syphilis) can occur in the vagina and may not be easily visible, while men may be more likely to notice sores on their penis.

5. STDs Can Lead to Serious Health Complications and Affect a Woman's Future Reproductive Plans.

- Untreated STDs can lead to pelvic inflammatory disease, which can result in infertility and ectopic pregnancy.

- Chlamydia (one of the most common STDs) results in few complications in men.

6. Women Who Are Pregnant Can Pass STDs to Their Babies.

- Genital herpes, syphilis and HIV can be passed to babies during pregnancy and at delivery.

- The harmful effects of STDs in babies may include stillbirth (a baby that is born dead), low birth weight (less than five pounds), brain damage, blindness and deafness.

7. Human Papillomavirus (HPV) Is the Most Common Sexually Transmitted Infection in Women, and Is the Main Cause of Cervical Cancer.

While HPV is also very common in men, most do not develop any serious health problems

8. Women Typically See Their Doctor More Often than Men

Women should use this time with their doctor as an opportunity to ask for STD testing, and not assume STD testing is part of their annual exam. While the Pap test screens for cervical cancer, it is not a good test for other types of cancer or STDs.

9. There Is a Vaccine to Prevent HPV; And Available Treatments for Other STDs Can Prevent Serious Health Consequences, Such as Infertility, If Diagnosed and Treated Early.

10. There Are Resources Available for Women to Learn More about Actions They Can Take to Protect Themselves and Their Partners from STDs, and Where to Receive Testing and Treatment.

- **Health care providers**—A doctor or physician can provide patient-specific information about STD prevention, protection and tests

- **1-800-CDC-INFO (232-4636)**—Operators can provide information about local STD testing sites and put callers in touch with trained professionals to answer questions about STDs

- **FindSTDTest.org**—This website provides users with locations for HIV and STD testing and STD vaccines around the United States

- **www.cdc.gov/std**—CDC's website includes comprehensive information about STDs, including fact sheets on STDs and Pregnancy (www.cdc.gov/std/ pregnancy) and STDs and Infertility (www.cdc.gov/std/ infertility)

Section 5.3

STDs in Women Who Have Sex with Women

This section includes text excerpted from "Lesbian and
Bisexual Health Fact Sheet," Office on Women's
Health (OWH), July 16, 2012. Reviewed April 2016.

What Does It Mean to Be a Lesbian?

A lesbian is a woman who is sexually attracted to another woman
or who has sex with another woman, even if it is only sometimes. A
lesbian is currently only having sex with a woman, even if she has had
sex with men in the past.

What Does It Mean to Be a Bisexual?

A bisexual person is sexually attracted to, or sexually active with,
both men and women.

There are a lot of things that can cause health problems for lesbians
and bisexual women. Some of these may be outside of your control.
Other things you can work to improve upon. These include:

Lack of fitness. Being obese and not exercising can raise your risk
of heart disease, some cancers, and early death.

Research shows that lesbian and bisexual women are more likely
to have a higher BMI if they:

- Are African American or Latina

- Are older

- Have poor health

- Have a lower level of education

- Don't exercise often

- Live with a female partner

Smoking. Smoking can lead to heart disease and cancers of the
lung, throat, stomach, colon, and cervix. The group of women most likely

41

to smoke is bisexual women. Lesbians are also more likely to smoke than heterosexual women are. Researchers think that higher rates of smoking among lesbians and bisexual women are due to:

- Tobacco ads aimed at gays and lesbians
- Differences in community norms
- Low self-esteem
- Stress from bias
- Anxiety from hiding one's sexual orientation

Alcohol and drug abuse. Substance abuse is a serious health problem for all people in the U.S. Recent data suggests that substance use among lesbians—mostly alcohol use—has gone down over the past two decades. Reasons for this may include:

- More general knowledge and concern about health
- More moderate drinking among women in general
- Some decrease in the social stigma and oppression of lesbians
- Changing norms around drinking in some lesbian groups

But, heavy drinking and drug abuse appear to be more common among lesbians (especially young women) than heterosexual women. Lesbian and bisexual women are also more likely to drink alcohol and smoke marijuana in moderation than other women are. Bisexual women are the most likely to have injected drugs, putting them at a higher risk for sexually transmitted infections (STIs).

Domestic violence. Also called intimate partner violence, this is when someone purposely causes either physical or mental harm to someone else. Domestic violence can occur in lesbian relationships (as it does in heterosexual ones). But, lesbian victims are more likely to stay silent about the violence. Some reasons include:

- Fewer services available to help lesbians and bisexual women
- Fear of discrimination
- Threats from the batterer to "out" the victim
- Fear of losing custody of children

There are many resources available to women who are victims of domestic violence. All women should seek help and safety from domestic violence.

Are Lesbian and Bisexual Women at Risk of Getting Sexually Transmitted Infections (STIs)?

Women who have sex with women are at risk for STIs. Lesbian and bisexual women can transmit STIs to each other through:

- Skin-to-skin contact
- Mucosa contact (e.g., mouth to vagina)
- Vaginal fluids
- Menstrual blood
- Sharing sex toys

Some STIs are more common among lesbians and bisexual women and may be passed easily from woman to woman (such as bacterial vaginosis). Other STIs are much less likely to be passed from woman to woman through sex (such as HIV). When lesbians get these less common STIs, it may be because they also have had sex with men, especially when they were younger. It is also important to remember that some of the less common STIs may not be passed between women during sex, but through sharing needles used to inject drugs. Bisexual women may be more likely to get infected with STIs that are less common for lesbians, since bisexuals have typically had sex with men in the past or are presently having sex with a man.

Common STIs That Can Be Passed between Women:

Bacterial vaginosis (BV). BV is more common in lesbian and bisexual women than in other women. The reason for this is unknown. BV often occurs in both members of lesbian couples.

The vagina normally has a balance of mostly "good" bacteria and fewer "harmful" bacteria. BV develops when the balance changes. With BV, there is an increase in harmful bacteria and a decrease in good bacteria.

Sometimes BV causes no symptoms. But over one-half of women with BV have vaginal itching or discharge with a fishy odor. BV can be treated with antibiotics.

Chlamydia. Chlamydia is caused by bacteria. It's spread through vaginal, oral, or anal sex. It can damage the reproductive organs, such as the uterus, ovaries, and fallopian tubes. The symptoms of chlamydia are often mild—in fact, it's known as a "silent infection." Because the symptoms are mild, you can pass it to someone else without even knowing you have it.

Chlamydia can be treated with antibiotics. Infections that are not treated, even if there are no symptoms, can lead to:

- Lower abdominal pain

- Lower back pain

- Nausea

- Fever

- Pain during sex

- Bleeding between periods

Genital herpes. Genital herpes is an STI caused by the herpes simplex viruses type 1 (HSV-1) or type 2 (HSV-2). Most genital herpes is caused by HSV-2. HSV-1 can cause genital herpes. But it more commonly causes infections of the mouth and lips, called "fever blisters" or "cold sores." You can spread oral herpes to the genitals through oral sex.

Most people have few or no symptoms from a genital herpes infection. When symptoms do occur, they usually appear as one or more blisters on or around the genitals or rectum. The blisters break, leaving tender sores that may take up to four weeks to heal. Another outbreak can appear weeks or months later. But it almost always is less severe and shorter than the first outbreak.

Although the infection can stay in the body forever, the outbreaks tend to become less severe and occur less often over time. You can pass genital herpes to someone else even when you have no symptoms.

There is no cure for herpes. Drugs can be used to shorten and prevent outbreaks or reduce the spread of the virus to others.

Human papillomavirus (HPV). HPV can cause genital warts. If left untreated, HPV can cause abnormal changes on the cervix that can lead to cancer. Most people don't know they're infected with HPV because they don't have symptoms. Usually the virus goes away on its own without causing harm. But not always. The Pap test checks for abnormal cell growths caused by HPV that can lead to cancer in women. If you are age 30 or older, your doctor may also do an HPV test with your Pap test. This is a DNA test that detects most of the high-risk types of HPV. It helps with cervical cancer screening. If you're younger than 30 years old and have had an abnormal Pap test result, your doctor may give you an HPV test. This test will show if HPV caused the abnormal cells on your cervix.

Both men and women can spread the virus to others whether or not they have any symptoms. Lesbians and bisexual women can transmit HPV through direct genital skin-to-skin contact, touching, or sex toys used with other women. Lesbians who have had sex with men are also at risk of HPV infection. This is why regular Pap tests are just as important for lesbian and bisexual women as they are for heterosexual women.

There is no treatment for HPV, but a healthy immune (body defense) system can usually fight off HPV infection. Two vaccines (Cervarix and Gardasil) can protect girls and young women against the types of HPV that cause most cervical cancers. The vaccines work best when given before a person's first sexual contact, when she could be exposed to HPV. Both vaccines are recommended for 11 and 12-year-old-girls. But the vaccines also can be used in girls as young as 9 and in women through age 26 who did not get any or all of the shots when they were younger. These vaccines are given in a series of 3 shots. It is best to use the same vaccine brand for all 3 doses. Ask your doctor which brand vaccine is best for you. Gardasil also has benefits for men in preventing genital warts and anal cancer caused by HPV. It is approved for use in boys as young as 9 and for young men through age 26. The vaccine does not replace the need to wear condoms to lower your risk of getting other types of HPV and other sexually transmitted infections. If you do get HPV, there are treatments for diseases caused by it. Genital warts can be removed with medicine you apply yourself or treatments performed by your doctor. Cervical and other cancers caused by HPV are most treatable when found early. There are many options for cancer treatment.

Pubic lice. Also known as crabs, pubic lice are small parasites that live in the genital areas and other areas with coarse hair. Pubic lice are spread through direct contact with the genital area. They can also be spread through sheets, towels, or clothes. Pubic lice can be treated with creams or shampoos you can buy at the drug store.

Trichomoniasis or **"Trich."** Trichomoniasis is caused by a parasite that can be spread during sex. You can also get trichomoniasis from contact with damp, moist objects, such as towels or wet clothes. Symptoms include:

- Yellow, green, or gray vaginal discharge (often foamy) with a strong odor
- Discomfort during sex and when urinating

45

- Irritation and itching of the genital area

- Lower abdominal pain (in rare cases)

Trichomoniasis can be treated with antibiotics.
Less Common STIs That May Affect Lesbians and Bisexual Women Include:

Gonorrhea. Gonorrhea is a common STI but is not commonly passed during woman to woman sex. However, it *could* be since it does live in vaginal fluid. It is caused by a type of bacteria that can grow in warm, moist areas of the reproductive tract, like the cervix, uterus, and fallopian tubes in women. It can grow in the urethra in men and women. It can also grow in the mouth, throat, eyes, and anus. Even when women have symptoms, they are often mild and are sometimes thought to be from a bladder or other vaginal infection.
Symptoms include:

- Pain or burning when urinating

- Yellowish and sometimes bloody vaginal discharge

- Bleeding between menstrual periods

Gonorrhea can be treated with antibiotics.

Hepatitis B. Hepatitis B is a liver disease caused by a virus. It is spread through bodily fluids, including blood, semen, and vaginal fluid. People can get hepatitis B through sexual contact, by sharing needles with an infected person, or through mother-to-child transmission at birth. Some women have no symptoms if they get infected with the virus.
Women with symptoms may have:

- Mild fever

- Headache and muscle aches

- Tiredness

- Loss of appetite

- Nausea or vomiting

- Diarrhea

- Dark-colored urine and pale bowel movements

- Stomach pain

- Yellow skin and whites of eyes

There is a vaccine that can protect you from hepatitis B.

HIV/AIDS. The human immunodeficiency virus (HIV) is spread through body fluids, such as blood, vaginal fluid, semen, and breast milk. It is primarily spread through sex with men or by sharing needles. Women who have sex with women can spread HIV, but this is rare. Some women with HIV may have no symptoms for 10 years or more.

Women with HIV symptoms may have:

- Extreme fatigue (tiredness)

- Rapid weight loss

- Frequent low-grade fevers and night sweats

- Frequent yeast infections (in the mouth)

- Vaginal yeast infections

- Other STIs

- Pelvic inflammatory disease (an infection of the uterus, ovaries, or fallopian tubes)

- Menstrual cycle changes

- Red, brown, or purplish blotches on or under the skin or inside the mouth, nose, or eyelids

AIDS, or acquired immunodeficiency syndrome, is the final stage of HIV infection. HIV infection turns to AIDS when you have one or more opportunistic infections, certain cancers, or a very low CD4 cell count.

Syphilis. Syphilis is an STI caused by bacteria. It's passed through direct contact with a syphilis sore during vaginal, anal, or oral sex. Untreated syphilis can infect other parts of the body. It is easily treated with antibiotics. Syphilis is very rare among lesbians. But, you should talk to your doctor if you have any sores that don't heal.

What Challenges Do Lesbian and Bisexual Women Face in the Health care System?

Lesbians and bisexual women face unique problems within the health care system that can hurt their health. Many health care professionals have not had enough training to know the specific health issues that lesbians and bisexuals face. They may not ask about sexual orientation when taking personal health histories. Health care professionals may not think that a lesbian or bisexual woman, like any woman, can be a healthy, normal female.

Things that can stop lesbians and bisexual women from getting good health care include:

- Being scared to tell your doctor about your sexuality or your sexual history

- Having a doctor who does not know your disease risks or the issues that affect lesbians and bisexual women

- Not having health insurance. Many lesbians and bisexuals don't have domestic partner benefits. This means that one person does not qualify to get health insurance through the plan that the partner has (a benefit usually available to married couples).

- Not knowing that lesbians are at risk for STIs and cancer

For these reasons, lesbian and bisexual women often avoid routine health exams. They sometimes even delay seeking health care when feeling sick. It is important to be proactive about your health, even if you have to try different doctors before you find the right one. Early detection—such as finding cancer early before it spreads—gives you the best chance to do something about it. That's one example of why it's important to find a doctor who will work with you to identify your health concerns and make a plan to address them.

Chapter 6

Sexually Transmitted Diseases in Men

Chapter Contents

Section 6.1

HIV/AIDS in Men

This section includes text excerpted from "HIV among
Men in the United States," Centers for Disease
Control and Prevention (CDC), April 15, 2015.

Quick Stats

- Men accounted for 76% of all adults and adolescents living with
  HIV infection at the end of 2010 in the United States.

- Men who have sex with men account for most new and existing
  HIV infections among men.

- By race/ethnicity, black men have the highest rates of new HIV
  infections among all men.

In 2010, an estimated 1.1 million people aged 13 years or older were
living with HIV infection in the United States. Most (76%) of those
living with HIV were male, and 69% of males were gay, bisexual, and
other men who have sex with men (MSM).

In 2010, the most recent year for which new HIV infection data
are available, men accounted for 80% (38,000) of the estimated 47,500
new HIV infections. Most infections occurred in adults aged 25 to 34
years, except among black/African American men, for whom 38% of
all new infections occurred in the youngest age group, 13 to 24 years.

HIV Infection in 2010

- There were an estimated 38,000 new HIV infections among men
  in the United States. Seventy-eight percent (29,800) of these
  were among MSM.

- Of the 38,000 total estimated new HIV infections in US men,
  39% (14,700) were in blacks, 35% (13,200) were in whites, and
  22% (8,500) were in Hispanics/Latinos.

- The rate of estimated new HIV infections among black men
  (per 100,000) was 103.6—six and a half times that of white

men (15.8) and more than twice the rate among Hispanic/Latino men (45.5).

HIV and AIDS Diagnoses and Deaths

- The Centers for Disease Control and Prevention (CDC) estimates that 1 in 51 men will receive a diagnosis of HIV infection at some point in their lifetimes. Over the course of their lifetimes, 1 in 16 black men will be diagnosed with HIV infection, as will 1 in 33 Native Hawaiian/Other Pacific Islander men, 1 in 36 Hispanic/ Latino men, 1 in 100 American Indian/Alaska Native men, 1 in 102 white men, and 1 in 145 Asian men.

- Overall, an estimated 16% of all adults and adolescents living with HIV infection in 2010 were undiagnosed. Among men, greater percentages of undiagnosed HIV infections were attributed to male-to-male sexual contact (19%) and heterosexual contact (19%)e compared to other transmission categories.

- In 2011, 79% (38,825) of the 49,273 estimated new diagnoses of HIV infection (including children) in the United States were among adult and adolescent men. Black/African American men had the highest rate of HIV diagnosis among all races/ethnicities.

- In 2011, 75% (24,088) of the 32,052 estimated AIDS diagnoses in the United States (including children) were among men. Men represent 79% (913,368) of the estimated 1,155,792 people (including children) diagnosed with AIDS in the United States through the end of 2011.

- In 2010, 74% (11,515) of the estimated 15,529 people with a diagnosis of AIDS who died in the United States (regardless of cause of death) were men.

- From 2000 to 2010, HIV infection was the 7th leading cause of death overall for black men, but was not a leading cause of death for other races/ethnicities.

Prevention Challenges

Like other populations affected by HIV, men face a number of risk factors that contribute to their risk for HIV infection.

Sexual contact: Most HIV infections in men are transmitted through sexual contact, especially anal sex.

Sexually transmitted infections (STIs): The presence of some STIs greatly increases the likelihood of acquiring or transmitting HIV. Rates of gonorrhea and syphilis are higher among black men than among white or Hispanic/Latino men. Rates of syphilis have increased in recent years among MSM.

Injection drug and other substance use: The use of injection drugs or other substances may increase the risk of HIV infection through sharing injection equipment contaminated with HIV or engaging in high-risk behaviors, such as unprotected sex, when under the influence of drugs or alcohol.

Section 6.2

STDs in Men Who Have Sex with Men

This section includes text excerpted from "CDC Fact Sheet: What Gay, Bisexual and Other Men Who Have Sex with Men Need to Know about Sexually Transmitted Diseases," Centers for Disease Control and Prevention (CDC), November 17, 2015.

What Are Sexually Transmitted Diseases?

Sexually transmitted diseases (STDs) are very common in the United States—half of all sexually active people will get an STD by age 25. These diseases can be passed from one person to another through intimate physical contact and sexual activity.

Am I at Risk for STDs?

While anyone who has sex can get an STD, sexually active gay, bisexual and other men who have sex with men (MSM) are at greater risk. In addition to having higher rates of syphilis, more than half of all new HIV infections occur among MSM. Many factors contribute to the higher rates of STDs among MSM:

- Higher rates of HIV and STDs among MSM increase a person's risk of coming into contact with an infected partner and becoming infected themselves.

- Certain behaviors, such as not using condoms regularly and having anal sex increase STD risk.

- Homophobia, stigma, and discrimination can negatively influence the health of gay, bisexual, and other men who have sex with men.

How Are STDs Spread?

STDs are spread through sexual contact with someone who has an STD. Sexual contact includes oral, anal, and vaginal sex, as well as genital skin-to-skin contact.

Some STDs—like HIV, chlamydia and gonorrhea—are spread through sexual fluids, like semen. Other STDs, including HIV and hepatitis B, are also spread through blood. Genital herpes, syphilis, and human papillomavirus (HPV) are most often spread through genital skin-to-skin contact.

How Will I Know If I Have an STD?

Most STDs have no signs or symptoms, so you (or your partner) could be infected and not know it. The only way to know your STD status is to get tested. Having an STD such as herpes makes it easier to get HIV, so it's important to get tested to protect your health and the health of your partner. CDC recommends sexually active gay, bisexual and other MSM test for:

- HIV at least once a year;

- Syphilis;

- Hepatitis B;

- Hepatitis C based on risk factors;

- Chlamydia and gonorrhea of the rectum if you've had receptive anal sex, or been a "bottom" in the past year;

- Chlamydia and gonorrhea of the penis (urethra) if you have had insertive anal sex or received oral sex in the past year;

- Gonorrhea of the throat if you've performed oral sex (i.e., your mouth on your partner's penis, vagina, or anus) in the past year;

- And sometimes your health care provider may suggest a herpes test.

Your health care provider can offer you the best care if you discuss your sexual history openly. You should have a provider you are comfortable with. CDC's Lesbian, Gay, Bisexual and Transgender Health Services page will help you find health services that are gay-friendly.

Can STDs Be Treated?

Some STDs (like gonorrhea, chlamydia and syphilis) can be cured with medication. If you are ever treated for an STD, be sure to finish all of your medicine, even if you feel better. Your partner should be tested and treated, too. It is important to remember that you are at risk for the same or a new STD every time you have unprotected sex (not using a condom) and/or have sex with someone who has an STD.

Other STDs like herpes and HIV cannot be cured, but medicines can be prescribed to manage symptoms.

How Can I Protect Myself?

For anyone, choosing to be sexually active means you are at risk for STDs. However, there are many things you can do to protect your health. You can learn about how STDs are spread and how you can reduce your risk of getting infected.

Get Vaccinated: Gay, bisexual and other MSM are at greater risk for hepatitis A, hepatitis B, and the human papillomavirus (HPV). For this reason, CDC recommends that you be vaccinated against hepatitis A and hepatitis B. The human papillomavirus (HPV) vaccine is also recommended for men up to age 26.

Be Safer: Getting tested regularly and getting vaccinated are both important, but there are other things you can do to reduce your risk for STDs.

- Get to know someone before having sex with them and talk honestly about STDs and getting tested—before you have sex.

- Use a condom correctly and use one every time you have sex.

- Think twice about mixing alcohol and/or recreational drugs with sex. They can reduce your ability to make good decisions and can lead to risky behavior—like having sex without a condom.

- Limit your number of partners. You can lower your risk for STDs if you only have sex with one person who only has sex with you.

Chapter 7

Child Sexual Abuse and STDs

Sexual Assault or Abuse of Children

These guidelines are limited to the identification and treatment of STDs in pre-pubertal children. Management of the psychosocial or legal aspects of the sexual assault or abuse of children is beyond the scope of these guidelines.

The identification of sexually transmissible agents in children beyond the neonatal period strongly suggests sexual abuse. The significance of the identification of a sexually transmitted organism in such children as evidence of possible child sexual abuse varies by pathogen. Postnatally acquired gonorrhea and syphilis; chlamydia infection; and nontransfusion, nonperinatally acquired HIV are indicative of sexual abuse. Chlamydia infection might be indicative of sexual abuse in children ≥3 years of age and among those aged <3 years when infection is not likely perinatally acquired. Sexual abuse should be suspected when genital herpes, *T. vaginalis*, or anogenital warts are diagnosed. The investigation of sexual abuse among children who have an infection that could have been transmitted sexually should be conducted in compliance with recommendations by clinicians who have experience and training in all elements of the evaluation of child abuse, neglect, and assault.

This chapter includes text excerpted from "Sexual Assault and Abuse and STDs," Centers for Disease Control and Prevention (CDC), June 4, 2015.

The social significance of an infection that might have been acquired sexually varies by the specific organism, as does the threshold for reporting suspected child sexual abuse. In cases in which any STD has been diagnosed in a child, efforts should be made in consultation with a specialist to evaluate the possibility of sexual abuse, including conducting a history and physical examination for evidence of abuse and diagnostic testing for other commonly occurring STDs.

The general rule that sexually transmissible infections beyond the neonatal period are evidence of sexual abuse has exceptions. For example, genital infection with *T. vaginalis* or rectal or genital infection with *C. trachomatis* among young children might be the result of perinatally acquired infection and has, in some cases of chlamydia infection, persisted for as long as 2–3 years, though perinatal CT infection is now uncommon because of prenatal screening and treatment of pregnant women. Genital warts have been diagnosed in children who have been sexually abused, but also in children who have no other evidence of sexual abuse. BV has been diagnosed in children who have been abused, but its presence alone does not prove sexual abuse. Most HBV infections in children result from household exposure to persons who have chronic HBV infection rather than sexual abuse.

Abbreviations: HIV=human immunodeficiency virus; SA=sexually associated; ST=sexually transmitted.

- If not likely to be perinatally acquired and rare vertical transmission is excluded.

- Reports should be made to the agency in the community mandated to receive reports of suspected child abuse or neglect.

- If not likely to be acquired perinatally or through transfusion.

- Unless a clear history of autoinoculation exists.

- Report if evidence exists to suspect abuse, including history, physical examination, or other identified infections.

Reporting

All U.S. states and territories have laws that require the reporting of child abuse. Although the exact requirements differ by state, if a health care provider has reasonable cause to suspect child abuse, a report must be made. Health-care providers should contact their state or local child-protection service agency regarding child-abuse reporting requirements in their states.

Evaluating Children for STDs

Evaluations of children for sexual assault or abuse should be conducted in a manner designed to minimize pain and trauma to the child. Examinations and collection of vaginal specimens in prepubertal children can be very uncomfortable and should be performed by an experienced clinician to avoid psychological and physical trauma to the child. The decision to obtain genital or other specimens from a child to evaluate for STDs must be made on an individual basis; however, children who received a diagnosis of one STD should be screened for all STDs. Because STDs are not common in prepubertal children or infants evaluated for abuse, testing all sites for all organisms is not routinely recommended. Factors that should lead the physician to consider screening for STD include:

1. Child has experienced penetration or has evidence of recent or healed penetrative injury to the genitals, anus, or oropharynx.

2. Child has been abused by a stranger.

3. Child has been abused by a perpetrator known to be infected with an STD or at high risk for STDs (e.g., intravenous drug abusers, MSM, persons with multiple sexual partners, and those with a history of STDs).

4. Child has a sibling, other relative, or another person in the household with an STD.

5. Child lives in an area with a high rate of STD in the community.

6. Child has signs or symptoms of STDs (e.g., vaginal discharge or pain, genital itching or odor, urinary symptoms, and genital lesions or ulcers).

7. Child or parent requests STD testing.

If a child has symptoms, signs, or evidence of an infection that might be sexually transmitted, the child should be tested for common STDs before the initiation of any treatment that could interfere with the diagnosis of those other STDs. Because of the legal and psychosocial consequences of a false-positive diagnosis, only tests with high specificities should be used. The potential benefit to the child of a reliable STD diagnosis justifies deferring presumptive treatment until specimens for highly specific tests are obtained by providers with experience in the evaluation of sexually abused and assaulted children.

Evaluations should be scheduled on a case-by-case basis according to history of assault or abuse and in a manner that minimizes the possibility for psychological trauma and social stigma. If the initial exposure was recent, the infectious organisms acquired through the exposure might not have produced sufficient concentrations of organisms to result in positive test results or examination findings. Alternatively, positive test results following a recent exposure might represent the assailant's secretions (but would nonetheless be an indication for treatment of the child). A second visit approximately 2 weeks after the most recent sexual exposure should be scheduled to include a repeat physical examination and collection of additional specimens to identify any infection that might not have been detected at the time of initial evaluation.

A single evaluation might be sufficient if the child was abused for an extended period of time and if a substantial amount of time elapsed between the last suspected episode of abuse and the medical evaluation. Compliance with follow-up appointments might be improved when law enforcement personnel or child protective services are involved.

Initial Examination

The following should be performed during the initial examination.

- Visual inspection of the genital, perianal, and oral areas for genital discharge, odor, bleeding, irritation, warts, and ulcerative lesions. The clinical manifestations of some STDs are different in children than in adults. For example, typical vesicular lesions might be absent even in the presence of HSV infection. Because HSV can be indicative of sexual abuse, specimens should be obtained from all vesicular or ulcerative genital or perianal lesions and then sent for viral culture or PCR.

- Culture for *N. gonorrhea* from specimens collected from the pharynx and anus in boys and girls, the vagina in girls, and the urethra in boys. Cervical specimens are not recommended for prepubertal girls. For boys with a urethral discharge, a meatal specimen discharge is an adequate substitute for an intraurethral swab specimen. Because of the legal implications of a diagnosis of *N. gonorrhea* infection in a child, if culture for the isolation of *N. gonorrhea* is done, only standard culture procedures should be performed. Gram stains are inadequate to evaluate prepubertal children for gonorrhea and should not be used to diagnose or exclude gonorrhea. Specimens from the vagina, urethra, pharynx, or rectum should be streaked onto selective media for isolation of *N. gonorrhoeae*, and all presumptive isolates of *N. gonorrhea* should be identified definitively by at least two tests that involve different approaches (e.g., biochemical, enzyme substrate, or serologic). Isolates should be preserved to enable additional or repeated testing. Data on use of NAAT for detection of *N. gonorrhoeae* in children are limited, and performance is test dependent. Consultation with an expert is necessary before using NAAT in this context, both to minimize the possibility of cross-reaction with nongonococcal *Neisseria* species and other commensals (e.g., *N. meningitidis, N. sicca, N. lactamica, N. cinerea,* and *Moraxella catarrhalis*) and to ensure appropriate interpretation of positive results. When testing vaginal secretions or urine from girls, NAAT can be used as an alternative to culture; however, culture remains the preferred method for testing urethral specimens or urine from boys and extragenital specimens (pharynx and rectum) from all children. All positive specimens should be retained for additional testing.

- Culture for *C. trachomatis* from specimens collected from the anus in both boys and girls and from the vagina in girls. The likelihood of recovering *C. trachomatis* from the urethra of prepubertal boys is too low to justify the trauma involved in obtaining an intraurethral specimen. However, a meatal specimen should be obtained if urethral discharge is present. Pharyngeal specimens for *C. trachomatis* are not recommended for children of either sex because the likelihood of recovering chlamydia is low, perinatally acquired infection might persist beyond infancy, and culture systems in some laboratories do not distinguish between *C. trachomatis* and *C. pneumoniae.* Only standard culture systems for the isolation of *C. trachomatis* should be used. The isolation of *C. trachomatis* should be confirmed by microscopic identification of inclusions by staining with fluorescein-conjugated monoclonal antibody specific for *C. trachomatis.* Isolates should be preserved for additional testing. Nonculture tests for chlamydia (e.g., DFA) are not specific enough for use in cases of possible child abuse or assault. NAATs can be used for detection of *C. trachomatis* in vaginal specimens or urine from girls. No data are available regarding the use of NAAT from urine in boys or for extragenital specimens (e.g., those obtained from the rectum) in boys and girls. Culture remains the preferred method for extragenital sites. All specimens should be retained for additional testing.

- Culture for *T. vaginalis* infection and wet mount of a vaginal swab specimen for *T. vaginalis* infection. Testing for *T. vaginalis* should not be limited to girls with vaginal discharge if other indications for vaginal testing exist, as there is some evidence to indicate that asymptomatic sexually abused children might be infected with *T. vaginalis* and might benefit from treatment. Data on use of NAAT for detection of *T. vaginalis* in children are too limited to inform recommendations, but no evidence suggests that performance of NAAT for detection of *T. vaginalis* in children would differ from that in adults.

- Wet mount of a vaginal swab specimen for BV.

- Collection of serum samples to be evaluated, preserved for subsequent analysis, and used as a baseline for comparison with follow-up serologic tests. Sera can be tested for antibodies to *T. pallidum*, HIV, and HBV. Decisions regarding the infectious agents for which to perform serologic tests should be made on a case-by-case basis.

Treatment

The risk of a child acquiring an STD as a result of sexual abuse or assault has not been well studied. Presumptive treatment for children who have been sexually assaulted or abused is not recommended because 1) the incidence of most STDs in children is low after abuse/assault, 2) prepubertal girls appear to be at lower risk for ascending infection than adolescent or adult women, and 3) regular follow-up of children usually can be ensured. However, some children or their parent(s) or guardian(s) might be concerned about the possibility of infection with an STD, even if the risk is perceived to be low by the health care provider. Such concerns might be an appropriate indication for presumptive treatment in some settings and might be considered after all relevant specimens for diagnostic tests have been collected.

Other Management Considerations

Because child sexual-assault survivors are at increased risk for future unsafe sexual practices that have been linked to higher risk of HPV acquisition and are more likely to engage in these behaviors at an earlier age, ACIP recommends vaccination of children who are victims of sexual abuse or assault at age ≥9 years who have not initiated or completed immunization. Although HPV vaccine will not protect against progression of infection already acquired or promote clearance of the infection, the vaccine protects against vaccine types not yet acquired.

Follow-Up

If no infections were identified at the initial examination after the last suspected sexual exposure and if this exposure was recent, a follow-up evaluation approximately 2 weeks after the last exposure can be considered. Likewise, if no physical examination or diagnostic testing was done at the initial visit, then a complete examination can be scheduled approximately 2 weeks after the last exposure to identify any evidence of STDs.

In circumstances in which transmission of syphilis, HIV, hepatitis B, or HPV is a concern but baseline tests for syphilis, HIV, and HBV are negative and examinations for genital warts are negative, follow-up serologic testing and an examination approximately 6 weeks and 3 months after the last suspected sexual exposure is recommended to allow time for antibodies to develop and signs of infection to appear. In addition, results of HBsAg testing must be interpreted carefully, because HBV can be transmitted nonsexually. Decisions regarding which tests should be performed must be made on an individual basis.

Risk for Acquiring HIV Infection

HIV infection has been reported in children for whom sexual abuse was the only known risk factor. Children might be at higher risk for HIV acquisition than adolescent and adult sexual assault or sexual abuse survivors because the sexual abuse of children is frequently associated with multiple episodes of assault and mucosal trauma might be more likely. Serologic testing for HIV infection should be considered for sexually abused children. The decision to test for HIV infection should involve the family, if possible, and be made on a case-by-case basis depending on the likelihood of infection among assailant(s). Although data are insufficient concerning the efficacy of nPEP among children, treatment is well tolerated by infants and children with and without HIV infection, and children have a minimal risk for serious adverse reactions because of the short period recommended for prophylaxis. In considering whether to offer nPEP, health care providers should consider whether the child can be treated soon after the sexual exposure (i.e., within 72 hours), the likelihood that the assailant is infected with HIV, and the likelihood of high compliance with the prophylactic regimen. The potential benefit of treating a sexually abused child should be weighed against the risk for adverse reactions. If nPEP is being considered, a provider specializing in evaluating or treating children with HIV infection should be consulted.

Chapter 8

STDs in Adolescents and Young Adults

How Are STDs Spread?

You can get an STD by having sex (vaginal, anal or oral) with someone who has an STD. Anyone who is sexually active can get an STD. You don't even have to "go all the way" (have anal or vaginal sex) to get an STD, since some STDs, like herpes and HPV, are spread by skin-to-skin contact.

How Common Are STDs?

STDs are common, especially among young people. There are about 20 million new cases of STDs each year in the United States, and about half of these are in people between the ages of 15 and 24. Young people are at greater risk of getting an STD for several reasons:

- Young women's bodies are biologically more susceptible to STDs.

- Some young people do not get the recommended STD tests.

- Many young people are hesitant to talk openly and honestly with a doctor or nurse about their sex lives.

This chapter includes text excerpted from "CDC Fact Sheet: Information for Teens and Young Adults: Staying Healthy and Preventing STDs," Centers for Disease Control and Prevention (CDC), November 17, 2015.

- Not having insurance or transportation can make it more difficult for young people to access STD testing.

- Some young people have more than one sex partner.

What Can I Do to Protect Myself?

- The surest way to protect yourself against STDs is to not have sex. That means not having any vaginal, anal, or oral sex ("abstinence"). There are many things to consider before having sex, and it's okay to say "no" if you don't want to have sex.

- If you do decide to have sex, you and your partner should get tested beforehand and make sure that you and your partner use a condom—every time you have oral, anal, or vaginal sex, from start to finish. Know where to get condoms and how to use them correctly. It is not safe to stop using condoms unless you've both been tested, know your status, and are in a mutually monogamous relationship.

- Mutual monogamy means that you and your partner both agree to only have sexual contact with each other. This can help protect against STDs, as long as you've both been tested and know you're STD-free.

- Before you have sex, talk with your partner about how you will prevent STDs and pregnancy. If you think you're ready to have sex, you need to be ready to protect your body and your future. You should also talk to your partner ahead of time about what you will and will not do sexually. Your partner should always respect your right to say no to anything that doesn't feel right.

- Make sure you get the health care you need. Ask a doctor or nurse about STD testing and about vaccines against HPV and hepatitis B.

- Girls and young women may have extra needs to protect their reproductive health. Talk to your doctor or nurse about regular cervical cancer screening and chlamydia testing. You may also want to discuss unintended pregnancy and birth control.

- Avoid using alcohol and drugs. If you use alcohol and drugs, you are more likely to take risks, like not using a condom or having sex with someone you normally wouldn't have sex with.

If I Get an STD, How Will I Know?

Many STDs don't cause any symptoms that you would notice, so the only way to know for sure if you have an STD is to get tested. You can get an STD from having sex with someone who has no symptoms. Just like you, that person might not even know he or she has an STD.

Where Can I Get Tested?

There are places that offer teen-friendly, confidential, and free STD tests. This means that no one has to find out you've been tested.

Can STDs Be Treated?

Your doctor can prescribe medicines to cure some STDs, like chlamydia and gonorrhea. Other STDs, like herpes, can't be cured, but you can take medicine to help with the symptoms.

If you are ever treated for an STD, be sure to finish all of your medicine, even if you feel better before you finish it all. Ask the doctor or nurse about testing and treatment for your partner, too. You and your partner should avoid having sex until you've both been treated. Otherwise, you may continue to pass the STD back and forth. It is possible to get an STD again (after you've been treated), if you have sex with someone who has an STD.

What Happens If I Don't Treat an STD?

Some curable STDs can be dangerous if they aren't treated. For example, if left untreated, chlamydia and gonorrhea can make it difficult—or even impossible—for a woman to get pregnant. You also increase your chances of getting HIV if you have an untreated STD. Some STDs, like HIV, can be fatal if left untreated.

What If My Partner or I Have an Incurable STD?

Some STDs like herpes and HIV aren't curable, but a doctor can prescribe medicine to treat the symptoms.

If you are living with an STD, it's important to tell your partner before you have sex. Although it may be uncomfortable to talk about your STD, open and honest conversation can help your partner make informed decisions to protect his or her health.

If I Have Questions, Who Can Answer Them?

If you have questions, talk to a parent or other trusted adult. Don't be afraid to be open and honest with them about your concerns. If you're ever confused or need advice, they're the first place to start. Remember, they were young once, too.

Talking about sex with a parent or another adult doesn't need to be a one-time conversation. It's best to leave the door open for conversations in the future.

It's also important to talk honestly with a doctor or nurse. Ask which STD tests and vaccines they recommend for you.

Chapter 9

STDs in Older Adults

Prevalence of STDs in Older Adults

Like most people, you probably have heard a lot about HIV and AIDS. You may have thought that these diseases aren't your problem and that only younger people have to worry about them. But, anyone at any age can get HIV/AIDS.

HIV and AIDS

HIV (human immunodeficiency virus) is a virus that damages and weakens the body's immune system—the system your body uses to fight off infection and disease. Having HIV puts a person in danger of getting other life-threatening diseases, infections, and cancers.

When the body cannot fight off the other diseases and infections anymore, HIV can lead to a much more serious illness called AIDS (acquired immunodeficiency syndrome). AIDS is the last stage of HIV infection. Not everyone with HIV will get AIDS.

If you think you may have HIV, it is very important to get tested. There are drugs that can help your body keep the HIV in check and fight against AIDS.

This chapter includes text excerpted from "HIV, AIDS, and Older People," U.S. Department of Health and Human Services (HHS), December 23, 2015.

How Do I Get Tested for HIV?

A small blood sample, mouth swab, or urine sample is used to test people for HIV. It can take as long as 3 to 6 months after the infection for the virus to show up in your blood.

You can be tested at a doctor's office, hospital, community health center, or other health clinic. Some places have mobile testing vans. AIDS services organizations also may provide testing.

Depending on where you go, testing may be free. In most states the tests are private, and you can choose to take the test without giving your name. Many providers or groups that offer HIV testing also provide counseling.

Another option is to test yourself for HIV at home. If you choose this option, make sure to use a test that has been approved by the U.S. Food and Drug Administration (FDA). If the test has not been approved by the FDA, it may not give accurate results. Home tests are sold at drugstores and online.

Finding a Place to Get Tested for HIV

Your doctor or other health care provider can test you for HIV or tell you where you can get tested. Or, the following resources can help you find a testing location:

- HIV Testing and Care Locator, locator.aids.gov

- Centers for Disease Control and Prevention, 1-800-232-4636 (toll-free) or gettested.cdc.gov

- Drugstores sell home testing kits (such as the Home Access™ HIV-1 Test System)

How Do You Get HIV/AIDS?

Anyone, at any age, can get HIV/AIDS. People usually get HIV from unprotected sex with someone who has HIV/AIDS, through contact with HIV-infected blood, or by sharing needles with an infected person. You may be at risk if:

- *You had sex without a latex or polyurethane condom.* The virus passes from the infected person to his or her partner in blood, semen, or vaginal fluid. During sex, HIV can get into your body through any opening, such as a tear or cut in the lining of the vagina, vulva, penis, rectum, or mouth. Latex condoms can help prevent an infected person from transferring the HIV virus to you. (Natural condoms are not as effective as latex and polyure-thane condoms at protecting against HIV/AIDS.)

- *You do not know your partner's drug and sexual history.* What you don't know *can* hurt you. Even though it may be hard to do, ask your partner about his or her sexual history and whether or not he or she has ever shared needles. Drug users are not the only people who might share needles. For example, people with diabetes who inject insulin or draw blood to test glucose levels could also share needles. You might ask: Have you been tested for HIV/AIDS? Have you had a number of different sex partners? Have you ever had unprotected sex with someone who has shared needles? Have you injected drugs or shared needles with someone else?

- *You had a blood transfusion or operation in a developing country at any time.*

- *You had a blood transfusion in the United States between 1978 and 1985.*

What Are Symptoms of HIV?

Many people have no symptoms when they first become infected with HIV. It can take as little as a few weeks for minor, flu-like symptoms to show up, or more than 10 years for more serious symptoms to appear, or any time in between. Signs of HIV include flu-like symptoms such as headache, cough, diarrhea, fevers, and/or sweats. Additional signs of HIV include swollen glands, lack of energy, loss of appetite, weight loss, repeated yeast infections, skin rashes, sores in the mouth or gen-ital area, pelvic and abdominal cramps, and short-term memory loss.

Is HIV/AIDS Different in Older Adults?

A growing number of older people have HIV/AIDS. One reason is because improved treatments are helping people with the disease live longer. Nearly one-fifth of people living with HIV in the United States are age 55 and older. Many of these people were diagnosed with HIV in their younger years. However, thousands of older people get HIV every year.

Many older people may not know they have HIV. Older people are less likely than younger people to get tested. Signs of HIV/AIDS can be mistaken for the aches and pains of normal aging. Older adults might be coping with other diseases common to aging that can mask the signs of HIV/AIDS.

Some older people may be ashamed or afraid of being tested. Plus, doctors do not always think to test older people for HIV/AIDS. By the time the older person is diagnosed, the virus may be in the late stages and more likely to progress to AIDS.

The number of HIV/AIDS cases among older people is growing every year because:

- Older Americans often know less about HIV/AIDS and how it spreads than younger people do. They may not know the importance of using condoms, not sharing needles, getting tested for HIV, and talking about HIV/AIDS with their doctor.

- Health care workers and educators often do not talk with middle-aged and older people about HIV/AIDS prevention.

- Older people are less likely than younger people to talk about their sex lives or drug use with their doctors.

- Doctors may not ask older patients about their sex lives or drug use or talk to them about risky behaviors.

- Remember, it is important to get tested for HIV/AIDS early. Early treatment may help prevent HIV turning into AIDS.

Facts about HIV/AIDS

You may have read or heard things that are not true about how you get HIV/AIDS. Here are the *facts:*

- You cannot get HIV through casual contact such as shaking hands or hugging a person with HIV/AIDS.

- You cannot get HIV from using a public telephone, drinking fountain, restroom, swimming pool, whirlpool, or hot tub.

- You cannot get HIV from sharing a drink.

- You cannot get HIV from being coughed or sneezed on by a person with HIV/AIDS.

- You cannot get HIV from giving blood.

- You cannot get HIV from a mosquito bite.

Caring for a Person with HIV/AIDS

As HIV/AIDS symptoms become worse, people may need help getting around and caring for themselves. This can be a special problem for older people who do not have a strong network of friends or family who can help. Your doctor may be able to direct you to groups that can help.

Sometimes, older people who don't have the virus become a caregiver for a child or grandchild with HIV/AIDS. They may provide financial support and/or nursing care. Being a caregiver can be mentally, physically, and financially difficult. This is especially true for older adults who are dealing with their own health problems. It is important that caregivers also take care of their own health needs.

Chapter 10

STDs in Racial and Ethnic Minorities

Public Health Impact

Centers for Disease Control and Prevention's (CDC) surveillance data show higher rates of reported STDs among some racial or ethnic minority groups when compared with rates among whites. Race and ethnicity in the United States are population characteristics that are correlated with other fundamental determinants of health status such as high rates of poverty, income inequality, unemployment and low educational attainment. People who struggle financially are often experiencing life circumstances that potentially increase their risk for STDs.

Those who cannot afford basic necessities may have trouble accessing and affording quality sexual health services. The overall U.S. poverty rate in 2013 was 14.5 (or 46.7 million) and remained the same in 2014 (the most recent year for which poverty statistics are available). Although the poverty rate did not change, many Americans continue to face economic challenges. For example, the poverty rate for whites was 10.1% (19.7 million), for blacks it was 26.2% (or 10.8 million), and for Hispanics it was 23.6% (or 13.1 million). Although the overall proportion of adults without health insurance decreased from 13.3% in 2013 to 10.4% (or 316 million) in 2014, many people in the U.S. may

---

This chapter includes text excerpted from "STDs in Racial and Ethnic Minorities," Centers for Disease Control and Prevention (CDC), November 17, 2015.

still not have access to health care. Among all races and ethnicities in the United States, Hispanics had the lowest rate of health insurance coverage in 2014 at 80.1% (or 55.6 million). Non-U.S. citizens (i.e., immigrants or undocumented persons) may face additional barriers in accessing care. In 2014, 31.2% (or 7 million) of persons not U.S. citizens did not have health insurance coverage. Even when health care is available, fear and distrust of health care institutions can negatively affect the health care-seeking experience for many racial/ethnic minorities when there is social discrimination, provider bias, or the perception that these may exist. Moreover, the quality of care may differ substantially for minority patients. These inequities in social and economic conditions are reflected in the profound disparities observed in the incidence of STDs among some racial and ethnic minorities.

STD Reporting Practices

CDC's surveillance data are based on cases of STDs reported to state and local health departments. In many state and local health jurisdictions, electronic laboratory reporting is increasingly a primary source of initial case notifications. These reports are often missing race and ethnicity of the patient; ascertainment of information on race and Hispanic ethnicity is often a function of active follow-up or dependent on previous information available about the patient in existing health department surveillance databases. Prevalence data from population-based surveys, such as National Health and Nutrition Examination Survey (NHANES) and the National Longitudinal Study of Adolescent Health, confirm the existence of marked STD disparities in some minority populations.

Method of Classifying Race and Hispanic Ethnicity

Interpretation of racial and ethnic disparities among persons with STDs is influenced by data collection methods, and by the categories by which these data are displayed. Race/ethnicity data are presented in Office of Management and Budget (OMB) race and ethnic categories, according to the 1997 revised OMB standards. However, NCHS bridged-race categories are used where OMB categories are not available (congenital syphilis). Forty-eight states collect and report data in formats compliant with these standards as of 2014. One additional jurisdiction reported cases of primary and secondary (P&S) syphilis by the appropriate standard, but did not report chlamydia and gonorrhea cases by this standard. Historical trend and rate data by race and

Hispanic ethnicity displayed in figures and interpreted in this report for 2010–2014 include only those jurisdictions (43 states for chlamydia/gonorrhea and 44 states for syphilis) reporting in the current standard consistently for years 2010 through 2014.

Completeness of Race/Ethnicity Data

Chlamydia—In 2014, 27.1% of chlamydia case reports were missing race or ethnicity data, ranging by state from 0.5% to 65.9%.

Gonorrhea—In 2014, 19.3% of gonorrhea case reports were missing information on race or ethnicity, ranging by state from 0.0% to 64.0%.

Syphilis—In 2014, 4.5% of P&S syphilis case reports were missing information on race or ethnicity, ranging from 0% to 31.3% among states with 10 or more cases of P&S syphilis.

Observations

Chlamydia

Among the 43 states that submitted data on race and Hispanic ethnicity for each year during 2010–2014 according to the OMB standards, rates of reported cases of chlamydia increased during 2010–2014 among all racial and ethnic groups except among blacks. During 2010–2014, chlamydia rates increased 12.6% among American Indians/Alaska Natives, 5.6% among Hispanics, 11.5% among Asians, 34.5% among Native Hawaiians/Other Pacific Islanders, and 26.9% among whites. During 2010–2014, rates of reported cases of chlamydia decreased 6.2% among blacks.

In 2014, 48 states submitted data on race and Hispanic ethnicity according to the OMB standards. The following data pertain to those jurisdictions:

Blacks—In 2014, the overall rate among blacks in the United States was 1,117.9 cases per 100,000 population. The rate of reported cases of chlamydia among black women was 5.7 times the rate among white women (1,432.6 and 253.3 per 100,000 females, respectively). The chlamydia rate among black men was 7.3 times the rate among white men (772.0 and 105.5 cases per 100,000 males, respectively).

Rates of reported cases of chlamydia were highest for blacks aged 15–19 and 20–24 years in 2014. The chlamydia rate among black females aged 15–19 years was 6,371.5 cases per 100,000 females, which was 4.9 times the rate among white females in the same age group (1,291.6 per 100,000 females). The rate among black women aged 20–24 years was 4.1 times the rate among white women in the same age group.

Similar racial disparities in reported chlamydia rates exist among men. Among males aged 15–19 years, the rate among blacks was nine times the rate among whites. The chlamydia rate among black men aged 20–24 years was 5.4 times the rate among white men of the same age group (3,241.2 and 603.5 cases per 100,000 males, respectively).

American Indians/Alaska Natives—In 2014, the chlamydia rate among American Indians/Alaska Natives was 668.8 cases per 100,000 population. Overall, the rate of chlamydia among American Indians/Alaska Natives in the United States was 3.7 times the rate among whites.

Native Hawaiians/Other Pacific Islanders—In 2014, the chlamydia rate among Native Hawaiians/Other Pacific Islanders was 625.1 cases per 100,000 population. The overall rate among Native Hawaiians/Other Pacific Islanders was 5.6 times the rate among whites and 3.5 times the rate among Asians.

Hispanics—In 2014, the chlamydia rate among Hispanics was 380.6 cases per 100,000 population which is 2.1 times the rate among whites.

Asians—In 2014, the chlamydia rate among Asians was 112.0 cases per 100,000 population. The overall rate among whites is 1.6 times the rate among Asians.

Gonorrhea

During 2010–2014, among the 43 states that submitted data for each year according to the OMB standards, rates of reported gonorrhea cases increased 100.4% among American Indians/Alaska Natives (84.7 to 169.7 per 100,000 population), 59.8% among whites (25.1 to 40.1 per 100,000), 51.1% among Hispanics (49.1 to 74.2 per 100,000), 44.8% among Asians (14.3 to 20.7 per 100,000), and 44.1% among Native Hawaiians/Other Pacific Islanders (74.3 to 107.1 per 100,000). The gonorrhea rate decreased 8.2% among blacks (466.4 to 428.1 per 100,000).

In 2014, 48 states submitted data in race and ethnicity categories according to the OMB standards. The following data pertain to those jurisdictions:

Blacks—In 2014, 55.4% of reported gonorrhea cases with known race/ethnicity occurred among blacks (excluding cases with missing information on race or ethnicity, and cases whose reported race or ethnicity was other). The rate of gonorrhea among blacks in 2014 was 405.4 cases per 100,000 population, which was 10.6 times the rate among whites (38.3 per 100,000). Although the calculated rate ratio for 2014 differs when considering the 43 jurisdictions that submitted data in race and ethnic categories according to the OMB standards for each year during 2010–2014, this disparity has decreased slightly in recent years. In 2014, this disparity was similar for black men (10.6 times the rate among white men) and black women (10.7 times the rate among white women).

As in previous years, the disparity in gonorrhea rates for blacks in 2014 was larger in the Midwest and Northeast than in the West or the South.

Considering all racial/ethnic and age categories, gonorrhea rates were highest for blacks aged 20–24, 15–19, and 25–29 years in 2014. Black women aged 20–24 had a gonorrhea rate of 1,799.9 cases per 100,000 women. This rate was 9.5 times the rate among white women in the same age group (188.7 per 100,000). Black women aged 15–19 years had a gonorrhea rate of 1,541.0 cases per 100,000 women, which was 12.7 times the rate among white women in the same age group (121.3 per 100,000).

Black men aged 20–24 years had a gonorrhea rate of 1,670.4 cases per 100,000 men, which was 10.7 times the rate among white men in the same age group (155.4 per 100,000). Black men aged 25–29 years had a gonorrhea rate of 1,291.6 cases per 100,000 men, which was 8.9 times the rate among white (men in the same age group (145.5 per 100,000).

American Indians/Alaska Natives—In 2014, the gonorrhea rate among American Indians/Alaska Natives was 159.4 cases per 100,000 population, which was 4.2 times the rate among whites. The disparity between gonorrhea rates for American Indians/Alaska Natives and whites was larger for American Indian/Alaska Native women (5.6 times the rate among white women) than for American Indian/Alaska Native men (2.9 times the rate among white men). The disparity in gonorrhea rates for American Indians/Alaska Natives in 2014 was larger in the Midwest than in the West, Northeast, and South.

Native Hawaiians/Other Pacific Islanders—In 2014, the gonorrhea rate among Native Hawaiians/Other Pacific Islanders was 102.1 cases per 100,00 population, which was 2.7 times the rate among whites. The disparity between gonorrhea rates for Native Hawaiians/Other Pacific Islanders and whites was the similar for Native Hawaiian/Other Pacific Islander women (2.9 times the rate among white women) and Native Hawaiian/Other Pacific Islander men (2.4 times the rate among white men). The disparity in gonorrhea rates for Native Hawaiians/Other Pacific Islanders in 2014 was lower in the West than in the Midwest, Northeast, and South.

Hispanics—In 2014, the gonorrhea rate among Hispanics was 73.3 cases per 100,000 population, which was 1.9 times the rate among whites. This disparity was similar for Hispanic women (1.8 times the rate among white women) and Hispanic men (2.0 times the rate among white men). The disparity in gonorrhea rates for Hispanics was highest in the Northeast and lowest in the West and Midwest.

Asians—In 2014, the gonorrhea rate among Asians was 19.3 cases per 100,000 population, which was lower than (0.5 times) the rate among whites. This difference is larger for Asian women than for Asian men. In 2014, rates among Asians were lower than rates among whites in all four regions of the United States.

Primary and Secondary (P&S) Syphilis

During 2010–2014, 44 states submitted syphilis data for each year according to the OMB standards. Among these states during 2010–2014, rates of reported P&S syphilis cases increased 152.6% among American Indians/Alaska Natives (3.1 to 7.9 per 100,000 population), 135.2% among Asians (1.2 to 2.9 per 100,000), 80.2% among Hispanics (4.2 to 7.5 per 100,000 population), 56.7% among whites (2.2 to 3.5 per 100,000), 38.2% among Native Hawaiians/Other Pacific Islanders (5.1 to 7.1 per 100,000), and 7.8% among blacks (17.8 to 19.2 per 100,000).

In 2014, 49 states submitted syphilis data by race and ethnicity according to the OMB standards. The following data pertain to those jurisdictions:

Blacks—In 2014, 38.1% of reported P&S syphilis cases with known race/ethnicity occurred among blacks (excluding cases with missing information on race or ethnicity, and cases whose reported race or ethnicity was other). The P&S syphilis rate among blacks in 2014 was 18.9 cases per 100,000 population, which was 5.4 times the rate among whites (3.5 per 100,000). This disparity was higher for black women (9.2 times the rate among white women) than for black men (5.3 times the rate among white men).

Considering all race/ethnicity, sex, and age categories, P&S syphilis rates were highest among black men aged 20–24 years and 25–29 years in 2014. Black men aged 20–24 years had a P&S syphilis rate of 106.3 cases per 100,000 men. This rate was 8.5 times the rate among white men in the same age group (12.5 per 100,000). Black men aged 25–29 years had a P&S syphilis rate of 121.3 cases per 100,000 men, which was 7.9 times the rate among white men in the same age group (15.4 per 100,000).

American Indians/Alaska Natives—In 2014, the P&S syphilis rate among American Indians/Alaska Natives was 7.6 cases per 100,000 population, 2.2 times the rate among whites. This disparity was larger for American Indian/Alaska Native women (9.6 times the rate among white women) than for American Indian/Alaska Native men (1.6 times the rate among white men).

Native Hawaiians/Other Pacific Islanders—In 2014, the P&S syphilis rate among Native Hawaiians/Other Pacific Islanders was 6.5 cases per 100,000 population, which was 1.9 times the rate among whites. This disparity was similar for Native Hawaiian/Other Pacific Islander women (1.6 times the rate among white women) and Native Hawaiian/Other Pacific Islander men (1.8 times the rate among white men).

Hispanics—In 2014, the P&S syphilis rate among Hispanics was 7.6 cases per 100,000 population, which was 2.2 times the rate among whites. This disparity was similar for Hispanic women (2.2 times the rate among white women) and Hispanic men (2.1 times the rate among white men).

Asians—In 2014, the P&S syphilis rate among Asians was 2.8 cases per 100,000 population, which was 0.8 times the rate among whites. This difference is larger for Asian women (0.4 times the rate among white women) than for Asian men (0.9 times the rate among white men).

Congenital Syphilis

Race/ethnicity for cases of congenital syphilis is based on the mother's race/ethnicity. During 2013–2014, rates of reported congenital syphilis cases increased 102.9% among Asians/Pacific Islanders, 32.1%

among whites, 21.7% among blacks, and 19.8% among Hispanics. The congenital syphilis rate did not change among American Indians/ Alaska Natives.

In 2014, 50.6% of congenital syphilis cases with known race/ethnicity occurred among blacks (excluding cases with missing information on race or ethnicity, and cases whose reported race or ethnicity was other). The rate of congenital syphilis among blacks in 2014 was 38.2 cases per 100,000 live births, which was 10.3 times the rate among whites (3.7 per 100,000 live births). The rate of congenital syphilis was 12.7 cases per 100,000 live births among American Indians/Alaska Natives (3.4 times the rate among whites), 12.1 cases per 100,000 live births among Hispanics (3.3 times the rate among whites), and 6.9 cases per 100,000 births among Asians/Pacific Islanders (1.9 times the rate among whites).

In 2014, 50.6% of congenital syphilis cases with known race/ethnicity occurred among blacks (excluding cases with missing information on race or ethnicity, and cases whose reported race or ethnicity was other). The rate of congenital syphilis among blacks in 2014 was 38.2 cases per 100,000 live births, which was 10.3 times the rate among whites (3.7 per 100,000 live births). The rate of congenital syphilis was 12.7 cases per 100,000 live births among American Indians/Alaska Natives (3.4 times the rate among whites), 12.1 cases per 100,000 live births among Hispanics (3.3 times the rate among whites), and 6.9 cases per 100,000 births among Asians/Pacific Islanders (1.9 times the rate among whites).

Chapter 11

STDs in People in Correctional Facilities

Quick Stats

- HIV is a serious health issue for correctional facilities and their incarcerated populations.

- Most incarcerated people with HIV got the virus before entering a correctional facility.

- HIV testing at a correctional facility may be the first time incarcerated people are tested and diagnosed with HIV.

More than 2 million people in the United States are incarcerated in federal, state, and local correctional facilities on any given day. In 2010, the rate of diagnosed HIV infection among inmates in state and federal prisons was more than five times greater than the rate among people who were not incarcerated. Most inmates with HIV acquire it in their communities, before they are incarcerated.

This chapter contains text excerpted from the following sources: Text beginning with the heading "Quick Stats" is excerpted from "HIV among Incarcerated Populations," Centers for Disease Control and Prevention (CDC), July 22, 2015; Text under the heading "Public Health Impact" is excerpted from "STDs in Persons Entering Corrections Facilities," Centers for Disease Control and Prevention (CDC), December 13, 2012. Reviewed April 2016.

- In 2012, 1.57 million people were incarcerated in state and federal prisons and at midyear 2013 there were 731,208 people detained in local jails.

- In 2010, there were 20,093 inmates with HIV/AIDS in state and federal prisons with 91% being men.

- Among state and federal jurisdictions reporting in 2010 there were 3,913 inmates living with an AIDS diagnosis.

- Rates of AIDS-related deaths among state and federal prisoners declined an average of 16% per year between 2001 and 2010, from 24 deaths/100,000 in 2001 to 5/100,000 in 2010.

- Among jail populations, African American men are 5 times as likely as white men, and twice as likely as Hispanic/Latino men, to be diagnosed with HIV.

- Among jail populations, African American women are more than twice as likely to be diagnosed with HIV as white or Hispanic/Latino women.

Prevention Challenges

- Lack of awareness about HIV and lack of resources for HIV testing and treatment in inmates' home communities. Most inmates with HIV become infected in their communities, where they may engage in high-risk behaviors or be unaware of available prevention and treatment resources.

- Lack of resources for HIV testing and treatment in correctional facilities. Prison and jail administrators must weigh the costs of HIV testing and treatment against other needs, and some correctional systems may not provide such services. HIV testing can identify inmates with HIV before they are released. Early diagnosis and treatment can potentially reduce the level of HIV in communities to which inmates return.

- Rapid turnover among jail populations. While most HIV programs in correctional facilities are in prisons, most incarcerated people are detained in jails. Nine out of ten jail inmates are released in under 72 hours, which makes it hard to test them for HIV and help them find treatment.

- Inmate concerns about privacy and fear of stigma. Many inmates do not disclose their high-risk behaviors, such as anal sex or injection drug use, because they fear being stigmatized. Health care providers should keep inmate's health care information confidential, know the public health confidentiality and reporting laws, and inform inmates about them.

Public Health Impact

Multiple studies and surveillance projects have demonstrated a high prevalence of STDs in persons entering jails and juvenile corrections facilities. Prevalence rates for chlamydia and gonorrhea in these settings are consistently among the highest observed in any venue. Screening for chlamydia, gonorrhea, and syphilis at intake offers an opportunity to identify infections, prevent complications, and reduce transmission in the general community.

For example, data from one study in a location with high syphilis incidence suggested that screening and treatment of female inmates for syphilis may reduce syphilis in the general community. In some locations, a substantial proportion of all early syphilis cases are reported from corrections facilities.

Description of Population

In 2011, STD screening data from corrections facilities were reported in 33 states and Puerto Rico for chlamydia and in 32 states and Puerto Rico for gonorrhea. Line-listed (i.e., case-specific) data for chlamydia and gonorrhea are provided to CDC through the regional infertility prevention infrastructure. The figures presented in this section represent 40,211 chlamydia tests of women (19,081 from juvenile corrections facilities and 21,130 from adult facilities), 96,917 chlamydia tests of men (64,350 from juvenile facilities and 32,567 from adult facilities), 37,754 gonorrhea tests of women (16,991 from juvenile facilities and 20,763 from adult facilities), and 93,193 gonorrhea tests of men (61,080 from juvenile facilities and 32,113 from adult facilities). Syphilis data from notifiable disease surveillance are reported to CDC by local and state STD prevention programs.

Chlamydia

Overall, chlamydia positivity was higher in women than in men for all age groups.

Males in Juvenile Corrections Facilities—Among males aged 12–18 years entering 118 juvenile corrections facilities, the overall chlamydia positivity was 7.4%. Chlamydia positivity ranged from 1.0% for adolescent males aged 12 years to 10.2% for those aged 18 years.

Females in Juvenile Corrections Facilities—Among females aged 12–18 years entering 63 juvenile corrections facilities, the overall chlamydia positivity was 15.7%. Positivity ranged from 5.4% for females aged 12 years to 17.3% for those aged 17 years.

Men in Adult Corrections Facilities—Among men entering 49 adult corrections facilities in 2011, positivity in men aged younger than 20 years (12.6%) was higher than the overall prevalence observed in adolescent males entering juvenile facilities (7.4%). Chlamydia positivity decreased with age, from 12.6% for those aged younger than 20 years to 1.6% for those aged older than 34 years. Overall chlamydia positivity among adult men entering corrections facilities in 2011 was 7.1%.

Women in Adult Corrections Facilities—Among women entering 34 adult corrections facilities in 2011, positivity was 7.4%. Chlamydia positivity decreased with age, from 16.8% for those aged younger than 20 years to 2.5% for those aged older than 34 years. Overall chlamydia positivity in women entering adult corrections facilities (7.4%) was substantially lower than that in adolescent females entering juvenile corrections facilities (15.7%). However, chlamydia positivity among women aged younger than 20 years entering adult corrections facilities was similar to that among females entering juvenile corrections facilities.

Gonorrhea

Overall, gonorrhea positivity in women was uniformly higher than in men for all age groups.

Males in Juvenile Corrections Facilities—The overall gonorrhea positivity for adolescent males entering 115 juvenile corrections facilities in 2011 was 1.2%. Positivity increased with age, from 0.1% for those aged 12 years to 2.3% for those aged 18 years.

Females in Juvenile Corrections Facilities—The overall gonorrhea positivity for adolescent females entering 57 juvenile corrections facilities in 2011 was 4.4%. Positivity ranged from 2.5% for those aged 13 years to 4.9% for those aged 16 years.

Men in Adult Corrections Facilities—The overall gonorrhea positivity for men entering 49 adult corrections facilities in 2011 was

1.0%. Positivity was highest in men aged younger than 20 years (1.7%) and declined with age to 0.4% in men aged older than 34 years. Men aged younger than 20 years entering adult facilities (1.7%) had a similar gonorrhea positivity compared with males entering juvenile corrections facilities (1.2%).

Women in Adult Corrections Facilities—Among women entering 32 adult corrections facilities in 2011, overall gonorrhea positivity was 1.8%. Positivity decreased with age, from 4.3% among those aged younger than 20 years to 0.8% among those aged older than 34 years. Women aged younger than 20 years entering adult facilities (4.3%) had a similar gonorrhea positivity compared with females entering juvenile corrections facilities (4.4%).

Syphilis

In 2011, reports of P&S syphilis cases from corrections facilities accounted for 6% of P&S syphilis among MSW, 3% among women, and 1% among MSM.

Chapter 12

Why STD Prevention Is Important

The Inside Story on Sexually Transmitted Diseases (STDs)

Too many people want to avoid the topic altogether, but public health data show us that there is a hidden STD epidemic in this nation. In fact, CDC estimates 20 million new STD infections occur each year in the United States, costing the healthcare system nearly $16 billion in direct medical costs. There are also now more than 110 million total sexually transmitted infections in U.S. men and women.

Why do we care?

For the first time in nearly a decade, rates for three of the most common STDs (chlamydia, gonorrhea, and syphilis) all increased at the same time. These infections can threaten immediate and longterm health and well-being. Untreated STDs can lead to reproductive complications such as infertility (inability to get pregnant) and ectopic

This chapter contains text excerpted from the following sources: Text under the heading "The Inside Story on STDs" is excerpted from "Sexually Transmitted Diseases (STDs): Other FAQs," National Institute of Child Health and Human Development (NICHD), May 28, 2013.

pregnancy (pregnancy outside the womb). They can also increase a person's risk for getting and giving HIV.

Young people aged 15–24 and gay, bisexual, and other men who have sex with men continue to be at greatest risk for infection. Why? It's complicated, but we know that individual risk behaviors aren't the only reason. Environmental, social, and cultural factors, including a high level of STDs in these populations and difficulty in accessing quality health care contribute to a higher STD burden.

The good news is that STDs are preventable!

There are steps everyone can take to avoid the negative health consequences and to reduce the overall burden of STDs. Let's breakdown how you can Talk. Test. Treat to protect your sexual health:

Talk. Talk openly with your partner(s) and your healthcare provider about sex and STDs.

- Talk with your partner before having sex. Not sure how? We've got a resource to help you get started. If you're going to have sex, discuss the many prevention options available, including the use of condoms.

- Talk with your healthcare provider about your sexual history, and ask what STD tests are right for you.

Test. Get tested. Many STDs have no symptoms, so getting tested is the only way to know for sure if you have an infection. See what tests CDC recommends, and find out where you can get tested.

Treat. If you test positive for an STD, work with your doctor to get the correct treatment. Some STDs can be cured with the right medication. Those that aren't curable can be treated. To ensure treatment is successful, be sure to

- Take all of the medicine your doctor prescribes for you, and don't share it with anyone.

- Don't have sex again until both you and your partner(s) have completed your treatment.

Healthcare providers can help too. Protecting your patient's health is also as easy as Talk. Test. Treat.

Talk. Providing the best care possible means talking with your patients about sexual health and safe sex practices.

- This involves taking an accurate sexual history. Uncomfortable asking questions about sex? Don't be—studies have shown that most patients want to be asked about their sexual health.

- Talking also means counseling your patients on how to have safe sex, and ensuring that they know about the many prevention options currently available.

Test. Test your patients as recommended by CDC. Pregnant women can get STDs, too. Protect mother and baby by testing all pregnant women for syphilis, HIV, chlamydia, and hepatitis B, as well as testing at-risk women for gonorrhea, starting early in pregnancy.

Am I at Risk for STDs/STIs?

STDs/STIs affect men and women of all races, backgrounds, sexual orientations, and economic levels. Anyone who is having or has had vaginal, anal, or oral sex has some degree of risk for an STD/STI. In fact, some STDs/STIs can be passed through sexual play that does not involve intercourse.

You can analyze your risk for STDs/STIs with the STD Wizard a free interactive online tool based on the Centers for Disease Control and Prevention's (CDC's) STD Treatment Guidelines. The STD Wizard recommends tests and vaccines based on your responses concerning some of your personal characteristics and behaviors. You can use these recommendations to start a discussion with your health care provider about your STD/STI risk and the tests you may need. The STD Wizard is available in both English and Spanish.

How Can I Avoid Getting a Sexually Transmitted Disease or Sexually Transmitted Infection (STD/STI)?

The most reliable ways to avoid STDs/STIs are to abstain from sexual contact or to be in a long-term monogamous relationship with a partner who has been tested and is uninfected. In addition, the following measures can also help you avoid STDs/STIs:

- Know your sexual partner's STD/STI and health history.

- Talk to your health care provider about your risk, and get tested for STDs/STIs.

• Get vaccinated against hepatitis A virus (HAV), hepatitis B virus (HBV), and human papillomavirus (HPV).

• Use latex condoms correctly and consistently.

Remember, however, that while condoms greatly reduce the chance of getting certain STDs/STIs, such as gonorrhea, condoms cannot fully protect against infection because viruses and some bacteria can be passed from person to person by skin-to-skin contact in the genital area not covered by a condom.

What Should I Do If I Have Been Diagnosed with an STD/STI?

You should see your health care provider for treatment as soon as possible after receiving a diagnosis of an STD/STI. You also should notify, either yourself or with the help of the local health department, all recent sex partners and advise them to see their health care providers and be treated. These steps will reduce your risk of becoming re-infected, help avoid spreading the STD/STI to other people, and decrease the risk that your previous sexual partners will develop serious complications from the STD/STI. You and all of your sex partners must avoid sex until treatment is complete and all symptoms have disappeared.

In the case of STDs/STIs caused by viruses with no cure (for example, HIV, genital herpes, or hepatitis), special care and preventive measures can help control the infection, limit symptoms, and help maximize health.

Are There Disorders or Conditions Associated with Sexually Transmitted Diseases and Sexually Transmitted Infections (STDs/STIs)?

STDs/STIs in women can cause pelvic inflammatory disease (PID), which may result in infertility (difficulty getting pregnant).

Men with STDs/STIs also can have problems with infertility.

Additionally, a person with an STD/STI other than HIV is two to five times more likely to contract the HIV virus than a person without an STD/STI. If a person is already HIV positive, having another STD/STI increases the chances that he or she will pass the virus on to his or her sexual partner.

Some STDs/STIs, such as human papillomavirus, viral hepatitis, and HIV, increase the risk of some forms of cancer.

Certain STDs/STIs can pass from a pregnant woman to the fetus in her womb. The effects can be life threatening, as is the case with HIV. Other STDs/STIs can cause a range of disorders in the infant, including deafness, blindness, and intellectual disability.

Can a Sexually Transmitted Disease or Sexually Transmitted Infection (STD/STI) Lead to Cancer?

Having an STD/STI increases a person's risk for several types of cancer.

Certain high-risk types of human papillomavirus (HPV) can cause cervical cancer in women. In men, HPV infection can lead to the development of penile cancers. HPV also can cause cancers of the mouth, throat, and anus in both sexes.

Acquiring viral hepatitis B or C puts a person at risk for liver cancer, and untreated HIV/AIDS increases risk for several types of rare cancers, including lymphomas, sarcomas, and cervical cancer.

If I Have a Sexually Transmitted Disease or Sexually Transmitted Infection (STD/STI), Will I Be Able to Get Pregnant?

Having an STD/STI will not prevent a woman from getting pregnant.

However, in some instances, women who have had STDs/STIs may have difficulty getting pregnant because of scarring and damage to their reproductive organs leading to infertility. This situation is particularly common in women who have had pelvic inflammatory disease. Additionally, early during pregnancy, STDs/STIs may increase the risk of miscarriage.

What Is the Link between Sexually Transmitted Diseases or Sexually Transmitted Infections (STDs/STIs) and Infertility?

In most cases, STDs/STIs are linked to infertility primarily when they are left untreated.

For instance, chlamydia and gonorrhea are sexually transmitted bacterial infections that can be cured easily with antibiotics. Left untreated, 10% to 20% of chlamydial and gonorrheal infections in women can result in pelvic inflammatory disease (PID)—a condition that can cause long-term complications, such as chronic pelvic pain, ectopic pregnancy (pregnancy outside of the uterus), and infertility.

Additionally, infections with gonorrhea and chlamydia may not cause symptoms and may go unnoticed. These undiagnosed and untreated infections can lead to severe health consequences, especially in women, causing permanent damage to reproductive organs.

The Centers for Disease Control and Prevention estimates that these infections cause infertility in at least 24,000 women each year. Although infertility is less common among men, it does occur. More commonly, untreated chlamydia and gonorrhea infections in men may cause epididymitis, a painful infection in the tissue surrounding the testicles, or urethritis, an infection of the urinary canal in the penis, which causes painful urination and fever.

What Are the Common Symptoms of STDs?

People with STDs/STIs may feel ill and notice some of the following signs and symptoms:

- Unusual discharge from the penis or vagina
- Sores or warts on the genital area
- Painful or frequent urination
- Itching and redness in the genital area
- Blisters or sores in or around the mouth
- Abnormal vaginal odor
- Anal itching, soreness, or bleeding
- Abdominal pain
- Fever

In some cases, people with STDs/STIs have no symptoms, and over time the symptoms, if present, can improve on their own. However, it is common for individuals to have an STD/STI and pass it on to others without knowing it.

If you are concerned that you or your sexual partner may have an STD/STI, talk to your health care provider. Even if you do not have symptoms, it is possible you may have an STD/STI that needs to be treated to ensure your and your partner's sexual health.

Part Two

Types of STDs

Chapter 13

Common Symptoms of STDs

Types of STDs (STIs)

Sexually transmitted diseases (STDs) are infections that you can get by having sex or skin-to-skin contact between genitals with someone who has an STD.

STDs are also sometimes called sexually transmitted infections or STIs. Whatever you call them, they can cause serious health problems. And they happen a lot to young people: About half of all new infections happen to people ages 15 to 24.

There are more than 25 STDs caused by many different bacteria and viruses. Each STD has its own symptoms, but some have similar symptoms. One thing is clear: If you get an unusual discharge, sore, or rash, especially in the pubic area, you should stop having sex and see a doctor right away.

Chlamydia

Chlamydia is a very common STD. Women who have chlamydia are much more likely to get HIV if they are exposed to it. Also, if it's not treated, chlamydia can cause serious problems, like pelvic inflammatory disease and not being able to have a baby.

This chapter includes text excerpted from "Types of STDs (STIs)," Office on Women's Health (OWH), April 15, 2014.

Symptoms can include:

- Unusual vaginal discharge (not the clear or slightly white fluid women often have)
- Burning when urinating
- Bleeding between periods
- Pain in your belly area
- Back pain
- Nausea
- Fever
- Pain during sex

Genital Herpes

Genital herpes is caused by a virus called herpes simplex virus (HSV). There are two types of herpes virus that cause genital herpes: HSV-1 and HSV-2. Usually, genital herpes are HSV-2. But a person with HSV-1—that's oral herpes or cold sores around a person's mouth—can pass the virus to another person's genitals during oral sex.

Genital herpes can increase the risk of HIV infection. That's because HIV can enter the body more easily where there's a break in the skin, such as a herpes sore.

Symptoms can include:

- Small red bumps, blisters, or open sores in the genital area or anus (bottom) that can hurt a lot
- Fever, headache, and muscle aches
- Swollen glands in the genital area
- Itching or burning in genital area
- Pain in legs, buttocks, or genital area
- Pain when urinating

Symptoms may go away and then come back. Sores usually heal after 2 to 4 weeks. If the sores are mild, a person might think they are just bug bites or other skin problem.

Gonorrhea

Gonorrhea is a common STD. Recently, it has gotten harder to treat successfully because germs have built up resistance (strength) in fighting the medicine used against them.

Having gonorrhea can make you more likely to get HIV if you're exposed to it. Untreated gonorrhea can cause serious problems, including not being able to get pregnant, even if you don't have symptoms. It can also sometimes spread to the blood, joints, heart, or even the brain. Any young person who has had sex should be tested for gonorrhea.

Symptoms can include:

- Yellow or green vaginal discharge that may smell bad

- Pain or burning when urinating (peeing)

- Pain during sex

- Vaginal bleeding between menstrual periods

Gonorrhea infection can also be in your throat, which may cause a sore throat. It can also spread to your eyes, causing symptoms like pain and sensitivity to light.

It can also be in your anus (bottom). Symptoms there include:

- Anal discharge

- Anal itching

- Soreness

- Bleeding

Hepatitis B

Hepatitis B is caused by a virus that attacks the liver. It's also called HBV. If hepatitis B doesn't go away, it can lead to liver cancer and other serious liver problems.

Most babies now get vaccinated for HBV. Talk to your doctor or look at your health records to see if you were vaccinated. If not, you should get the shots now to help prevent this serious illness.

Symptoms can include:

- Yellow skin or yellowing of the whites of the eyes

- Tiredness

- Dark-colored urine

- Stomach pain

- Loss of appetite

- Nausea and vomiting

- Diarrhea

- Low fever

- Headache or muscle aches

- Hives or skin rash

- Joint pain and swelling

Symptoms usually appear about 6 to 12 weeks after you get infected.

HIV / AIDS

Human immunodeficiency virus, or HIV, is the virus that can cause AIDS (acquired immunodeficiency syndrome). HIV and AIDS weaken the body's ability to fight infections and diseases.

Symptoms of AIDS include:

Women and girls with HIV may have no symptoms for years. Even if HIV causes no symptoms, it is still causing problems with your body's immune system that need treatment as early as possible. HIV can lead to AIDS.

Some people have flu-like symptoms within the first few weeks or months after they get infected with HIV.

Some people have flu-like symptoms within the first few weeks or months after they get infected with HIV.

- Weight loss

- Fevers, chills, and night sweats

- Being very tired

- Headache

- Diarrhea, vomiting, and nausea

- Mouth, genital, or anal sores

- Dry cough

- Rash

- Swollen lymph nodes

- Other STDs (STIs), vaginal yeast infections, and other vaginal infections

- Pelvic inflammatory disease (PID) that does not get better with treatment

- Menstrual cycle changes, like not having periods or having heavy bleeding

- Human papillomavirus (HPV) infections, which can cause genital warts and cervical cancer

You cannot rely on symptoms to know whether you have HIV. More than half of young people with HIV don't know they have it.

You have to get tested to know if you have HIV. Get tested at least once if you are 13 or older.

You may need to get tested more often if you do things that increase your risk of HIV, such as having unprotected sex or using injection drugs. Find a place to get tested.

Human Papillomavirus (HPV)

Human papillomavirus, or HPV, is the most common STD in the United States. In fact, most people who have sex get it at some point in their lives. HPV often goes away on its own. But some types of HPV can cause genital warts, cervical cancer, and other types of cancer.

The HPV vaccine can help prevent the types of HPV that cause most cases of cervical cancer and genital warts. Ask your parents or doctor about getting vaccinated. Keep in mind that the vaccine works much better if you get it before you ever have sex.

Symptoms can include:

Some people have no symptoms.

- Warts on the genitals or inner thighs or around the anus (bottom). These can be flat or raised and alone or in groups. Some genital warts are so small you cannot see them. They may cause itching, burning, or pain.

- Growths on the cervix and vagina that the person often can't see.

HPV can be passed to a partner even if the infected person has no symptoms.

Pubic lice

Lice (a kind of tiny insect) that feed on human blood. Also known as "crabs."

Symptoms can include:

- Itching in the pubic area
- Finding lice or eggs attached to your pubic hair
- Sores from bites or scratching
- Rust-colored spots on your underwear
- Mild fever and tiredness if you've been bitten by a large number of lice

Syphilis

Syphilis that is not treated can lead to serious problems and even death. Also, the sores caused by syphilis make it easier to get or give someone HIV during sex.

Symptoms can include:

An infected person may not have any symptoms for years, but he or she can still give the disease to someone else. Different stages have different symptoms.

Symptoms in the first (primary) stage appear 10 to 90 days after getting infected. They include:

- A painless sore, usually in the genital area, but possibly on the lips or other parts of the body that had contact with a syphilis sore from another person.
- Swollen lymph glands

Sores heal on their own in around 3 to 6 weeks. But if the infection is not treated, a secondary stage follows. Symptoms of that stage include:

- Rash on the palms, stomach, or soles of the feet that usually doesn't itch and goes away on its own

- Fever

- Swollen lymph glands and sore throat

- Patchy hair loss

- Raised gray, warty-looking areas in moist places, such as your genital area, armpits, and anus (bottom)

- Headaches and muscle aches

- Weight loss

- Tiredness

If the infection is still not treated, it moves on to a hidden (latent) stage. Then it can possibly enter a last stage. During this stage there can be damage to the brain, nerves, eyes, heart, and blood vessels. Some people may even die.

Trichomoniasis

Trichomoniasis is caused by a parasite (a tiny organism that feeds off you). It is sometimes called "trich." Trichomoniasis is very common in sexually active young women. Having trichomoniasis increases your chances of getting HIV if you're exposed to it.

Symptoms can include:

Some women don't have symptoms, but those who do can have symptoms appear between 5 and 28 days after getting infected. Symptoms can include:

- Foamy, yellow-green vaginal discharge with a strong odor

- Discomfort during sex and when urinating

- Irritation and itching of the genital area

- Sometimes, lower abdominal pain

Chapter 14

Chancroid

Risk of Chancroid

The prevalence of chancroid has declined in the United States. When infection does occur, it is usually associated with sporadic outbreaks. Worldwide, chancroid appears to have declined as well, although infection might still occur in some regions of Africa and the Caribbean. Like genital herpes and syphilis, chancroid is a risk factor in the transmission and acquisition of HIV infection

Diagnostic Considerations

A definitive diagnosis of chancroid requires the identification of *H. Ducreyi* on special culture media that is not widely available from commercial sources; even when these media are used, sensitivity is <80%. No FDA-cleared PCR test for *H. Ducreyi* is available in the United States, but such testing can be performed by clinical laboratories that have developed their own PCR test and have conducted CLIA verification studies in genital specimens.

The combination of a painful genital ulcer and tender suppurative inguinal adenopathy suggests the diagnosis of chancroid. For both clinical and surveillance purposes, a probable diagnosis of chancroid can be made if all of the following criteria are met:

1. the patient has one or more painful genital ulcers;

This chapter includes text excerpted from "Chancroid," Centers for Disease Control and Prevention (CDC), June 4, 2015.

2. the clinical presentation, appearance of genital ulcers and, if present, regional lymphadenopathy are typical for chancroid;

3. the patient has no evidence of *T. Pallidum* infection by dark-field examination of ulcer exudate or by a serologic test for syphilis performed at least 7 days after onset of ulcers; and

4. an HSV PCR test or HSV culture performed on the ulcer exudate is negative.

Treatment

Successful treatment for chancroid cures the infection, resolves the clinical symptoms, and prevents transmission to others. In advanced cases, scarring can result despite successful therapy.

Azithromycin and ceftriaxone offer the advantage of single-dose therapy. Worldwide, several isolates with intermediate resistance to either ciprofloxacin or erythromycin have been reported. However, because cultures are not routinely performed, data are limited regarding the current prevalence of antimicrobial resistance.

Other Management Considerations

Men who are uncircumcised and patients with HIV infection do not respond as well to treatment as persons who are circumcised or HIV-negative. Patients should be tested for HIV infection at the time chancroid is diagnosed. If the initial test results were negative, a serologic test for syphilis and HIV infection should be performed 3 months after the diagnosis of chancroid.

Follow-Up

Patients should be re-examined 3–7 days after initiation of therapy. If treatment is successful, ulcers usually improve symptomatically within 3 days and objectively within 7 days after therapy. If no clinical improvement is evident, the clinician must consider whether

1. the diagnosis is correct,

2. the patient is co-infected with another STD,

3. the patient is infected with HIV,

4. the treatment was not used as instructed, or

5. the *H. Ducreyi* strain causing the infection is resistant to the prescribed antimicrobial.

The time required for complete healing depends on the size of the ulcer; large ulcers might require >2 weeks. In addition, healing is slower for some uncircumcised men who have ulcers under the foreskin. Clinical resolution of fluctuant lymphadenopathy is slower than that of ulcers and might require needle aspiration or incision and drainage, despite otherwise successful therapy. Although needle aspiration of buboes is a simpler procedure, incision and drainage might be preferred because of reduced need for subsequent drainage procedures.

Management of Sex Partners

Regardless of whether symptoms of the disease are present, sex partners of patients who have chancroid should be examined and treated if they had sexual contact with the patient during the 10 days preceding the patient's onset of symptoms.

Special Considerations

Pregnancy

Data suggest ciprofloxacin presents a low risk to the fetus during pregnancy, with a potential for toxicity during breastfeeding. Alternate drugs should be used during pregnancy and lactation. No adverse effects of chancroid on pregnancy outcome have been reported.

HIV Infection

Persons with HIV infection who have chancroid should be monitored closely because they are more likely to experience treatment failure and to have ulcers that heal slowly. Persons with HIV infection might require repeated or longer courses of therapy, and treatment failures can occur with any regimen. Data are limited concerning the therapeutic efficacy of the recommended single-dose azithromycin and ceftriaxone regimens in persons with HIV infection.

Chapter 15

Chlamydia

Chapter Contents

107

Section 15.1

What Is Chlamydia?

This section includes text excerpted from "Chlamydia—
CDC Fact Sheet (Detailed)," Centers for Disease Control
and Prevention (CDC), September 24, 2015.

Chlamydia is a common sexually transmitted disease (STD) caused by infection with *Chlamydia trachomatis*. It can cause cervicitis in women and urethritis and proctitis in both men and women. Chlamydial infections in women can lead to serious consequences including pelvic inflammatory disease (PID), tubal factor infertility, ectopic pregnancy, and chronic pelvic pain. Lymphogranuloma venereum (LGV), another type of STD caused by different serovars of the same bacterium, occurs commonly in the developing world, and has more recently emerged as a cause of outbreaks of proctitis among men who have sex with men (MSM) worldwide.

How Common Is Chlamydia?

Chlamydia is the most frequently reported bacterial sexually transmitted infection in the United States. In 2014, 1,441,789 cases of chlamydia were reported to CDC from 50 states and the District of Columbia, but an estimated 2.86 million infections occur annually. A large number of cases are not reported because most people with chlamydia are asymptomatic and do not seek testing. Chlamydia is most common among young people. Almost two-thirds of new chlamydia infections occur among youth aged 15–24 years. It is estimated that 1 in 20 sexually active young women aged 14–24 years has chlamydia.

Substantial racial/ethnic disparities in chlamydial infection exist, with prevalence among non-Hispanic blacks 6.7 times the prevalence among non-Hispanic whites. Chlamydia is also common among men who have sex with men (MSM). Among MSM screened for rectal chlamydial infection, positivity has ranged from 3.0% to 10.5%. Among MSM screened for pharyngeal chlamydial infection, positivity has ranged from 0.5% to 2.3%.

How Do People Get Chlamydia?

Chlamydia is transmitted through sexual contact with the penis, vagina, mouth, or anus of an infected partner. Ejaculation does not have to occur for chlamydia to be transmitted or acquired. Chlamydia can also be spread prenatally from an untreated mother to her baby during childbirth, resulting in ophthalmia neonatorum (conjunctivitis) or pneumonia in some exposed infants.

In published prospective studies, chlamydial conjunctivitis has been identified in 18–44% and chlamydial pneumonia in 3–16% of infants born to women with untreated chlamydial cervical infection at the time of delivery. While rectal or genital chlamydial infection has been shown to persist one year or longer in infants infected at birth, the possibility of sexual abuse should be considered in prepubertal children beyond the neonatal period with vaginal, urethral, or rectal chlamydial infection.

People who have had chlamydia and have been treated may get infected again if they have sexual contact with a person infected with chlamydia.

Who Is at Risk for Chlamydia?

Any sexually active person can be infected with chlamydia. It is a very common STD, especially among young people. It is estimated that 1 in 20 sexually active young women aged 14–19 years has chlamydia.

Sexually active young people are at high risk of acquiring chlamydia for a combination of behavioral, biological, and cultural reasons. Some young people don't use condoms consistently. Some adolescents may move from one monogamous relationship to the next more rapidly than the likely infectivity period of chlamydia, thus increasing risk of transmission.

Teenage girls and young women may have cervical ectopy (where cells from the endocervix are present on the ectocervix). Cervical ectopy may increase susceptibility to chlamydial infection. The higher prevalence of chlamydia among young people also may reflect multiple barriers to accessing STD prevention services, such as lack of transportation, cost, and perceived stigma.

Men who have sex with men (MSM) are also at risk for chlamydial infection since chlamydia can be transmitted by oral or anal sex. Among MSM screened for rectal chlamydial infection, positivity has ranged from 3.0% to 10.5%. Among MSM screened for pharyngeal chlamydial infection, positivity has ranged from 0.5% to 2.3%.

What Are the Symptoms of Chlamydia?

Chlamydia is known as a 'silent' infection because most infected people are asymptomatic and lack abnormal physical examination findings. Estimates of the proportion of chlamydia-infected people who develop symptoms vary by setting and study methodology; two published studies that incorporated modeling techniques to address limitations of point prevalence surveys estimated that only about 10% of men and 5–30% of women with laboratory-confirmed chlamydial infection develop symptoms. The incubation period of chlamydia is poorly defined. However, given the relatively slow replication cycle of the organism, symptoms may not appear until several weeks after exposure in those persons who develop symptoms.

In women, the bacteria initially infect the cervix, where the infection may cause signs and symptoms of cervicitis (e.g., mucopurulent endocervical discharge, easily induced endocervical bleeding), and sometimes the urethra, which may result in signs and symptoms of urethritis (e.g., pyuria, dysuria, urinary frequency). Infection can spread from the cervix to the upper reproductive tract (i.e., uterus, fallopian tubes), causing pelvic inflammatory disease (PID), which may be asymptomatic ("subclinical PID") or acute, with typical symptoms of abdominal and/or pelvic pain, along with signs of cervical motion tenderness, and uterine or adnexal tenderness on examination.

Men who are symptomatic typically have urethritis, with a mucoid or watery urethral discharge and dysuria. A minority of infected men develop epididymitis (with or without symptomatic urethritis), presenting with unilateral testicular pain, tenderness, and swelling.

Chlamydia can infect the rectum in men and women, either directly (through receptive anal sex), or possibly via spread from the cervix and vagina in a woman with cervical chlamydial infection. While these infections are often asymptomatic, they can cause symptoms of proctitis (e.g., rectal pain, discharge, and/or bleeding).

Sexually acquired chlamydial conjunctivitis can occur in both men and women through contact with infected genital secretions. While chlamydia can also be found in the throats of women and men having oral sex with an infected partner, it is typically asymptomatic and not thought to be an important cause of pharyngitis.

What Complications Can Result from Chlamydia Infection?

The initial damage that chlamydia causes often goes unnoticed. However, chlamydial infections can lead to serious health problems with both short- and long-term consequences.

In women, untreated chlamydia can spread into the uterus or fallopian tubes and cause pelvic inflammatory disease (PID). Symptomatic PID occurs in about 10 to 15 percent of women with untreated chlamydia. However, chlamydia can also cause subclinical inflammation of the upper genital tract ("subclinical PID"). Both acute and subclinical PID can cause permanent damage to the fallopian tubes, uterus, and surrounding tissues. The damage can lead to chronic pelvic pain, tubal factor infertility, and potentially fatal ectopic pregnancy.

Some patients with chlamydial PID develop perihepatitis, or "Fritz-Hugh-Curtis Syndrome", an inflammation of the liver capsule and surrounding peritoneum, which is associated with right upper quadrant pain.

In pregnant women, untreated chlamydia has been associated with pre-term delivery, as well as ophthalmia neonatorum (conjunctivitis) and pneumonia in the newborn.

Reactive arthritis can occur in men and women following symptomatic or asymptomatic chlamydial infection, sometimes as part of a triad of symptoms (with urethritis and conjunctivitis) formerly referred to as Reiter's Syndrome.

What about Chlamydia and HIV?

Untreated chlamydia may increase a person's chances of acquiring or transmitting HIV–the virus that causes AIDS.

How Does Chlamydia Affect a Pregnant Woman and Her Baby?

In pregnant women, untreated chlamydia has been associated with pre-term delivery, as well as ophthalmia neonatorum (conjunctivitis) and pneumonia in the newborn. In published prospective studies, chlamydial conjunctivitis has been identified in 18–44% and chlamydial pneumonia in 3–16% of infants born to women with untreated chlamydial cervical infection at the time of delivery. Neonatal prophylaxis against gonococcal conjunctivitis routinely performed at birth does not effectively prevent chlamydial conjunctivitis.

Screening and treatment of chlamydia in pregnant women is the best method for preventing neonatal chlamydial disease. All pregnant women should be screened for chlamydia at their first prenatal visit. Pregnant women under 25 and those at increased risk for chlamydia (e.g., women who have a new or more than one sex partner) should be screened again in their third trimester. Pregnant women with chlamydial infection should be retested 3 weeks and 3 months after completion of recommended therapy.

Who Should Be Tested for Chlamydia?

Any sexually active person can be infected with chlamydia. Anyone with genital symptoms such as discharge, burning during urination, unusual sores, or rash should refrain from having sex until they are able to see a healthcare provider about their symptoms.

Also, anyone with an oral, anal, or vaginal sex partner who has been recently diagnosed with an STD should see a healthcare provider for evaluation.

Because chlamydia is usually asymptomatic, screening is necessary to identify most infections. Screening programs have been demonstrated to reduce rates of adverse sequelae in women. CDC recommends yearly chlamydia screening of all sexually active women younger than 25, as well as older women with risk factors such as new or multiple partners, or a sex partner who has a sexually transmitted infection.

Pregnant women should be screened during their first prenatal care visit. Pregnant women under 25 or at increased risk for chlamydia (e.g., women who have a new or more than one sex partner) should be screened again in their third trimester. Women diagnosed with chlamydial infection should be retested approximately 3 months after treatment. Any woman who is sexually active should discuss her risk factors with a health care provider who can then determine if more frequent screening is necessary.

Routine screening is not recommended for men. However, the screening of sexually active young men should be considered in clinical settings with a high prevalence of chlamydia (e.g., adolescent clinics, correctional facilities, and STD clinics) when resources permit and do not hinder screening efforts in women.

Sexually active men who have sex with men (MSM) who had insertive intercourse should be screened for urethral chlamydial infection and MSM who had receptive anal intercourse should be screened for rectal infection at least annually; screening for pharyngeal infection is not recommended. More frequent chlamydia screening at 3-month intervals is indicated for MSM, including those with HIV infection, if risk behaviors persist or if they or their sexual partners have multiple partners.

At the initial HIV care visit, providers should test all sexually active persons with HIV infection for chlamydia and perform testing at least annually during the course of HIV care. A patient's health care provider might determine more frequent screening is necessary, based on the patient's risk factors.

How Is Chlamydia Diagnosed?

There are a number of diagnostic tests for chlamydia, including nucleic acid amplification tests (NAATs), cell culture, and others. NAATs are the most sensitive tests, and can be performed on easily obtainable specimens such as vaginal swabs (either clinician-or patient-collected) or urine.

Vaginal swabs, either patient- or clinician-collected, are the optimal specimen to screen for genital chlamydia using NAATs in women; urine is the specimen of choice for men, and is an effective alternative specimen type for women. Self-collected vaginal swab specimens perform at least as well as other approved specimens using NAATs. In addition, patients may prefer self-collected vaginal swabs or urine-based screening to the more invasive endocervical or urethral swab specimens. Adolescent girls may be particularly good candidates for self-collected vaginal swab- or urine-based screening because pelvic exams are not indicated if they are asymptomatic.

Chlamydial culture can be used for rectal or pharyngeal specimens, but is not widely available. NAATs have demonstrated improved sensitivity and specificity compared with culture for the detection of *C. Trachomatis* at non-genital sites. Most tests, including NAATs, are not FDA-cleared for use with rectal or pharyngeal swab specimens; however, NAATS have demonstrated improved sensitivity and specificity compared with culture for the detection of *C. Trachomatis* at rectal sites and however, some laboratories have met regulatory requirements and have validated NAAT testing on rectal and pharyngeal swab specimens.

What about Partners?

If a person has been diagnosed and treated for chlamydia, he or she should tell all recent anal, vaginal, or oral sex partners (all sex partners within 60 days before the onset of symptoms or diagnosis) so they can see a health care provider and be treated. This will reduce the risk that the sex partners will develop serious complications from chlamydia and will also reduce the person's risk of becoming re-infected. A person with chlamydia and all of his or her sex partners must avoid having sex until they have completed their treatment for chlamydia (i.e., seven days after single dose antibiotics or until completion of a seven-day course of antibiotics) and until they no longer have symptoms.

To help get partners treated quickly, healthcare providers in some states may give infected individuals extra medicine or prescriptions to give to their sex partners. This is called expedited partner therapy or EPT. In published clinical trials comparing EPT to traditional patient referral (i.e., asking the patient to refer their partners in for treatment), EPT was associated with fewer persistent or recurrent chlamydial infections in the index patient, and a larger reported number of partners treated. For providers, EPT represents an additional strategy for partner management of persons with chlamydial infection; partners should still be encouraged to seek medical evaluation, regardless of whether they receive EPT.

How Can Chlamydia Be Prevented?

Latex male condoms, when used consistently and correctly, can reduce the risk of getting or giving chlamydia. The surest way to avoid chlamydia is to abstain from vaginal, anal, and oral sex, or to be in a long-term mutually monogamous relationship with a partner who has been tested and is known to be uninfected.

Section 15.2

Chlamydia Treatment

This section includes text excerpted from "Chlamydial Infections," Centers for Disease Control and Prevention (CDC), June 4, 2015.

Chlamydial Infections in Adolescents and Adults

Chlamydial infection is the most frequently reported infectious disease in the United States, and prevalence is highest in persons aged ≤24 years. Several sequelae can result from *C. Trachomatis* infection in women, the most serious of which include PID, ectopic pregnancy, and infertility. Some women who receive a diagnosis of uncomplicated cervical infection already have subclinical upper-reproductive–tract infection.

Asymptomatic infection is common among both men and women. To detect chlamydial infections, health-care providers frequently rely on screening tests. Annual screening of all sexually active women aged <25 years is recommended, as is screening of older women at increased risk for infection (e.g., those who have a new sex partner, more than one sex partner, a sex partner with concurrent partners, or a sex partner who has a sexually transmitted infection. Although CT incidence might be higher in some women aged ≥25 years in some communities, overall the largest burden of infection is among women aged <25 years.

Chlamydia screening programs have been demonstrated to reduce the rates of PID in women. Although evidence is insufficient to recommend routine screening for *C. Trachomatis* in sexually active young men because of several factors (e.g., feasibility, efficacy, and cost-effectiveness), the screening of sexually active young men should be considered in clinical settings with a high prevalence of chlamydia (e.g., adolescent clinics, correctional facilities, and STD clinics) or in populations with high burden of infection (e.g., MSM).

Among women, the primary focus of chlamydia screening efforts should be to detect chlamydia, prevent complications, and test and treat their partners, whereas targeted chlamydia screening in men should only be considered when resources permit, prevalence is high, and such screening does not hinder chlamydia screening efforts in women. More frequent screening for some women (e.g., adolescents) or certain men (e.g., MSM) might be indicated.

Diagnostic Considerations of Chlamydia

C. trachomatis urogenital infection can be diagnosed in women by testing first-catch urine or collecting swab specimens from the endocervix or vagina. Diagnosis of *C. Trachomatis* urethral infection in men can be made by testing a urethral swab or first-catch urine specimen. NAATs are the most sensitive tests for these specimens and therefore are recommended for detecting *C. Trachomatis* infection. NAATs that are FDA-cleared for use with vaginal swab specimens can be collected by a provider or self-collected in a clinical setting. Self-collected vaginal swab specimens are equivalent in sensitivity and specificity to those collected by a clinician using NAATs, and women find this screening strategy highly acceptable. Optimal urogenital specimen types for chlamydia screening using NAAT include first catch-urine (men) and vaginal swabs (women). Rectal and oropharyngeal *C. Trachomatis* infection in persons engaging in receptive anal or oral intercourse can be diagnosed by testing at the anatomic site of exposure.

NAATs are not FDA-cleared for use with rectal or oropharyngeal swab specimens. However, NAATs have been demonstrated to have improved sensitivity and specificity compared with culture for the detection of *C. Trachomatis* at rectal sites and at oropharyngeal sites among men. Some laboratories have established CLIA-defined performance specifications when evaluating rectal and oropharyngeal swab specimens for *C. Trachomatis,* thereby allowing results to be used for clinical management. Most persons with *C. Trachomatis* detected at oropharyngeal sites do not have oropharyngeal symptoms. However, when gonorrhea testing is performed at the oropharyngeal site, chlamydia test results might be reported as well because some NAATs detect both bacteria from a single specimen.

Data indicate that performance of NAATs on self-collected rectal swabs is comparable to clinician-collected rectal swabs, and this specimen collection strategy for rectal *C. Trachomatis* screening is highly acceptable. Self-collected rectal swabs are a reasonable alternative to clinician-collected rectal swabs for *C. Trachomatis* screening by NAAT, especially when clinicians are not available or when self collection is preferred over clinician collection. Previous evidence suggests that the liquid-based cytology specimens collected for Pap smears might be acceptable specimens for NAAT testing, although test sensitivity using these specimens might be lower than that associated with use of cervical or vaginal swab specimens; regardless, certain NAATs have been FDA-cleared for use on liquid-based cytology specimens.

Treatment of Chlamydia

Treating persons infected with *C. Trachomatis* prevents adverse reproductive health complications and continued sexual transmission, and treating their sex partners can prevent reinfection and infection of other partners. Treating pregnant women usually prevents transmission of *C. Trachomatis* to neonates during birth. Chlamydia treatment should be provided promptly for all persons testing positive for infection; treatment delays have been associated with complications (e.g., PID) in a limited proportion of women.

A meta-analysis of 12 randomized clinical trials of azithromycin versus doxycycline for the treatment of urogenital chlamydial infection demonstrated that the treatments were equally efficacious, with microbial cure rates of 97% and 98%, respectively. These studies were conducted primarily in populations with urethral and cervical infection in which follow-up was encouraged, adherence to a 7-day regimen was effective, and culture or EIA (rather than the more sensitive NAAT) was used for determining microbiological outcome. More recent retrospective studies have raised concern about the efficacy of azithromycin for rectal *C. Trachomatis* infection, however, these studies have limitations, and prospective clinical trials comparing azithromycin versus doxycycline regimens for rectal *C. Trachomatis* infection are needed.

Although the clinical significance of oropharyngeal *C. Trachomatis* infection is unclear and routine oropharyngeal screening for CT is not recommended, available evidence suggests oropharyngeal *C. Trachomatis* can be sexually transmitted to genital sites; therefore, detection of *C. Trachomatis* from an oropharyngeal specimen should be treated with azithromycin or doxycycline. The efficacy of alternative antimicrobial regimens in resolving oropharyngeal chlamydia remains unknown.

In a double-blinded randomized control trial, a doxycycline delayed-release 200 mg tablet administered daily for 7 days was as effective as generic doxycycline 100 mg twice daily for 7 days for treatment of urogenital *C. Trachomatis* infection in men and women and had a lower frequency of gastrointestinal side effects. However, this regimen is more costly than those that involve multiple daily doses.

Delayed-release doxycycline (Doryx) 200 mg daily for 7 days might be an alternative regimen to the doxycycline 100 mg twice daily for 7 days for treatment of urogenital *C. Trachomatis* infection. Erythromycin might be less efficacious than either azithromycin or doxycycline, mainly because of the frequent occurrence of gastrointestinal side effects that can lead to nonadherence with treatment. Levofloxacin and ofloxacin are effective treatment alternatives, but they are more expensive and offer no advantage in the dosage regimen. Other quinolones either are not reliably effective against chlamydial infection or have not been evaluated adequately.

Other Management Considerations

To maximize adherence with recommended therapies, onsite, directly observed single-dose therapy with azithromycin should always be available for persons for whom adherence with multiday dosing is a concern. In addition, for multidose regimens, the first dose should be dispensed on site and directly observed. To minimize disease transmission to sex partners, persons treated for chlamydia should be instructed to abstain from sexual intercourse for 7 days after single-dose therapy or until completion of a 7-day regimen and resolution of symptoms if present. To minimize risk for reinfection, patients also should be instructed to abstain from sexual intercourse until all of their sex partners are treated. Persons who receive a diagnosis of chlamydia should be tested for HIV, GC, and syphilis.

Follow-Up

Test-of-cure to detect therapeutic failure (i.e., repeat testing 3–4 weeks after completing therapy) is not advised for persons treated with the recommended or alternative regimens, unless therapeutic adherence is in question, symptoms persist, or reinfection is suspected. Moreover, the use of chlamydial NAATs at <3 weeks after completion of therapy is not recommended because the continued presence of nonviable organisms can lead to false-positive results.

A high prevalence of *C. Trachomatis* infection has been observed in women and men who were treated for chlamydial infection during the preceding several months. Most post-treatment infections do not result from treatment failure, but rather from reinfection caused by failure of sex partners to receive treatment or the initiation of sexual activity with a new infected partner, indicating a need for improved education and treatment of sex partners. Repeat infections confer an elevated risk for PID and other complications in women.

Men and women who have been treated for chlamydia should be retested approximately 3 months after treatment, regardless of whether they believe that their sex partners were treated. If retesting at 3 months is not possible, clinicians should retest whenever persons next present for medical care in the 12-month period following initial treatment.

Treatment during Pregnancy

Doxycycline is contraindicated in the second and third trimesters of pregnancy. Human data suggest ofloxacin and levofloxacin present a low risk to the fetus during pregnancy, with a potential for toxicity during breastfeeding; however, data from animal studies raise concerns about cartilage damage to neonates. Thus, alternative drugs should be used to treat chlamydia in pregnancy. Clinical experience and published studies suggest that azithromycin is safe and effective. Test-of-cure to document chlamydial eradication (preferably by NAAT) 3–4 weeks after completion of therapy is recommended because severe sequelae can occur in mothers and neonates if the infection persists. In addition, all pregnant women who have chlamydial infection diagnosed should be retested 3 months after treatment. Detection of *C. Trachomatis* infection at repeat screening during the third semester is not uncommon in adolescent and young adult women, including in those without *C. Trachomatis* detected at the time of initial prenatal screening. Women aged <25 years and those at increased risk for chlamydia (e.g., those who have a new sex partner, more than one sex partner, a sex partner with concurrent partners, or a sex partner who has a sexually transmitted infection) should be rescreened during the third trimester to prevent maternal postnatal complications and chlamydial infection in the infant.

Because of concerns about chlamydia persistence following exposure to penicillin-class antibiotics that has been demonstrated in animal and in vitro studies, amoxicillin is now considered an alternative therapy for *C. Trachomatis* in pregnant women.

The frequent gastrointestinal side effects associated with erythromycin can result in nonadherence with these alternative regimens. The lower dose 14-day erythromycin regimens can be considered if gastrointestinal tolerance is a concern. Erythromycin estolate is contraindicated during pregnancy because of drug-related hepatotoxicity.

Diagnostic Considerations of Chlamydia during Pregnancy

Sensitive and specific methods used to diagnose chlamydial ophthalmia in the neonate include both tissue culture and nonculture tests (e.g., direct fluorescence antibody [DFA] tests and NAAT). DFA is the only nonculture FDA-cleared test for the detection of chlamydia from conjunctival swabs; NAATs are not FDA-cleared for the detection of chlamydia from conjunctival swabs, and clinical laboratories must verify the procedure according to CLIA regulations. Specimens for culture isolation and nonculture tests should be obtained from the everted eyelid using a dacron-tipped swab or the swab specified by the manufacturer's test kit; for culture and DFA, specimens must contain conjunctival cells, not exudate alone. Ocular specimens from neonates being evaluated for chlamydial conjunctivitis also should be tested for *N. Gonorrhoeae.*

Treatment of Ophthalmia Neonatorum

Although data on the use of azithromycin for the treatment of neonatal chlamydia infection are limited, available data suggest a short course of therapy might be effective. Topical antibiotic therapy alone is inadequate for treatment for ophthalmia neonatorum caused by chlamydia and is unnecessary when systemic treatment is administered.

Follow-Up

Because the efficacy of erythromycin treatment for ophthalmia neonatorum is approximately 80%, a second course of therapy might be required. Data on the efficacy of azithromycin for ophthalmia neonatorum are limited. Therefore, follow-up of infants is recommended to determine whether initial treatment was effective. The possibility of concomitant chlamydial pneumonia should be considered.

Section 15.3

Chlamydial Infections among Neonates

This section includes text excerpted from "Chlamydial Infections," Centers for Disease Control and Prevention (CDC), June 4, 2015.

Prenatal screening and treatment of pregnant women is the best method for preventing chlamydial infection among neonates. *C. Trachomatis* infection of neonates results from perinatal exposure to the mother's infected cervix. Although the efficacy of neonatal ocular prophylaxis with erythromycin ophthalmic ointments to prevent chlamydia ophthalmia is not clear, ocular prophylaxis with these agents prevents gonococcal ophthalmia and therefore should be administered.

Initial *C. Trachomatis* neonatal infection involves the mucous membranes of the eye, oropharynx, urogenital tract, and rectum, although infection might be asymptomatic in these locations. Instead, *C. Trachomatis* infection in neonates is most frequently recognized by conjunctivitis that develops 5–12 days after birth. *C. Trachomatis* also can cause a subacute, afebrile pneumonia with onset at ages 1–3 months. Although *C. Trachomatis* has been the most frequent identifiable infectious cause of ophthalmia neonatorum, neonatal chlamydial infections (including ophthalmia and pneumonia) have occurred less frequently since the institution of widespread prenatal screening and treatment of pregnant women.

Ophthalmia Neonatorum Caused by C. Trachomatis

A chlamydial etiology should be considered for all infants aged ≤30 days that have conjunctivitis, especially if the mother has a history of chlamydia infection. These infants should receive evaluation and appropriate care and treatment.

Diagnostic Considerations of Chlamydial Ophthalmia

Sensitive and specific methods used to diagnose chlamydial ophthalmia in the neonate include both tissue culture and nonculture tests (e.g., direct fluorescence antibody [DFA] tests and NAAT). DFA is the only nonculture FDA-cleared test for the detection of chlamydia from conjunctival swabs; NAATs are not FDA-cleared for the detection of chlamydia from conjunctival swabs, and clinical laboratories must verify the procedure according to CLIA regulations. Specimens for culture isolation and nonculture tests should be obtained from the everted eyelid using a dacron-tipped swab or the swab specified by the manufacturer's test kit; for culture and DFA, specimens must contain conjunctival cells, not exudate alone. Ocular specimens from neonates being evaluated for chlamydial conjunctivitis also should be tested for *N. Gonorrhoeae*.

Treatment of Ophthalmia Neonatorum

Although data on the use of azithromycin for the treatment of neonatal chlamydia infection are limited, available data suggest a short course of therapy might be effective. Topical antibiotic therapy alone is inadequate for treatment for ophthalmia neonatorum caused by chlamydia and is unnecessary when systemic treatment is administered.

Follow-Up

Because the efficacy of erythromycin treatment for ophthalmia neonatorum is approximately 80%, a second course of therapy might be required. Data on the efficacy of azithromycin for ophthalmia neonatorum are limited. Therefore, follow-up of infants is recommended to determine whether initial treatment was effective. The possibility of concomitant chlamydial pneumonia should be considered.

Diagnostic Considerations of Chlamydial Pneumonia

Specimens for chlamydial testing should be collected from the nasopharynx. Tissue culture is the definitive standard diagnostic test for chlamydial pneumonia. Nonculture tests (e.g., DFA and NAAT) can be used. DFA is the only nonculture FDA-cleared test for the detection of *C. Trachomatis* from nasopharyngeal specimens, but DFA of nasopharyngeal specimens has a lower sensitivity and specificity than culture. NAATs are not FDA-cleared for the detection of chlamydia from nasopharyngeal specimens, and clinical laboratories must verify the procedure according to CLIA regulations. Tracheal aspirates and lung biopsy specimens, if collected, should be tested for *C. Trachomatis*.

Treatment of Chlamydial Pneumonia

Because test results for chlamydia often are not available at the time that initial treatment decisions must be made, treatment for *C. Trachomatis* pneumonia must frequently be based on clinical and radiologic findings, age of the infant (i.e., 1–3 months), and risk of chlamydia in the mother (i.e., age <25, multiple partners, and history of chlamydial infection). The results of tests for chlamydial infection assist in the management of an infant's illness.

Follow-Up

Because the effectiveness of erythromycin in treating pneumonia caused by *C. Trachomatis* is approximately 80%, a second course of therapy might be required. Data on the effectiveness of azithromycin in treating chlamydial pneumonia are limited. Follow-up of infants is recommended to determine whether the pneumonia has resolved, although some infants with chlamydial pneumonia continue to have abnormal pulmonary function tests later in childhood.

Diagnostic Considerations

NAAT can be used for vaginal and urine specimens from girls, although data are insufficient to recommend the use of NAAT in boys. Data also are lacking regarding use of NAAT for specimens from extragenital sites (rectum and pharynx) in boys and girls; other nonculture tests (e.g., DFA) are not recommended because of specificity concerns. Culture is still the preferred method for detection of urogenital *C. Trachomatis* in boys and at extragenital sites in boys and girls.

Sexual Assault or Abuse of Children

These guidelines are limited to the identification and treatment of STDs in pre-pubertal children. Management of the psychosocial or legal aspects of the sexual assault or abuse of children is beyond the scope of these guidelines.

The identification of sexually transmissible agents in children beyond the neonatal period strongly suggests sexual abuse. The significance of the identification of a sexually transmitted organism in such children as evidence of possible child sexual abuse varies by pathogen. Postnatally acquired gonorrhea and syphilis; chlamydia infection; and nontransfusion, non-prenatally acquired HIV are indicative of sexual abuse. Chlamydia infection might be indicative of sexual abuse in children ≥3 years of age and among those aged <3 years when infection is not likely prenatally acquired.

Sexual abuse should be suspected when genital herpes, *T. Vaginalis*, or anogenital warts are diagnosed. The investigation of sexual abuse among children who have an infection that could have been transmitted sexually should be conducted in compliance with recommendations by clinicians who have experience and training in all elements of the evaluation of child abuse, neglect, and assault. The social significance of an infection that might have been acquired sexually varies by the specific organism, as does the threshold for reporting suspected child sexual abuse. In cases in which any STD has been diagnosed in a child, efforts should be made in consultation with a specialist to evaluate the possibility of sexual abuse, including conducting a history and physical examination for evidence of abuse and diagnostic testing for other commonly occurring STDs.

The general rule that sexually transmissible infections beyond the neonatal period are evidence of sexual abuse has exceptions. For example, genital infection with *T. Vaginalis* or rectal or genital infection with *C. Trachomatis* among young children might be the result of prenatally acquired infection and has, in some cases of chlamydia infection, persisted for as long as 2–3 years, though perinatal CT infection is now uncommon because of prenatal screening and treatment of pregnant women.

Genital warts have been diagnosed in children who have been sexually abused, but also in children who have no other evidence of sexual abuse. BV has been diagnosed in children who have been abused, but its presence alone does not prove sexual abuse. Most HBV infections in children result from household exposure to persons who have chronic HBV infection rather than sexual abuse.

Follow-Up

A test-of-cure culture (repeat testing after completion of therapy) to detect therapeutic failure ensures treatment effectiveness. Therefore, this culture with should be obtained at a follow-up visit approximately 2 weeks after treatment is completed.

Chapter 16

Granuloma Inguinale (Donovanosis)

What Is Granuloma Inguinale?

Granuloma inguinale is a genital ulcerative disease caused by the intracellular gram-negative bacterium *Klebsiella granulomatis* (formerly known as *Calymmatobacterium granulomatis*). The disease occurs rarely in the United States, although it is endemic in some tropical and developing areas, including India; Papua, New Guinea; the Caribbean; central Australia; and southern Africa. Clinically, the disease is commonly characterized as painless, slowly progressive ulcerative lesions on the genitals or perineum without regional lymphadenopathy; subcutaneous granulomas (pseudobuboes) also might occur. The lesions are highly vascular (i.e., beefy red appearance) and bleed. Extragenital infection can occur with extension of infection to the pelvis, or it can disseminate to intra-abdominal organs, bones, or the mouth. The lesions also can develop secondary bacterial infection and can coexist with other sexually transmitted pathogens.

Diagnostic Considerations

The causative organism of granuloma inguinale is difficult to culture, and diagnosis requires visualization of dark-staining Donovan

This chapter includes text excerpted from "Granuloma Inguinale (Donovanosis)," Centers for Disease Control and Prevention (CDC), June 4, 2015.

bodies on tissue crush preparation or biopsy. No FDA-cleared molecular tests for the detection of *K. Granulomatis* DNA exist, but such an assay might be useful when undertaken by laboratories that have conducted a CLIA verification study.

Treatment

Several antimicrobial regimens have been effective, but only a limited number of controlled trials have been published. Treatment has been shown to halt progression of lesions, and healing typically proceeds inward from the ulcer margins; prolonged therapy is usually required to permit granulation and re-epithelialization of the ulcers. Relapse can occur 6–18 months after apparently effective therapy.

The addition of another antibiotic to these regimens can be considered if improvement is not evident within the first few days of therapy. Addition of an aminoglycoside to these regimens is an option (gentamicin 1 mg/kg IV every 8 hours).

Recommended Regimen

Azithromycin 1 g orally once per week or 500 mg daily for at least 3 weeks and until all lesions have completely healed

Alternative Regimens

- Doxycycline 100 mg orally twice a day for at least 3 weeks and until all lesions have completely healed

  Or

- Ciprofloxacin 750 mg orally twice a day for at least 3 weeks and until all lesions have completely healed

  Or

- Erythromycin base 500 mg orally four times a day for at least 3 weeks and until all lesions have completely healed

  Or

- Trimethoprim-sulfamethoxazole one double-strength (160 mg/800 mg) tablet orally twice a day for at least 3 weeks and until all lesions have completely healed

Other Management Considerations

Persons should be followed clinically until signs and symptoms have resolved. All persons who receive a diagnosis of granuloma inguinale should be tested for HIV.

Follow-Up

Patients should be followed clinically until signs and symptoms resolve.

Chapter 17

Gonorrhea

Chapter Contents

Section 17.1

What Is Gonorrhea?

This section includes text excerpted from "Gonorrhea—CDC
Fact Sheet (Detailed Version)," Centers for Disease Control and
Prevention (CDC), November 17, 2015.

Gonorrhea is a sexually transmitted disease (STD) caused by infection with the *Neisseria gonorrhoeae* bacterium. *N. gonorrhoeae* infects the mucous membranes of the reproductive tract, including the cervix, uterus, and fallopian tubes in women, and the urethra in women and men. *N. gonorrhoeae* can also infect the mucous membranes of the mouth, throat, eyes, and rectum.

How Common Is Gonorrhea?

Gonorrhea is a very common infectious disease. CDC estimates that approximately 820,000 new gonorrheal infections occur in the United States each year, and that less than half of these infections are detected and reported to CDC. CDC estimates that 570,000 of them were among young people 15–24 years of age. In 2014, 350,062 cases of gonorrhea were reported to CDC.

How Do People Get Gonorrhea?

Gonorrhea is transmitted through sexual contact with the penis, vagina, mouth, or anus of an infected partner. Ejaculation does not have to occur for gonorrhea to be transmitted or acquired. Gonorrhea can also be spread perinatally from mother to baby during childbirth.

People who have had gonorrhea and received treatment may be reinfected if they have sexual contact with a person infected with gonorrhea.

Who Is at Risk for Gonorrhea?

Any sexually active person can be infected with gonorrhea. In the United States, the highest reported rates of infection are among sexually active teenagers, young adults, and African Americans.

130

What Are the Signs and Symptoms of Gonorrhea?

Many men with gonorrhea are asymptomatic. When present, signs and symptoms of urethral infection in men include dysuria or a white, yellow, or green urethral discharge that usually appears one to fourteen days after infection. In cases where urethral infection is complicated by epididymitis, men with gonorrhea may also complain of testicular or scrotal pain.

Most women with gonorrhea are asymptomatic. Even when a woman has symptoms, they are often so mild and nonspecific that they are mistaken for a bladder or vaginal infection. The initial symptoms and signs in women include dysuria, increased vaginal discharge, or vaginal bleeding between periods. Women with gonorrhea are at risk of developing serious complications from the infection, regardless of the presence or severity of symptoms.

Symptoms of rectal infection in both men and women may include discharge, anal itching, soreness, bleeding, or painful bowel movements. Rectal infection also may be asymptomatic. Pharyngeal infection may cause a sore throat, but usually is asymptomatic.

What Are the Complications of Gonorrhea?

Untreated gonorrhea can cause serious and permanent health problems in both women and men.

In women, gonorrhea can spread into the uterus or fallopian tubes and cause pelvic inflammatory disease (PID). The symptoms may be quite mild or can be very severe and can include abdominal pain and fever. PID can lead to internal abscesses and chronic pelvic pain. PID can also damage the fallopian tubes enough to cause infertility or increase the risk of ectopic pregnancy.

In men, gonorrhea may be complicated by epididymitis. In rare cases, this may lead to infertility.

If left untreated, gonorrhea can also spread to the blood and cause disseminated gonococcal infection (DGI). DGI is usually characterized by arthritis, tenosynovitis, and/or dermatitis. This condition can be life threatening.

What about Gonorrhea and HIV?

Untreated gonorrhea can increase a person's risk of acquiring or transmitting HIV, the virus that causes AIDS.

How Does Gonorrhea Affect a Pregnant Woman and Her Baby?

If a pregnant woman has gonorrhea, she may give the infection to her baby as the baby passes through the birth canal during delivery. This can cause blindness, joint infection, or a life-threatening blood infection in the baby. Treatment of gonorrhea as soon as it is detected in pregnant women will reduce the risk of these complications. Pregnant women should consult a healthcare provider for appropriate examination, testing, and treatment, as necessary.

Who Should Be Tested for Gonorrhea?

Any sexually active person can be infected with gonorrhea. Anyone with genital symptoms such as discharge, burning during urination, unusual sores, or rash should stop having sex and see a health care provider immediately.

Also, anyone with an oral, anal, or vaginal sex partner who has been recently diagnosed with an STD should see a healthcare provider for evaluation.

Some people should be tested (screened) for gonorrhea even if they do not have symptoms or know of a sex partner who has gonorrhea. Anyone who is sexually active should discuss his or her risk factors with a health care provider and ask whether he or she should be tested for gonorrhea or other STDs.

CDC recommends yearly gonorrhea screening for all sexually active women younger than 25 years, as well as older women with risk factors such as new or multiple sex partners, or a sex partner who has a sexually transmitted infection.

People who have gonorrhea should also be tested for other STDs.

How Is Gonorrhea Diagnosed?

Urogenital gonorrhea can be diagnosed by testing urine, urethral (for men), or endocervical or vaginal (for women) specimens using nucleic acid amplification testing (NAAT). It can also be diagnosed using gonorrhea culture, which requires endocervical or urethral swab specimens.

If a person has had oral and/or anal sex, pharyngeal and/or rectal swab specimens should be collected either for culture or for NAAT (if the local laboratory has validated the use of NAAT for extra-genital specimens).

What Is the Treatment for Gonorrhea?

Gonorrhea can be cured with the right treatment. CDC now recommends dual therapy (i.e., using two drugs) for the treatment of gonorrhea. It is important to take all of the medication prescribed to cure gonorrhea. Medication for gonorrhea should not be shared with anyone. Although medication will stop the infection, it will not repair any permanent damage done by the disease. Antimicrobial resistance in gonorrhea is of increasing concern, and successful treatment of gonorrhea is becoming more difficult. If a person's symptoms continue for more than a few days after receiving treatment, he or she should return to a health care provider to be reevaluated.

What about Partners?

If a person has been diagnosed and treated for gonorrhea, he or she should tell all recent anal, vaginal, or oral sex partners (all sex partners within 60 days before the onset of symptoms or diagnosis) so they can see a health provider and be treated. This will reduce the risk that the sex partners will develop serious complications from gonorrhea and will also reduce the person's risk of becoming reinfected. A person with gonorrhea and all of his or her sex partners must avoid having sex until they have completed their treatment for gonorrhea and until they no longer have symptoms.

How Can Gonorrhea Be Prevented?

Latex condoms, when used consistently and correctly, can reduce the risk of transmission of gonorrhea. The surest way to avoid transmission of gonorrhea or other STDs is to abstain from vaginal, anal, and oral sex, or to be in a long-term mutually monogamous relationship with a partner who has been tested and is known to be uninfected.

Section 17.2

Gonorrhea Treatment

This section includes text excerpted from "Gonococcal Infections," Centers for Disease Control and Prevention (CDC), June 4, 2015.

Gonococcal Infections in Adolescents and Adults

In the United States, an estimated 820,000 new *N. gonorrhoeae* infections occur each year. Gonorrhea is the second most commonly reported communicable disease. Urethral infections caused by *N. gonorrhoeae* among men can produce symptoms that cause them to seek curative treatment soon enough to prevent sequelae, but often not soon enough to prevent transmission to others. Among women, gonococcal infections are commonly asymptomatic or might not produce recognizable symptoms until complications (e.g., PID) have occurred. PID can result in tubal scarring that can lead to infertility and ectopic pregnancy.

Annual screening for *N. gonorrhoeae* infection is recommended for all sexually active women aged <25 years and for older women at increased risk for infection (e.g., those who have a new sex partner, more than one sex partner, a sex partner with concurrent partners, or a sex partner who has an STI). Additional risk factors for gonorrhea include inconsistent condom use among persons who are not in mutually monogamous relationships, previous or coexisting sexually transmitted infections, and exchanging sex for money or drugs.

Clinicians should consider the communities they serve and might opt to consult local public health authorities for guidance on identifying groups at increased risk. Gonococcal infection, in particular, is concentrated in specific geographic locations and communities. Subgroups of MSM are at high risk for gonorrhea infection and should be screened at sites of exposure. Screening for gonorrhea in men and older women who are at low risk for infection is not recommended. A recent travel history with sexual contacts outside of the United States should be part of any gonorrhea evaluation.

Diagnostic Considerations

Specific microbiologic diagnosis of infection with *N. gonorrhoeae* should be performed in all persons at risk for or suspected to have gonorrhea; a specific diagnosis can potentially reduce complications, reinfections, and transmission. Culture and NAAT are available for the detection of genitourinary infection with *N. gonorrhoeae*; culture requires endocervical (women) or urethral (men) swab specimens. NAAT allows for the widest variety of FDA-cleared specimen types, including endocervical swabs, vaginal swabs, urethral swabs (men), and urine (from both men and women). However, product inserts for each NAAT manufacturer must be carefully consulted because collection methods and specimen types vary. Culture is available for detection of rectal, oropharyngeal, and conjunctival gonococcal infection, but NAAT is not FDA-cleared for use with these specimens.

Some laboratories have met CLIA regulatory requirements and established performance specifications for using NAAT with rectal and oropharyngeal swab specimens that can inform clinical management. Certain NAATs that have been demonstrated to detect commensal *Neisseria* species might have comparable low specificity when testing oropharyngeal specimens for *N gonorrhoeae*.

The sensitivity of NAAT for the detection of *N. Gonorrhoeae* in urogenital and nongenital anatomic sites is superior to culture, but varies by NAAT type. In cases of suspected or documented treatment failure, clinicians should perform both culture and antimicrobial susceptibility testing because nonculture tests cannot provide antimicrobial susceptibility results. Because *N. gonorrhoeae* has demanding nutritional and environmental growth requirements, optimal recovery rates are achieved when specimens are inoculated directly and when the growth medium is promptly incubated in an increased CO_2 environment. Several non-nutritive swab transport systems are available that might maintain gonococcal viability for up to 48 hours in ambient temperatures.

Because of its high specificity (>99%) and sensitivity (>95%), a Gram stain of urethral secretions that demonstrates polymorphonuclear leukocytes with intracellular Gram-negative diplococci can be considered diagnostic for infection with *N. gonorrhoeae* in symptomatic men. However, because of lower sensitivity, a negative Gram stain should not be considered sufficient for ruling out infection in asymptomatic men. Detection of infection using Gram stain of endocervical, pharyngeal, and rectal specimens also is insufficient and is not recommended. MB/GV stain of urethral secretions is an alternative point-of-care diagnostic test with performance characteristics similar to Gram stain. Presumed gonococcal infection is established by documenting the presence of WBC containing intracellular purple diplococci in MB/GV smears.

Antimicrobial-Resistant N. gonorrhoeae

Gonorrhea treatment is complicated by the ability of *N. gonorrhoeae* to develop resistance to antimicrobials. In 1986, the Gonococcal Isolate Surveillance Project (GISP), a national sentinel surveillance system, was established to monitor trends in antimicrobial susceptibilities of urethral *N. gonorrhoeae* strains in the United States. The epidemiology of antimicrobial resistance guides decisions about gonococcal treatment recommendations and has evolved because of shifts in antimicrobial resistance patterns.

In 2007, emergence of fluoroquinolone-resistant *N. gonorrhoeae* in the United States prompted CDC to cease recommending fluoroquinolones for treatment of gonorrhea, leaving cephalosporins as the only remaining class of antimicrobials available for treatment of gonorrhea in the United States. Reflecting concern about emerging gonococcal resistance, CDC's 2010 STD treatment guidelines recommended dual therapy for gonorrhea with a cephalosporin plus either azithromycin or doxycycline, even if NAAT for *C.Trachomatis* was negative at the time of treatment. However, during 2006–2011, the minimum concentrations of cefixime needed to inhibit in vitro growth of the *N. gonorrhoeae* strains circulating in the United States and many other countries increased, suggesting that the effectiveness of cefixime might be waning.

In addition, treatment failures with cefixime or other oral cephalosporins have been reported in Asia, Europe, South Africa, and Canada. Ceftriaxone treatment failures for pharyngeal infections have been reported in Australia, Japan, and Europe. As a result, CDC no longer recommends the routine use of cefixime as a first-line regimen for treatment of gonorrhea in the United States. In addition, U.S. gonococcal strains with elevated MICs to cefixime also are likely to be resistant to tetracyclines but susceptible to azithromycin. Consequently, only one regimen, dual treatment with ceftriaxone and azithromycin, is recommended for treatment of gonorrhea in the United States. CDC and state health departments can provide the most current information on gonococcal susceptibility.

Criteria for resistance to cefixime and ceftriaxone have not been defined by the Clinical and Laboratory Standards Institute (CLSI). However, isolates with cefixime or ceftriaxone MICs ≥ 0.5 $\mu g/mL$ are considered to have decreased susceptibility. In the United States, the proportion of isolates in GISP demonstrating decreased susceptibility to ceftriaxone or cefixime has remained low; during 2013, no isolates with decreased susceptibility (MIC >0.5 ug/mL) to ceftriaxone or cefixime were identified. Because increasing MICs might predict the emergence of resistance, GISP established lower cephalosporin MIC breakpoints than those set by CLSI to provide greater sensitivity in detecting declining gonococcal susceptibility for surveillance purposes.

The percentage of isolates with cefixime MICs ≥0.25 μg/mL increased from 0.1% in 2006 to 1.4% in 2011, and declined to 0.4% in 2013. The percentage of isolates with ceftriaxone MICs ≥0.125 μg/mL increased from <0.1% in 2006 to 0.4% in 2011 and decreased to 0.05% in 2013. Isolates with high-level cefixime and ceftriaxone MICs (cefixime MICs 1.5–8 μg/mL and ceftriaxone MICs 1.5–4 μg/mL) have been identified in Japan, France, and Spain. Decreased susceptibility of *N. gonorrhoeae* to cephalosporins and other antimicrobials is expected to continue; state and local surveillance for antimicrobial resistance is crucial for guiding local therapy recommendations.

Although approximately 3% of all U.S. men who have gonococcal infections are sampled through GISP, surveillance by clinicians also is critical. Clinicians who diagnose *N. gonorrhoeae* infection in a person with suspected cephalosporin treatment failure should perform culture and antimicrobial susceptibility testing (AST) of relevant clinical specimens, consult an infectious-disease specialist for guidance in clinical management, and report the case to CDC through state and local public health authorities. Isolates should be saved and sent to CDC through local and state public health laboratory mechanisms. Health departments should prioritize notification and culture evaluation for sexual partner(s) of persons with *N. gonorrhoeae* infection thought to be associated with cephalosporin treatment failure or persons whose isolates demonstrate decreased susceptibility to cephalosporin.

Dual Therapy for Gonococcal Infections

On the basis of experience with other microbes that have developed antimicrobial resistance rapidly, a theoretical basis exists for combination therapy using two antimicrobials with different mechanisms of action (e.g., a cephalosporin plus azithromycin) to improve treatment efficacy and potentially slow the emergence and spread of resistance to cephalosporins. Use of azithromycin as the second antimicrobial is preferred to doxycycline because of the convenience and compliance advantages of single-dose therapy and the substantially higher prevalence of gonococcal resistance to tetracycline than to azithromycin among GISP isolates, particularly in strains with elevated cefixime MICs. In addition, clinical trials have demonstrated the efficacy of azithromycin 1 g for the treatment of uncomplicated urogenital GC.

Limited data suggest that dual treatment with azithromycin might enhance treatment efficacy for pharyngeal infection when using oral cephalosporins. In addition, persons infected with *N. gonorrhoeae* frequently are coinfected with *C.Trachomatis*; this finding has led to the longstanding recommendation that persons treated for gonococcal infection also be treated with a regimen that is effective against uncomplicated genital *C.Trachomatis* infection, further supporting the use of dual therapy that includes azithromycin.

Other Management Considerations

To maximize adherence with recommended therapies and reduce complications and transmission, medication for gonococcal infection should be provided on site and directly observed. If medications are not available when treatment is indicated, linkage to an STD treatment facility should be provided for same-day treatment. To minimize disease transmission, persons treated for gonorrhea should be instructed to abstain from sexual activity for 7 days after treatment and until all sex partners are adequately treated (7 days after receiving treatment and resolution of symptoms, if present). All persons who receive a diagnosis of gonorrhea should be tested for other STDs, including chlamydia, syphilis, and HIV.

Follow-Up

A test-of-cure is not needed for persons who receive a diagnosis of uncomplicated urogenital or rectal gonorrhea who are treated with any of the recommended or alternative regimens; however, any person with pharyngeal gonorrhea who is treated with an alternative regimen should return 14 days after treatment for a test-of cure using either culture or NAAT. If the NAAT is positive, effort should be made to perform a confirmatory culture before retreatment. All positive cultures for test-of-cure should undergo antimicrobial susceptibility testing.

Symptoms that persist after treatment should be evaluated by culture for *N. gonorrhoeae* (with or without simultaneous NAAT), and any gonococci isolated should be tested for antimicrobial susceptibility.

Persistent urethritis, cervicitis, or proctitis also might be caused by other organisms.

A high prevalence of *N. gonorrhoeae* infection has been observed among men and women previously treated for gonorrhea. Rather than signaling treatment failure, most of these infections result from reinfection caused by failure of sex partners to receive treatment or the initiation of sexual activity with a new infected partner, indicating a need for improved patient education and treatment of sex partners. Men or women who have been treated for gonorrhea should be retested 3 months after treatment regardless of whether they believe their sex partners were treated. If retesting at 3 months is not possible, clinicians should retest whenever persons next present for medical care within 12 months following initial treatment.

Treatments during Special Considerations

Allergy, Intolerance, and Adverse Reactions

Allergic reactions to first-generation cephalosporins occur in <2.5% of persons with a history of penicillin allergy and are uncommon with third-generation cephalosporins (e.g., ceftriaxone and cefixime). Use of ceftriaxone or cefixime is contraindicated in persons with a history of an IgE-mediated penicillin allergy (e.g., anaphylaxis, Stevens Johnson syndrome, and toxic epidermal necrolysis). Data are limited regarding alternative regimens for treating gonorrhea among persons who have either a cephalosporin or IgE-mediated penicillin allergy. Potential therapeutic options are dual treatment with single doses of oral gemifloxacin 320 mg plus oral azithromycin 2 g or dual treatment with single doses of intramuscular gentamicin 240 mg plus oral azithromycin 2 g. Spectinomycin for treatment of urogenital and anorectal gonorrhea can be considered when available. Providers treating persons with cephalosporin or IgE-mediated penicillin allergy should consult an infectious-disease specialist.

Pregnancy

Pregnant women infected with *N. gonorrhoeae* should be treated with dual therapy consisting of ceftriaxone 250 mg in a single IM dose and azithromycin 1 g orally as a single dose. When cephalosporin allergy or other considerations preclude treatment with this regimen and spectinomycin is not available, consultation with an infectious-disease specialist is recommended.

139

HIV Infection

Persons who have gonorrhea and HIV infection should receive the same treatment regimen as those who are HIV negative.

Gonococcal Infections among Infants and Children

Neonates born to mothers who have untreated gonorrhea are at high risk for infection. Neonates should be tested for gonorrhea at exposed sites and treated presumptively for gonorrhea as recommended in these guidelines. No data exist on the use of dual therapy to treat neonates born to mothers who have gonococcal infection.

Other Management Considerations

Appropriate chlamydial testing should be done simultaneously in neonates with gonococcal infection. Follow-up examination is not required.

Management of Mothers and Their Sex Partners

Mothers who have gonorrhea and their sex partners should be evaluated, tested, and presumptively treated for gonorrhea.

Diagnostic Considerations

NAAT can be used to test vaginal and urine specimens from girls, although data are insufficient to recommend the use of these tests in boys and from extragenital sites (rectum and pharynx) in boys and girls. Culture remains the preferred method for diagnosing boys and for detecting infection in specimens obtained from extragenital sites regardless of gender. Gram stains are inadequate for evaluating prepubertal children for gonorrhea and should not be used to diagnose or exclude gonorrhea. If evidence of disseminated gonococcal infection exists, gonorrhea culture and antimicrobial susceptibility testing should be obtained from relevant clinical sites.

No data exist regarding the use of dual therapy for treating children with gonococcal infection.

Other Management Considerations

Follow-up cultures are unnecessary. Only parenteral cephalosporins (i.e., ceftriaxone) are recommended for use in children. All children found to have gonococcal infections should be tested for *C.Trachomatis*, syphilis, and HIV. For a discussion of concerns regarding sexual assault.

Section 17.3

Antibiotic-Resistant Gonorrhea Infections

This section includes text excerpted from "Antibiotic-Resistant Gonorrhea Basic Information," Centers for Disease Control and Prevention (CDC), November 17, 2015.

Antibiotic resistance (AR) is the ability of bacteria to resist the effects of the drugs used to treat them. This means the germs are not killed and they will continue to reproduce. *Neisseria (N.) gonorrhoeae*, the bacteria that cause the STD gonorrhea, has developed resistance to nearly all of the antibiotics used for gonorrhea treatment: sulfonilamides, penicillin, tetracycline, and fluoroquinolones, such as ciprofloxacin. The Centers for Disease Control and Prevention (CDC) is currently down to one last effective class of antibiotics, cephalosporins, to treat this common infection. This is an urgent public health threat because gonorrhea control in the United States largely relies on effective antibiotic therapy.

Given the bacteria's ability to adapt and survive antibiotics, it is critical to continuously monitor for antibiotic resistance and encourage research and development of new treatment regimens for gonorrhea.

Surveillance

Surveillance for antimicrobial resistance in *N. gonorrhoeae* in the United States is conducted through the Gonococcal Isolate Surveillance Project (GISP). Each year, 25–30 sites and 4–5 regional laboratories across the United States participate in GISP and collect thousands of *N. gonorrhoeae* samples from men with urethral gonorrhea at STD clinics. Isolates from these samples are then used by researchers to determine the bacteria's susceptibility to a given set of antibiotics.

Clinicians are asked to report any *N. gonorrhoeae* specimen with decreased cephalosporin susceptibility and any gonorrhea cephalosporin treatment failure to CDC through their state or local public health authority. Bacteria have decreased susceptibility to a given antibiotic when laboratory results indicate that higher-than-expected antibiotic concentrations are needed to stop their growth.

Trends and Treatment

In 1993, ciprofloxacin, a fluoroquinolone, and cephalosporins ceftriaxone and cefixime were the recommended treatments for gonorrhea. However, in the late 1990s and early 2000s, ciprofloxacin resistance was detected in Hawaii and the West Coast, and by 2004 ciprofloxacin resistance was detected among men who have sex with men (MSM) with gonorrhea. By 2006, 13.8% of isolates exhibited resistance to ciprofloxacin, and ciprofloxacin resistance was present in all regions of the country, and in the heterosexual population. On April 13, 2007, CDC stopped recommending fluoroquinolones as empiric treatment for gonococcal infections for all people in the United States. The cephalosporins, either cefixime or ceftriaxone, were the only remaining recommended treatments.

Similar to trends observed elsewhere in the world, CDC has observed recent worrisome trends of decreasing cephalosporin susceptibility, especially to the oral cephalosporin cefixime. To preserve cephalosporins for as long as possible, CDC has since then made the following changes to its STD Treatment Guidelines:

- In 2010, CDC changed its treatment recommendations to recommend dual therapy for the treatment of gonorrhea and increased the recommended dose of ceftriaxone to 250 mg.

- Following continued declines in cefixime susceptibility, CDC updated its recommendations in 2012 to recommend ceftriaxone plus either azithromycin or doxycycline as the only first-line treatment.

- CDC's 2015 STD Treatment Guidelines now recommend only one regimen of dual therapy for the treatment of gonorrhea—the injectable cephalosporin ceftriaxone, plus oral azithromycin. Dual therapy is recommended to address the potential emergence of gonococcal cephalosporin resistance.

In 2012 and 2013, there were dramatic decreases in resistance to cefixime. However, resistance levels increased in 2014. CDC has not received any reports of verified clinical treatment failures to any cephalosporin in the United States.

Challenges

A major challenge to monitoring emerging antimicrobial resistance of *N. gonorrhoeae* is the substantial decline in the use of gonorrhea culture by many clinicians, as well as the reduced capability of many laboratories to perform gonorrhea culture techniques required for antibiotic susceptibility testing. Culture testing is when the bacteria is first grown on a nutrient plate and is then exposed to known amounts of an antibiotic to determine the bacteria's susceptibility to the antibiotic. The decline in culture testing results from an increased use of newer nonculture-based laboratory technology, such as a diagnostic test called the Nucleic Acid Amplification Test (NAAT). Currently, there is no well-studied reliable technology that allows for antibiotic susceptibility testing from nonculture specimens. Increased laboratory culture capacity is needed.

Laboratory Issues

CDC recommends that all state and local health department labs maintain or develop the capacity to perform gonorrhea culture, or form partnerships with experienced laboratories that can perform this type of testing.

Chapter 18

Herpes

Chapter Contents

Section 18.1

Genital Herpes

This section includes text excerpted from "Genital
Herpes—CDC Fact Sheet (Detailed)," Centers for Disease
Control and Prevention (CDC), September 24, 2015.

What Is Genital Herpes?

Genital herpes is a sexually transmitted disease (STD) caused by
the herpes simplex viruses type 1 (HSV-1) or type 2 (HSV-2).

How Common Is Genital Herpes?

Genital herpes infection is common in the United States. CDC
estimates that, annually, 776,000 people in the United States get
new herpes infections. Nationwide, 15.5 % of persons aged 14 to 49
years have HSV-2 infection. The overall prevalence of genital herpes
is likely higher than 15.5% because an increasing number of genital
herpes infections are caused by HSV-1. HSV-1 is typically acquired in
childhood; as the prevalence of HSV-1 infection has declined in recent
decades, people may have become more susceptible to genital herpes
from HSV-1.

HSV-2 infection is more common among women than among men
(20.3% versus 10.6% in 14 to 49 year olds). Infection is more easily
transmitted from men to women than from women to men. HSV-2
infection is more common among non-Hispanic blacks (41.8%) than
among non-Hispanic whites (11.3%). This disparity remains even
among persons with similar numbers of lifetime sexual partners. For
example, among persons with 2–4 lifetime sexual partners, HSV-2 is
still more prevalent among non-Hispanic blacks (34.3%) than among
non-Hispanic whites (9.1%) or Mexican Americans (13%). Most infected
persons are unaware of their infection. In the United States, an estimated 87.4% of 14–49 year olds infected with HSV-2 have never
received a clinical diagnosis.

The percentage of persons in the United States who are infected
with HSV-2 decreased from 21.2% in 1988–1994 to 15.5% in 2007–2010.

How Do People Get Genital Herpes?

Infections are transmitted through contact with lesions, mucosal surfaces, genital secretions, or oral secretions. HSV-1 and HSV-2 can also be shed from skin that looks normal. Generally, a person can only get HSV-2 infection during sexual contact with someone who has a genital HSV-2 infection. Transmission most commonly occurs from an infected partner who does not have visible sores and who may not know that he or she is infected. In persons with asymptomatic HSV-2 infections, genital HSV shedding occurs on 10% of days, and on most of those days the person has no signs or symptoms.

What Are the Symptoms of Genital Herpes?

Most individuals infected with HSV-1 or HSV-2 are asymptomatic or have very mild symptoms that go unnoticed or are mistaken for another skin condition. As a result, 87.4% of infected individuals remain unaware of their infection. When symptoms do occur, they typically appear as one or more vesicles on or around the genitals, rectum or mouth. The average incubation period after exposure is 4 days (range, 2 to 12). The vesicles break and leave painful ulcers that may take two to four weeks to heal. Experiencing these symptoms is referred to as having an "outbreak" or episode.

Clinical manifestations of genital herpes differ between the first and recurrent outbreaks of HSV. The first outbreak of herpes is often associated with a longer duration of herpetic lesions, increased viral shedding (making HSV transmission more likely) and systemic symptoms including fever, body aches, swollen lymph nodes, or headache. Recurrent outbreaks of genital herpes are common, in particular during the first year of infection. Approximately half of patients who recognize recurrences have prodromal symptoms, such as mild tingling or shooting pains in the legs, hips or buttocks, which occur hours to days before the eruption of herpetic lesions. Symptoms of recurrent outbreaks are typically shorter in duration and less severe than the first outbreak of genital herpes. Although the infection can stay in the body indefinitely, the number of outbreaks tends to decrease over time. Recurrences and subclinical shedding are much less frequent for genital HSV-1 infection than for genital HSV-2 infection.

What Are the Complications of Genital Herpes?

Genital herpes may cause painful genital ulcers that can be severe and persistent in persons with suppressed immune systems, such as

HIV-infected persons. Both HSV-1 and HSV-2 can also cause rare but serious complications such as blindness, encephalitis (inflammation of the brain), and aseptic meningitis (inflammation of the linings of the brain). Development of extragenital lesions in the buttocks, groin, thigh, finger, or eye may occur during the course of infection.

Some persons who contract genital herpes have concerns about how it will impact their overall health, sex life, and relationships. There can be can be considerable embarrassment, shame, and stigma associated with a herpes diagnosis that can substantially interfere with a patient's relationships. Clinicians can address these concerns by encouraging patients to recognize that while herpes is not curable, it is a manageable condition. Three important steps that providers can take for their newly-diagnosed patients are, giving information, providing support resources, and helping define options. Since a diagnosis of genital herpes may affect perceptions about existing or future sexual relationships, it is important for patients to understand how to talk to sexual partners about STDs.

There are also potential complications for a pregnant woman and her unborn child.

What Is the Link between Genital Herpes and HIV?

Genital ulcerative disease caused by herpes make it easier to transmit and acquire HIV infection sexually. There is an estimated 2- to 4-fold increased risk of acquiring HIV, if exposed to HIV when genital herpes is present. Ulcers or breaks in the skin or mucous membranes (lining of the mouth, vagina, and rectum) from a herpes infection may compromise the protection normally provided by the skin and mucous membranes against infections, including HIV. Herpetic genital ulcers can bleed easily, and when they come into contact with the mouth, vagina, or rectum during sex, they may increase the risk of HIV transmission.

How Does Genital Herpes Affect a Pregnant Woman and Her Baby?

Neonatal herpes is one of the most serious complications of genital herpes. Healthcare providers should ask all pregnant women if they have a history of genital herpes. Herpes infection can be passed from mother to child during pregnancy, childbirth, or in the newborn period, resulting in a potentially fatal neonatal herpes infection. During pregnancy there is a higher risk of perinatal transmission during the first outbreak than with a recurrent outbreak, thus it is important that women avoid contracting herpes during pregnancy. Women should be counseled to abstain from intercourse during the third trimester with partners known to have or suspected of having genital herpes.

A woman with genital herpes may be offered antiviral medication from 36 weeks gestation through delivery to reduce the risk of a recurrent outbreak. Routine HSV screening of pregnant women is not recommended. However, at onset of labor, all women should undergo careful examination and questioning to evaluate for presence of prodromal symptoms or herpetic lesions. If herpes symptoms are present a cesarean delivery is recommended to prevent HSV transmission to the infant.

How Is Genital Herpes Diagnosed?

The preferred HSV tests for patients with active genital ulcers include viral culture or detection of HSV DNA by polymerase chain reaction (PCR). HSV culture requires collection of a sample from the sore and, once viral growth is seen, specific cell staining to differentiate between HSV-1 and HSV-2. However, culture sensitivity is low, especially for recurrent lesions, and declines as lesions heal. PCR is more sensitive, allows for more rapid and accurate results, and is increasingly being used. Because viral shedding is intermittent, failure to detect HSV by culture or PCR does not indicate and absence of HSV infection. Tzanck preparations are insensitive and nonspecific and should not be used.

Serologic tests are blood tests that detect antibodies to the herpes virus. Several ELISA-based serologic tests are FDA approved and available commercially. Older assays that do not accurately distinguish HSV-1 from HSV-2 antibody remain on the market, so providers should specifically request serologic type-specific assays when blood tests are performed for their patients. The sensitivities of type-specific serologic tests for HSV-2 vary from 80–98%; false-negative results might be more frequent at early stages of infection. Additionally, false positive results may occur at low index values and should be confirmed with another test such as Biokit or the Western Blot. Negative HSV-1 results should be interpreted with caution because some ELISA-based serologic tests are insensitive for detection of HSV-1 antibody.

For the symptomatic patient, testing with both virologic and serologic assays can determine whether it is a new infection or a newly-recognized old infection. A primary infection would be supported by a positive virologic test and a negative serologic test, while the diagnosis of recurrent disease would be supported by positive virologic and serologic test results.

CDC does not recommend screening for HSV-1 or HSV-2 in the general population. Several scenarios where type-specific serologic HSV tests may be useful include:

- Patients with recurrent genital symptoms or atypical symptoms and negative HSV PCR or culture;

- Patients with a clinical diagnosis of genital herpes but no laboratory confirmation;

- Patients who report having a partner with genital herpes;

- Patients presenting for an STD evaluation (especially those with multiple sex partners);

- Persons with HIV infection; and

- MSM at increased risk for HIV acquisition.

Is There a Cure or Treatment for Herpes?

There is no cure for herpes. Antiviral medications can, however, prevent or shorten outbreaks during the period of time the person takes the medication. In addition, daily suppressive therapy (i.e. daily use of antiviral medication) for herpes can reduce the likelihood of transmission to partners.

Several clinical trials have tested vaccines against genital herpes infection, but there is currently no commercially available vaccine that is protective against genital herpes infection. One vaccine trial showed efficacy among women whose partners were HSV-2 infected, but only among women who were not infected with HSV-1. No efficacy was observed among men whose partners were HSV-2 infected. A subsequent trial testing the same vaccine showed some protection from genital HSV-1 infection, but no protection from HSV-2 infection.

How Can Herpes Be Prevented?

Correct and consistent use of latex condoms can reduce the risk of genital herpes. However, outbreaks can occur in areas that are not covered by a condom.

The surest way to avoid transmission of sexually transmitted diseases, including genital herpes, is to abstain from sexual contact, or to be in a long-term mutually monogamous relationship with a partner who has been tested and is known to be uninfected.

Persons with herpes should abstain from sexual activity with partners when sores or other symptoms of herpes are present. It is important to know that even if a person does not have any symptoms, he or she can still infect sex partners. Sex partners of infected persons should be advised that they may become infected and they should use condoms to reduce the risk. Sex partners can seek testing to determine if they are infected with HSV.

Section 18.2

Treating and Managing Herpes

This section contains text excerpted from the following sources:
Text under the heading "Is There a Cure or Treatment for Herpes?"
is excerpted from "Genital Herpes Treatment and Care," Centers
for Disease Control and Prevention (CDC), December 2, 2015; Text
under the heading "Genital HSV Infections" is excerpted from
"Genital HSV Infections," Centers for Disease
Control and Prevention (CDC), June 4, 2015.

Is There a Cure or Treatment for Herpes?

There is no cure for herpes. Antiviral medications can, however, prevent or shorten outbreaks during the period of time the person takes the medication. In addition, daily suppressive therapy (i.e. daily use of antiviral medication) for herpes can reduce the likelihood of transmission to partners.

Several clinical trials have tested vaccines against genital herpes infection, but there is currently no commercially available vaccine that is protective against genital herpes infection. One vaccine trial showed efficacy among women whose partners were HSV-2 infected, but only among women who were not infected with HSV-1. No efficacy was observed among men whose partners were HSV-2 infected. A subsequent trial testing the same vaccine showed some protection from genital HSV-1 infection, but no protection from HSV-2 infection.

Genital HSV Infections

Genital herpes is a chronic, life-long viral infection. Two types of HSV can cause genital herpes: HSV-1 and HSV-2. Most cases of recurrent genital herpes are caused by HSV-2, and approximately 50 million persons in the United States are infected with this type of genital herpes. However, an increasing proportion of anogenital herpetic infections have been attributed to HSV-1 infection, which is especially prominent among young women and MSM.

Most persons infected with HSV-2 have not had the condition diagnosed. Many such persons have mild or unrecognized infections but shed virus intermittently in the anogenital area. As a result, most genital herpes infections are transmitted by persons unaware that they have the infection or who are asymptomatic when transmission occurs. Management of genital HSV should address the chronic nature of the disease rather than focusing solely on treatment of acute episodes of genital lesions.

Diagnostic Considerations

The clinical diagnosis of genital herpes can be difficult, because the painful multiple vesicular or ulcerative lesions typically associated with HSV are absent in many infected persons. Recurrences and subclinical shedding are much more frequent for genital HSV-2 infection than for genital HSV-1 infection. A patient's prognosis and the type of counseling needed depend on the type of genital herpes (HSV-1 or HSV-2) causing the infection; therefore, the clinical diagnosis of genital herpes should be confirmed by type-specific laboratory testing. Both type-specific virologic and type-specific serologic tests for HSV should be available in clinical settings that provide care to persons with or at risk for STDs. Persons with genital herpes should be tested for HIV infection.

Virologic Tests

Cell culture and PCR are the preferred HSV tests for persons who seek medical treatment for genital ulcers or other mucocutaneous lesions. The sensitivity of viral culture is low, especially for recurrent lesions, and declines rapidly as lesions begin to heal. Nucleic acid amplification methods, including PCR assays for HSV DNA, are more sensitive and are increasingly available. PCR is the test of choice for diagnosing HSV infections affecting the central nervous system and systemic infections (e.g., meningitis, encephalitis, and neonatal herpes). Viral culture isolates and PCR amplicons should be typed to determine which type of HSV is causing the infection. Failure to detect HSV by culture or PCR, especially in the absence of active lesions, does not indicate an absence of HSV infection because viral shedding is intermittent. Cytologic detection of cellular changes associated with HSV infection is an insensitive and nonspecific method of diagnosing genital lesions (i.e., Tzanck preparation) and therefore should not be relied on. Although a direct immunofluorescence (IF) assay using fluorescein-labeled monoclonal antibodies is also available to detect HSV antigen from genital specimens, this assay lacks sensitivity.

Type-Specific Serologic Tests

Both type-specific and type-common antibodies to HSV develop during the first several weeks after infection and persist indefinitely. Accurate type-specific HSV serologic assays are based on the HSV-specific glycoprotein G2 (HSV-2) and glycoprotein G1 (HSV-1). Providers should only request type-specific glycoprotein G (gG)-based serologic assays when serology is performed for their patients.

Both laboratory-based assays and point-of-care tests that provide results for HSV-2 antibodies from capillary blood or serum during a clinic visit are available. The sensitivities of these glycoprotein G type-specific tests for the detection of HSV-2 antibody vary from 80%–98%; false-negative results might be more frequent at early stages of infection. The most commonly used test, HerpeSelect HSV-2 Elisa might be falsely positive at low index values (1.1–3.5). Such low values should be confirmed with another test, such as Biokit or the Western blot. The HerpeSelect HSV-2 Immunoblot should not be used for confirmation, because it uses the same antigen as the HSV-2 Elisa. Repeat testing is indicated if recent acquisition of genital herpes is suspected. The HerpeSelect HSV-1 Elisa is insensitive for detection of HSV-1 antibody. IgM testing for HSV 1 or HSV-2 is not useful, because IgM tests are not type-specific and might be positive during recurrent genital or oral episodes of herpes.

Because nearly all HSV-2 infections are sexually acquired, the presence of type-specific HSV-2 antibody implies anogenital infection. In this instance, education and counseling appropriate for persons with genital HSV infections should be provided. The presence of HSV-1 antibody alone is more difficult to interpret. Many persons with HSV-1 antibody have oral HSV infection acquired during childhood, which might be asymptomatic. However, acquisition of genital HSV-1 is increasing, and genital HSV-1 also can be asymptomatic. Lack of symptoms in a person who is HSV-1 seropositive does not distinguish anogenital from orolabial or cutaneous infection, and regardless of site of infection, these persons remain at risk for acquiring HSV-2.

Type-specific HSV serologic assays might be useful in the following scenarios:

1. recurrent genital symptoms or atypical symptoms with negative HSV PCR or culture

2. clinical diagnosis of genital herpes without laboratory confirmation; and

3. a patient whose partner has genital herpes. HSV serologic testing should be considered for persons presenting for an STD evaluation (especially for those persons with multiple sex partners), persons with HIV infection, and MSM at increased risk for HIV acquisition. Screening for HSV-1 and HSV-2 in the general population is not indicated.

Management of Genital Herpes

Antiviral chemotherapy offers clinical benefits to most symptomatic patients and is the mainstay of management. Counseling regarding the natural history of genital herpes, sexual and perinatal transmission, and methods to reduce transmission is integral to clinical management.

Systemic antiviral drugs can partially control the signs and symptoms of genital herpes when used to treat first clinical and recurrent episodes or when used as daily suppressive therapy. However, these drugs neither eradicate latent virus nor affect the risk, frequency, or severity of recurrences after the drug is discontinued. Randomized trials have indicated that three antiviral medications provide clinical benefit for genital herpes: acyclovir, valacyclovir, and famciclovir. Valacyclovir is the valine ester of acyclovir and has enhanced absorption after oral administration. Famciclovir also has high oral bioavailability. Topical therapy with antiviral drugs offers minimal clinical benefit and is discouraged.

First Clinical Episode of Genital Herpes

Newly acquired genital herpes can cause a prolonged clinical illness with severe genital ulcerations and neurologic involvement. Even persons with first-episode herpes who have mild clinical manifestations initially can develop severe or prolonged symptoms. Therefore, all patients with first episodes of genital herpes should receive antiviral therapy.

Established HSV-2 Infection

Almost all persons with symptomatic first-episode genital HSV-2 infection subsequently experience recurrent episodes of genital lesions; recurrences are less frequent after initial genital HSV-1 infection. Intermittent asymptomatic shedding occurs in persons with genital HSV-2 infection, even in those with longstanding or clinically silent infection. Antiviral therapy for recurrent genital herpes can be administered either as suppressive therapy to reduce the frequency of recurrences or episodically to ameliorate or shorten the duration of lesions. Some persons, including those with mild or infrequent recurrent outbreaks, benefit from antiviral therapy; therefore, options for treatment should be discussed. Many persons prefer suppressive therapy, which has the additional advantage of decreasing the risk for genital HSV-2 transmission to susceptible partners.

Suppressive Therapy for Recurrent Genital Herpes

Suppressive therapy reduces the frequency of genital herpes recurrences by 70%–80% in patients who have frequent recurrences; many persons receiving such therapy report having experienced no symptomatic outbreaks. Treatment also is effective in patients with less frequent recurrences. Safety and efficacy have been documented among patients receiving daily therapy with acyclovir for as long as 6 years and with valacyclovir or famciclovir for 1 year. Quality of life is improved in many patients with frequent recurrences who receive suppressive therapy rather than episodic treatment.

The frequency of genital herpes recurrences diminishes over time in many persons, potentially resulting in psychological adjustment to the disease. Therefore, periodically during suppressive treatment (e.g., once a year), providers should discuss the need to continue therapy. However, neither treatment discontinuation nor laboratory monitoring in a healthy person is necessary.

Treatment with valacyclovir 500 mg daily decreases the rate of HSV-2 transmission in discordant, heterosexual couples in which the source partner has a history of genital HSV-2 infection. Such couples should be encouraged to consider suppressive antiviral therapy as part of a strategy to prevent transmission, in addition to consistent condom use and avoidance of sexual activity during recurrences. Suppressive antiviral therapy also is likely to reduce transmission when used by persons who have multiple partners (including MSM) and by those who are HSV-2 seropositive without a history of genital herpes.

Acyclovir, famciclovir, and valacyclovir appear equally effective for episodic treatment of genital herpes, but famciclovir appears somewhat less effective for suppression of viral shedding. Ease of administration and cost also are important considerations for prolonged treatment.

Episodic Therapy for Recurrent Genital Herpes

Effective episodic treatment of recurrent herpes requires initiation of therapy within 1 day of lesion onset or during the prodrome that precedes some outbreaks. The patient should be provided with a supply of drug or a prescription for the medication with instructions to initiate treatment immediately when symptoms begin.

Severe Disease

Intravenous (IV) acyclovir therapy should be provided for patients who have severe HSV disease or complications that necessitate hospitalization (e.g., disseminated infection, pneumonitis, or hepatitis) or CNS complications (e.g., meningoencephalitis). The recommended regimen is acyclovir 5–10 mg/kg IV every 8 hours for 2–7 days or until clinical improvement is observed, followed by oral antiviral therapy to complete at least 10 days of total therapy. HSV encephalitis requires 21 days of intravenous therapy. Impaired renal function warrants an adjustment in acyclovir dosage.

Counseling

Counseling of infected persons and their sex partners is critical to the management of genital herpes. The goals of counseling include helping patients cope with the infection and preventing sexual and perinatal transmission. Although initial counseling can be provided at the first visit, many patients benefit from learning about the chronic aspects of the disease after the acute illness subsides. Multiple resources, including websites (http://www.ashasexualhealth.org) and printed materials, are available to assist patients, their partners, and clinicians who become involved in counseling.

Although the psychological effect of a serologic diagnosis of HSV-2 infection in a person with asymptomatic or unrecognized genital herpes appears minimal and transient, some HSV-infected persons might express anxiety concerning genital herpes that does not reflect the actual clinical severity of their disease; the psychological effect of HSV infection can be substantial. Common concerns regarding genital herpes include the severity of initial clinical manifestations, recurrent episodes, sexual relationships and transmission to sex partners, and ability to bear healthy children. The misconception that HSV causes cancer should be dispelled.

The following topics should be discussed when counseling persons with genital HSV infection:

- the natural history of the disease, with emphasis on the potential for recurrent episodes, asymptomatic viral shedding, and the attendant risks of sexual transmission;

- the effectiveness of suppressive therapy for persons experiencing a first episode of genital herpes in preventing symptomatic recurrent episodes;

- use of episodic therapy to shorten the duration of recurrent episodes;

- importance of informing current sex partners about genital herpes and informing future partners before initiating a sexual relationship;

- potential for sexual transmission of HSV to occur during asymptomatic periods (asymptomatic viral shedding is more frequent in genital HSV-2 infection than genital HSV-1 infection and is most frequent during the first 12 months after acquiring HSV-2);

- importance of abstaining from sexual activity with uninfected partners when lesions or prodromal symptoms are present;

- effectiveness of daily use of valacyclovir in reducing risk for transmission of HSV-2, and the lack of effectiveness of episodic or suppressive therapy in persons with HIV and HSV infection in reducing risk for transmission to partners who might be at risk for HSV-2 acquisition;

- effectiveness of male latex condoms, which when used consistently and correctly can reduce (but not eliminate) the risk for genital herpes transmission;

- HSV infection in the absence of symptoms (type-specific serologic testing of the asymptomatic partners of persons with genital herpes is recommended to determine whether such partners are already HSV seropositive or whether risk for acquiring HSV exists);

- risk for neonatal HSV infection; and

- increased risk for HIV acquisition among HSV-2 seropositive persons who are exposed to HIV (suppressive antiviral therapy does not reduce the increased risk for HIV acquisition associated with HSV-2 infection).

Asymptomatic persons who receive a diagnosis of HSV-2 infection by type-specific serologic testing should receive the same counseling messages as persons with symptomatic infection. In addition, such persons should be educated about the clinical manifestations of genital herpes.

Pregnant women and women of childbearing age who have genital herpes should inform the providers who care for them during pregnancy and those who will care for their newborn infant about their infection.

Special Considerations

Allergy, Intolerance, and Adverse Reactions

Allergic and other adverse reactions to oral acyclovir, valacyclovir, and famciclovir are rare. Desensitization to acyclovir has been described.

HIV Infection

Immunocompromised patients can have prolonged or severe episodes of genital, perianal, or oral herpes. Lesions caused by HSV are common among persons with HIV infection and might be severe, painful, and atypical. HSV shedding is increased in persons with HIV infection. Whereas antiretroviral therapy reduces the severity and frequency of symptomatic genital herpes, frequent subclinical shedding still occurs. Clinical manifestations of genital herpes might worsen during immune reconstitution early after initiation of antiretroviral therapy.

Suppressive or episodic therapy with oral antiviral agents is effective in decreasing the clinical manifestations of HSV among persons with HIV infection. HSV type-specific serologic testing can be offered to persons with HIV infection during their initial evaluation if infection status is unknown, and suppressive antiviral therapy can be considered in those who have HSV-2 infection. Suppressive anti-HSV therapy in persons with HIV infection does not reduce the risk for either HIV transmission or HSV-2 transmission to susceptible sex partners.

For severe HSV disease, initiating therapy with acyclovir 5–10 mg/ kg IV every 8 hours might be necessary.

Antiviral Resistant HSV

If lesions persist or recur in a patient receiving antiviral treatment, HSV resistance should be suspected and a viral isolate obtained for sensitivity testing. Such persons should be managed in consultation with an infectious-disease specialist, and alternate therapy should be administered. All acyclovir-resistant strains are also resistant to valacyclovir, and most are resistant to famciclovir. Foscarnet (40–80 mg/kg IV every 8 hours until clinical resolution is attained) is often effective for treatment of acyclovir-resistant genital herpes. Intravenous cidofovir 5 mg/kg once weekly might also be effective. Imiquimod is a topical alternative, as is topical cidofovir gel 1%; however, cidofovir must be compounded at a pharmacy. These topical preparations should be applied to the lesions once daily for 5 consecutive days.

Clinical management of antiviral resistance remains challenging among persons with HIV infection, necessitating other preventative approaches. However, experience with another group of immunocompromised persons (hematopoietic stem-cell recipients) demonstrated that persons receiving daily suppressive antiviral therapy were less likely to develop acyclovir-resistant HSV compared with those who received episodic therapy for outbreaks.

Genital Herpes in Pregnancy

Most mothers of newborns who acquire neonatal herpes lack histories of clinically evident genital herpes. The risk for transmission to the neonate from an infected mother is high (30%–50%) among women who acquire genital herpes near the time of delivery and low (<1%) among women with prenatal histories of recurrent herpes or who acquire genital HSV during the first half of pregnancy.

Prevention of neonatal herpes depends both on preventing acquisition of genital HSV infection during late pregnancy and avoiding exposure of the neonate to herpetic lesions and viral shedding during delivery. Because the risk for herpes is highest in newborn infants of women who acquire genital HSV during late pregnancy, these women should be managed in consultation with maternal-fetal medicine and infectious-disease specialists.

Women without known genital herpes should be counseled to abstain from vaginal intercourse during the third trimester with partners known or suspected of having genital herpes. In addition, pregnant women without known orolabial herpes should be advised to abstain from receptive oral sex during the third trimester with partners known or suspected to have orolabial herpes. Type-specific serologic tests may be useful for identifying pregnant women at risk for HSV infection and guiding counseling regarding the risk for acquiring genital herpes during pregnancy. For example, such testing could be offered to women with no history of genital herpes whose sex partner has HSV infection. However, the effectiveness of antiviral therapy to decrease the risk for HSV transmission to pregnant women by infected partners has not been studied. Routine HSV-2 serologic screening of pregnant women is not recommended.

All pregnant women should be asked whether they have a history of genital herpes. At the onset of labor, all women should be questioned carefully about symptoms of genital herpes, including prodromal symptoms, and all women should be examined carefully for herpetic lesions. Women without symptoms or signs of genital herpes or its prodrome can deliver vaginally. Although cesarean delivery does not completely eliminate the risk for HSV transmission to the neonate, women with recurrent genital herpetic lesions at the onset of labor should deliver by cesarean delivery to reduce the risk for neonatal HSV infection.

Many infants are exposed to acyclovir each year, and no adverse effects in the fetus or newborn attributable to the use of this drug during pregnancy have been reported. Acyclovir can be safely used to treat women in all stages of pregnancy, along with those who are breastfeeding. Although data regarding prenatal exposure to valacyclovir and famciclovir are limited, data from animal trials suggest these drugs also pose a low risk in pregnant women. Acyclovir can be administered orally to pregnant women with first-episode genital herpes or recurrent herpes and should be administered IV to pregnant women with severe HSV infection. Suppressive acyclovir treatment late in pregnancy reduces the frequency of cesarean delivery among women who have recurrent genital herpes by diminishing the frequency of recurrences at term. However, such treatment may not protect against transmission to neonates in all cases. No data support use of antiviral therapy among HSV-seropositive women without a history of genital herpes.

Neonatal Herpes

Newborn infants exposed to HSV during birth, as documented by maternal virologic testing of maternal lesions at delivery or presumed by observation of maternal lesions, should be followed carefully in consultation with a pediatric infectious-disease specialist. Guidance is available on management of neonates who are delivered vaginally in the presence of maternal genital HSV lesions.

Surveillance cultures or PCR of mucosal surfaces of the neonate to detect HSV infection might be considered before the development of clinical signs of neonatal herpes to guide initiation of treatment. In addition, administration of acyclovir might be considered for neonates born to women who acquired HSV near term because the risk for neonatal herpes is high for these infants. All infants who have neonatal herpes should be promptly evaluated and treated with systemic acyclovir. The recommended regimen for infants treated for known or suspected neonatal herpes is acyclovir 20 mg/kg IV every 8 hours for 14 days if disease is limited to the skin and mucous membranes, or for 21 days for disseminated disease and that involving the central nervous system.

Chapter 19

Hepatitis

Chapter Contents

Section 19.1

What Is Hepatitis?

This section includes text excerpted from
"Hepatitis-Women's Health Guide," U.S. Department
of Veterans Affairs (VA), June 3, 2015.

Hepatitis means that the liver is inflamed. This inflammation (swelling) can be caused by germs, viruses, some medicines, some diseases, or heavy alcohol use.

Three Common Types of Hepatitis Are Caused by Viruses

1. Hepatitis A virus causes hepatitis A.

2. Hepatitis B virus causes hepatitis B.

3. Hepatitis C virus causes hepatitis C.

These three kinds of hepatitis can be acute. Hepatitis B and C can become chronic.
Chronic hepatitis B and C are serious health problems.

Hepatitis A

Hepatitis A is a disease of the liver caused by hepatitis A virus. It may make you sick for a few weeks to a few months. Most recover with no lasting liver damage.

How Is It Spread?

Hepatitis A is spread by coming in contact with the hepatitis A virus. This includes:

- Contact with any person infected with the hepatitis A virus

- Sexual contact with an infected person

- Touching contaminated surfaces and then placing your hands near or in your mouth

- Sharing eating utensils that have virus on them
- Eating food or drinking water that has been contaminated by feces that contain the virus. The food and drinks most likely to be contaminated are:
  - Fruits
  - Vegetables
  - Shellfish
  - Ice
  - Water

In the United States, chlorine in the water kills hepatitis A virus. But infected food workers can still spread hepatitis A directly to food. This occurs when hands are not washed or cleaned before food is handled.

Infected people can spread the virus to others a few weeks before they begin to feel bad.

Who Is at Risk of Hepatitis A?

Anyone can get hepatitis A if they have not been vaccinated. In the United States., you are at a higher risk if you:

- Use illegal drugs, whether injected or not
- Live with someone who has hepatitis A
- Have bleeding problems and take clotting factors
- Have oral-anal sexual contact with someone who has hepatitis A
- Travel to areas that have high rates of hepatitis A

Travel to Africa, Asia, Eastern Europe, or Central and South America, including Mexico, increases the risk of getting hepatitis A.

What Are Signs of Hepatitis A?

Hepatitis A does not always cause people to feel bad. It may make you sick for a few weeks to a few months. Older people can get sicker when they have hepatitis A. Young children with hepatitis A usually do not show any signs. Signs of hepatitis A include:

- Yellow skin or eyes (jaundice)
- Tiredness

- Fever
- Nausea
- Vomiting
- Loss of appetite
- Stomach pain
- Light stools
- Dark urine
- Diarrhea

How Do You Know If You Have Hepatitis A?

The only way to know if you have hepatitis A is by a medical exam. Your health care provider can examine and test you for hepatitis A.

How Is It Treated?

There are no medicines for treating hepatitis A. If you have been exposed to hepatitis A virus, tell your health care provider. They may be able to give you a protein that fights hepatitis A virus to help keep you from getting sick. Most people with hepatitis A recover without treatment in a few months. A few people will need to be hospitalized for hepatitis A.

What Can Happen If You Have Hepatitis a for a Long Time?

People with hepatitis A usually improve without treatment and have no lasting liver damage. Symptoms usually last less than 2 months. A few people can be ill for as long as 6 months. Hepatitis A can sometimes cause liver failure and death. This is usually occurs in:

- People 50 years of age or older
- People with other liver diseases, such as hepatitis B or C

If You Have Hepatitis A

- Get plenty of rest.
- Eat healthy foods.
- Drink plenty of fluids.
- Avoid drinking any alcohol.
- Check with your health care provider before taking:
  - Medicines
  - Supplements and herbal medicines
  - Over-the-counter drugs

- Clean hands often, especially after using the bathroom.

  - Avoid preparing food, if possible, while you are sick.

  - Talk to those listed below about having hepatitis A so they can get more information to protect themselves:

    - Household contacts

    - Sexual contacts

    - Playmates/attendees at childcare centers

    - Persons sharing illegal drugs

    - Persons sharing food or drink

    - Coworkers and/or restaurant patrons where there is an infected food worker

    - If you have hepatitis A, avoid drinking alcohol.

How Can You Avoid Hepatitis A?

The best way to prevent hepatitis A is to be vaccinated. People with certain risk factors and health problems need this vaccine. Ask your doctor if the vaccine is right for you. You cannot get hepatitis A from the vaccine. Hepatitis A vaccination is recommended for:

- All children at age 1 year

- People who use injection and non-injection illegal drugs

- People with chronic (lifelong) liver diseases, such as hepatitis B or hepatitis C

- People with bleeding problems who take clotting factors

- People whose work has a risk for hepatitis A infection

- People who live in areas with high rates of hepatitis A infection

- Travelers to countries that have high rates of hepatitis A. These include:

  - Africa

  - Asia

  - Latin America

  - South America

  - Eastern Europe

Getting vaccinated is the best way to prevent hepatitis A. Other ways to avoid hepatitis A:

- Boil water or drink bottled water in places where the water may not be clean.

- Eat cooked foods and fruits that you can peel. Avoid eating uncooked vegetables or fruits that could have been washed with dirty water, such as lettuce.

- Avoid eating raw or steamed shellfish such as oysters. Shellfish may live in dirty water.

- Use condoms correctly and every time you have sex.

- Clean hands often.

What about Pregnancy?

Hepatitis A vaccine does not contain live virus, so the risk to the baby is expected to be low. However, the safety of hepatitis A vaccination during pregnancy is not known. The risk of the vaccination should be weighed against the risk for hepatitis A in pregnant women. Ask your health care provider if the vaccine is right for you.

Hepatitis B

Hepatitis B is a disease of the liver caused by hepatitis B virus. Most adults who have hepatitis B will recover on their own. However, children and some adults can develop chronic (lifelong) hepatitis B.

How Is It Spread?

Hepatitis B virus is spread by contact with body fluids that carry the virus, such as:

- Blood

- Semen

- Vaginal fluids

- Other body fluids

Hepatitis B is spread by contact with infected body fluids, mostly by:

- Sexual contact: (This is the most common way it is spread in the United States)

- Vaginal and anal sex
- Sharing unclean sex toys
- Body fluids with hepatitis B can enter tiny breaks or rips in the linings of the vagina, vulva, rectum,or mouth. Rips and tears in these areas can be common and often unnoticed.

- Needle sharing:
  - Used or unclean needle
  - During illegal drug or drug equipment use
- Contact with blood:
  - Open sores of an infected person.
  - Sharing items such as razors or toothbrushes with an infected person
  - Being tattooed or pierced with tools that were not properly cleaned
- Pregnancy and birth:
  - Hepatitis B can spread to babies during pregnancy and birth.

Infected mothers can pass hepatitis B to their babies during childbirth.

Hepatitis B is rarely spread from a blood transfusion because:

- Hepatitis B tests are done on all donated blood.
- Blood and blood products that test positive for hepatitis B are safely destroyed. None are used for transfusions.
- There is no risk of getting hepatitis B when donating or giving blood.

Who Is at Risk of Hepatitis B?

Anyone can get hepatitis B if not vaccinated. However, in the United States, you may be at a higher risk if you:

- Have sex partners that have hepatitis B
- Have HIV or another STD
- Inject drugs or share needles, syringes, or other drug-injection equipment

- Live with someone who has hepatitis B

- Are undergoing dialysis

- Have diabetes

- Travel to areas that have moderate to high rates of hepatitis B

- Work in health care or public safety and are exposed to blood or body fluids on the job

- Are an infant born to an infected mother

What Are Signs of Hepatitis B?

When you first get hepatitis B, it is called acute hepatitis B. Most adults who have hepatitis B will recover on their own. However, children and some adults can develop chronic (lifelong) hepatitis B.

Acute hepatitis B: Signs of acute hepatitis B can appear within 3 months after you get the virus. These signs may last from several weeks to 6 months. Up to 50% of adults have signs of acute hepatitis B virus infection. Many young children do not show any signs. Signs include:

- Yellow skin or eyes (jaundice)
- Loss of appetite

- Tiredness
- Stomach pain

- Fever
- Light stools

- Nausea
- Dark urine

- Vomiting
- Joint pain

Chronic hepatitis B: Hepatitis B is chronic when the body can't get rid of the virus. Children, mostly infants, are more likely to get chronic hepatitis B than adults. People with chronic hepatitis B may have no signs for as long as 20 or 30 years. Signs may be the same as acute hepatitis B. There may also be signs of liver damage and cirrhosis such as:

- Weakness

- Weight loss

- Small, red, spider-like blood vessels on the skin

- Confusion or problems thinking

- Loss of interest in sex

- Swollen stomach or ankles

  - A longer than normal amount of time for bleeding to stop

How Do You Know If You Have Hepatitis B?

The only way to know if you have hepatitis B is by a medical exam. There are several blood tests your health care provider can use to diagnose hepatitis B. These tests can tell you:

- If it is an acute or a chronic infection

- If you have recovered from infection

- If you are immune to hepatitis B

- If you could benefit from vaccination

How Is It Treated?

Acute hepatitis B: There are no drugs to treat acute hepatitis B. Doctors usually suggest rest, good nutrition, and fluids. Some people may need to be in the hospital.

Chronic hepatitis B: People with chronic hepatitis B virus infection should receive care from a provider who has experience treating hepatitis B. These providers can be:

- Some internists or family medicine providers

- Infection specialists

- Gastroenterologists (digestive system specialists)

- Hepatologists (liver specialists)

If you have chronic hepatitis B, get checked regularly for signs of liver disease. Discuss treatment with your health care provider. Not every person with chronic hepatitis B needs treatment. If you show no signs of liver damage, your provider will continue to check you for liver disease.

What Can Happen If Chronic Hepatitis B Is Not Treated?

Chronic hepatitis B is a serious disease that can result in long-term health problems. Up to 1 in 4 people with chronic hepatitis B develop serious liver problems. These include:

- Liver damage and scarring (cirrhosis)

- Liver failure

- Liver cancer
  - Death

If You Have Hepatitis B

- See your health care provider regularly.
- Tell current and recent sex partners that you have hepatitis B.
- Get plenty of rest.
- Eat healthy foods.
- Drink plenty of fluids.
- Avoid drinking any alcohol.
- Check with your health care provider before taking:
  - Prescription medicines
  - Supplements or herbal medicines
  - Over-the-counter drugs
- Avoid spreading hepatitis B to others by:
  - Having safer sex and using condoms during all sexual contact.
  - Not sharing used or unclean needles and sex toys.
  - Not donating blood, blood products, or organs.
  - Cleaning all blood spills – even those that have already dried. Use a mixture of bleach and water (one part household bleach to 10 parts water). Even dried blood is a risk to others.
  - Not sharing personal care items like razors, toothbrushes, nail clippers or earrings.
  - Not sharing glucose-monitoring equipment.
  - Asking sexual partner(s) and people living in close contact with you to be tested and vaccinated.

How Can You Avoid Hepatitis B?

Getting the vaccine for hepatitis B is the best way to prevent hepatitis B. The hepatitis B vaccine is safe and effective. It is usually given as 3–4 shots over a 6-month period. You will not get hepatitis B from the vaccine. Ask your health care provider if you should get this vaccine. The hepatitis B vaccine is the best way to prevent hepatitis B. It is recommended for:

- All infants, starting with the first dose of hepatitis B vaccine at birth
- Everyone under the age of 19 who has not been vaccinated
- People whose sex partners have hepatitis B
- Sexually active people who are not in a long-term, faithful relationship
- People with a sexually transmitted disease
- People who share needles, syringes, or other drug-injection equipment
- People who have close household contact with someone infected with the hepatitis B virus
- Health care and public safety workers at risk for exposure to blood or body fluids on the job
- People with kidney disease. This includes all those on dialysis and those being considered for dialysis.
- Adults with diabetes
- Residents and staff of facilities for disabled persons
- People with chronic liver disease
- People with HIV infection
- Travelers to regions with moderate or high rates of hepatitis B

Travelers at increased risk for infection include:

- Adventure travelers
- Peace Corps volunteers
- Missionaries
- Military personnel

Certain events may increase the risk for hepatitis B for travelers:

- An injury or illness that requires certain types of treatment. These include anything that breaks the skin such as shots, fluids in the vein, transfusion, stitches, and surgery.

- Dental treatment
- Unprotected sexual contact
- Sharing drug injection equipment
- Tattooing, ear piercing, acupuncture and other practices that break the skin
- Practices with risk for breaking the skin such as manicures and pedicures
- Sharing certain items such as earrings, razors, toothbrushes and nail clippers

Other ways to avoid hepatitis B:

- Avoid sexual contact.
- Have safer sex:
  - Reduce the number of sexual partners.
  - Condoms, when used correctly, can reduce the risk of getting hepatitis B. Each time you have sex use a condom (male or female type):
    - Before vaginal sex
    - Before anal sex
    - Before oral sex
- Have sex with only one partner who does not have sex with others and does not have hepatitis B.
- Know that other forms of birth control do not protect against hepatitis B.
- Not using or injecting drugs.
- Not reusing or sharing syringes, or drug equipment (works).
- Wear gloves if you have to touch another person's blood.
- Do not use another person's toothbrush, razor, nail clippers or any other item that might have even a tiny bit of blood on it. Make sure any tattoos or body piercings are done under good conditions, using:
  - Sterile tools
  - Clean hands and gloves
  - Disinfected work surfaces

What about Pregnancy?

If you have hepatitis B, your baby has a very high chance of getting it. Pregnant women should be checked for hepatitis B by a health care provider. If you are at risk for hepatitis B, ask your provider about getting vaccinated. The hepatitis B vaccine is safe for pregnant women and their baby. The vaccine can help your baby if:

- It is given to the baby within 12 hours of birth.

- The baby finishes the vaccine series. Note: babies should be tested after the last vaccine shot to make sure they are protected from the disease.

Don't breastfeed until you have discussed it with your health care provider. Avoid breastfeeding if your nipples are cracking or bleeding until the sores heal. Until they heal, you can pump your milk to keep up your milk supply. Do not feed this milk to your baby. Throw it away.

Hepatitis B is a very serious disease for babies. 9 out of 10 babies infected develop chronic hepatitis B.

Hepatitis C

Hepatitis C is a disease of the liver caused by hepatitis C virus. Hepatitis C infection can lead to chronic viral hepatitis, including liver damage, cirrhosis (scarring of the liver), and liver cancer.

How Is It Spread?

Hepatitis C virus is mostly spread by blood from an infected person when:

- Sharing needles or other equipment to inject drugs. This is the most common way people get hepatitis C in the United States

- Getting a needle stick with a needle that was used on an infected person

- Sharing items that may have come in contact with another person's blood, such as razors, nail clippers, pierced earrings, toothbrushes

- Being tattooed or pierced with tools that were used on an infected person

- Having sexual contact with a person infected with the hepatitis C virus. The risk of getting hepatitis C from sexual contact is thought to be low.

Hepatitis C is rarely spread from a blood transfusion because:

- Hepatitis C tests are done on all donated blood.

- Blood and blood products that test positive for hepatitis C are safely destroyed. None are used for transfusions.

- There is no risk of getting hepatitis C when donating or giving blood.

Hepatitis C is not spread by kissing,hugging, coughing, or sharing food and eating utensils.

Who Is at Risk of Hepatitis C?

Anyone can get hepatitis C. It is important for people at high risk of infection to be tested and treated for hepatitis C. In the United States, you are at a higher risk if you:

- Have ever used a needle to inject drugs, even if once and long ago

- Had a blood transfusion or organ transplant before 1992

- Are a health care worker who had blood exposure to mucous membranes or to non-intact skin, or a needlestick injury

- Have ever been on kidney dialysis

- Were born of a mother who had hepatitis C at the time

- Are a Vietnam-era Veteran

- Had contact with hepatitis-C-positive blood to nonintact skin or to mucous membranes

- Received tattoos or body piercings in non-regulated settings

- Have ever snorted drugs or shared drug equipment

- Have liver disease Have abnormal liver tests

- Have a history of alcohol abuse

- Have hemophilia and received clotting factor before 1987

- Have had a sexual partner with hepatitis C, now or in the past

- Have had 10 or more lifetime sexual partners

- Have HIV infection

The only way to know if you have Hepatitis C is to be tested. VA offers hepatitis C testing and treatment to enrolled Veterans.

What Are Signs of Hepatitis C?

When you first get hepatitis C, it is called acute hepatitis C. About 15% of people who have acute hepatitis C infection clear the virus from their bodies. The other 85% of people develop a chronic (lifelong) hepatitis C infection. Of these, 50 to 80%, if treated, may be cured.

Acute hepatitis C: Most people with acute hepatitis C do not have any signs. If signs occur, the average time is 6–7 weeks after exposure, but can be less or more. Some people can have mild to severe signs including:

- Yellow skin or eyes (jaundice)
- Tiredness
- Fever
- Nausea
- Vomiting
- Loss of appetite
- Stomach pain
- Light stools
- Dark urine

Chronic hepatitis C: 3–5 million persons in the United States have chronic hepatitis C infection. Most people do not know they are infected. They don't look or feel sick until the virus causes liver damage. This can take 10 years or more to happen. Signs may be the same as acute hepatitis C. There may also be signs of liver damage and cirrhosis such as:

- Weakness
- Weight loss
- Small, red, spider-like blood vessels on the skin
- Confusion or problems thinking
- Loss of interest in sex
- Swollen stomach or ankles
- A longer than normal amount of time for bleeding to stop

How Do You Know If You Have Hepatitis C?

The only way to know if you have hepatitis C is by a medical exam. There are several blood tests your health care provider can use to diagnose hepatitis C. These tests can tell you:

- If it is acute or chronic infection

- If you have recovered from infection
- If you could benefit from vaccination for hepatitis A and B

In some cases, your health care provider may suggest a liver biopsy. A liver biopsy is a test for liver damage. A needle is used to remove a tiny piece of liver, which is then sent for tests.

How Is It Treated?

If you have chronic hepatitis C infection, your health care provider will examine you for liver problems and may prescribe drugs to help control the disease. Hepatitis C drugs can help to:

- Clear the virus from the body
- Slow down or prevent liver damage
- Lower the chance of getting cirrhosis and liver cancer

Before starting treatment it is important to discuss your options with your health care provider. Treatment for hepatitis C may not be for everyone. Some patients might not need treatment. Other patients might not be able to be treated due to other medical problems.

What Can Happen If Hepatitis C Is Not Treated?

For every 100 people infected with hepatitis C:

- About 15 will clear the virus from their bodies.
- About 85 will develop chronic (long-term) infection. Of these 85 people:
  - 66 will get only minor liver damage
  - 17 will develop cirrhosis and may have symptoms of severe liver disease
  - 2 will develop liver cancer

Chronic hepatitis C infection is the leading cause of liver cancer and cirrhosis in the United States. Cirrhosis is scarring of the liver which causes it to not work properly. Both liver cancer and cirrhosis can be fatal. A liver transplant may be necessary if chronic hepatitis C causes the liver to fail.

If You Have Hepatitis C

- See your health care provider regularly.
- Tell current and recent sex partners that you have hepatitis C.
- Get vaccinated against hepatitis A and hepatitis B.
- Get plenty of rest.
- Eat healthy foods.
- Drink plenty of fluids
- Avoid drinking any alcohol. Alcohol use speeds up the damage hepatitis C causes in your liver. Drinking alcohol before starting hepatitis C treatment makes treatment less likely to work.
- Check with your health care provider before taking:
  - Prescription medicines
  - Supplements
  - Over-the-counter drugs
  - Avoid spreading hepatitis C to others by:
    - Having safer sex and using condoms during all sexual contact.
    - Not sharing used or unclean needles and sex toys.
    - Not donating blood, blood products, or organs.
    - Cleaning all blood spills – even those that have already dried. Use a mixture of bleach and water (one part household bleach to 10 parts water). Even dried blood is a risk to others.
    - Not sharing personal care items like razors, toothbrushes, nail clippers or earrings.
    - Not sharing glucose-monitoring equipment.
    - Asking your sexual partner(s) to be tested for hepatitis C (and perhaps other infections).

If you have hepatitis C, you can prevent liver damage by not drinking alcohol and by getting vaccinated for hepatitis A and hepatitis B.

How Can You Avoid Hepatitis C?

Right now there is no vaccination to protect you against hepatitis C. However, you can take steps to protect yourself from becoming infected:

- Don't use injectable drugs.

- If you use drugs, get vaccinated against hepatitis A and hepatitis B and enter a treatment program.

- Never share needles, syringes, water, or "works" for intravenous drug use, to inject steroids, or cosmetic substances.

- Handle needles and other sharp objects safely.

- Do not use personal items that may have come into contact with an infected person's blood.

- Do not get tattoos or body piercings from an unlicensed facility or in an informal setting.

- Wear gloves if you have to touch another person's blood.

- Always clean hands after removing gloves.

- Have safer sex. Each time you have sex use a condom.

What about Pregnancy?

It is possible to get pregnant if you or your partner has hepatitis C. If you are a pregnant woman who already has hepatitis C (or gets hepatitis C during the pregnancy), the chance of passing the virus to your baby is 4 out of 100. The risk becomes greater if the mother has both hepatitis C and HIV. With good prenatal care, babies born to mothers or fathers with hepatitis C are usually quite healthy. The chance of your baby being infected with hepatitis C is the same whether your baby is born by vaginal delivery or C-section. Before breastfeeding, talk to your health care provider.

Section 19.2

Hepatitis and HIV Coinfection

This section includes text excerpted from "Hepatitis-Women's Health Guide," U.S. Department of Veterans Affairs (VA), June 3, 2015.

The management of hepatitis C virus (HCV)-infected patients is rapidly evolving. Data suggest that HIV/HCV-coinfected patients treated with all-oral HCV regimens have sustained virologic response rates comparable to those of HCV-monoinfected patients. The purpose of this section is to discuss hepatic safety and drug-drug interaction issues related to HIV/HCV coinfection and the concomitant use of antiretroviral (ARV) agents and HCV drugs.

Among patients with chronic HCV infection, approximately one-third progress to cirrhosis, at a median time of less than 20 years. The rate of progression increases with older age, alcoholism, male sex, and HIV infection. A meta-analysis found that HIV/HCV-coinfected patients had a threefold greater risk of progression to cirrhosis or decompensated liver disease than HCV-monoinfected patients. The risk of progression is even greater in HIV/HCV-coinfected patients with low CD4 T lymphocyte (CD4) cell counts. Although antiretroviral therapy (ART) appears to slow the rate of HCV disease progression in HIV/HCV-coinfected patients, several studies have demonstrated that the rate continues to exceed that observed in those without HIV infection. Whether HCV infection accelerates HIV progression, as measured by AIDS-related opportunistic infections (OIs) or death, is unclear. Although some older ARV drugs that are no longer commonly used have been associated with higher rates of hepatotoxicity in patients with chronic HCV infection, newer ARV agents currently in use appear to be less hepatotoxic.

For more than a decade, the mainstay of treatment for HCV infection was a combination regimen of peginterferon and ribavirin (PegIFN/RBV), but this regimen was associated with a poor rate of sustained virologic response (SVR), especially in HIV/HCV-coinfected patients. Rapid advances in HCV drug development led to the discovery of new classes of direct acting antiviral (DAA) agents that target the HCV replication cycle. These new agents, when used with or without PegIFN and RBV, have been shown to achieve high SVR rates. The first DAA agents approved for the treatment of HCV infection in combination with PegIFN/RBV were the HCV protease inhibitors (PI), boceprevir and telaprevir. In HCV genotype 1 infected patients, the combined use of either boceprevir or telaprevir with PegIFN/RBV was associated with higher rates of SVR than use of PegIFN/RBV alone. However, combined use of these drugs was associated with a large pill burden, increased dosing frequency, and adverse effects. Subsequently approved DAA agents in the same class and in newer classes that are used with or without RBV have higher SVR rates, reduced pill burden, less frequent dosing, fewer side effects, and shorter durations of therapy. Therefore, the combination of boceprevir or telaprevir and PegIFN/RBV **is no longer recommended**, and has been replaced by newer combination regimens.

Assessment of HIV/Hepatitis C Virus Coinfection

* All HIV-infected patients should be screened for HCV infection using sensitive immunoassays licensed for detection of antibody to HCV in blood. At risk HCV-seronegative patients should undergo repeat testing annually. HCV-seropositive patients should be tested for HCV RNA using a sensitive quantitative assay to confirm the presence of active infection. Patients who test HCV RNA-positive should undergo HCV genotyping and liver disease staging as recommended by the most updated HCV guidelines.

* Patients with HIV/HCV coinfection should be counseled to avoid consuming alcohol and to use appropriate precautions to prevent transmission of HIV and/or HCV to others. HIV/HCV-coinfected patients who are susceptible to hepatitis A virus (HAV) or hepatitis B virus (HBV) infection should be vaccinated against these viruses.

* All patients with HIV/HCV coinfection should be evaluated for HCV therapy.

Antiretroviral Therapy in HIV/Hepatitis C Virus Coinfection

When to Start Antiretroviral Therapy

The rate of liver disease (liver fibrosis) progression is accelerated in HIV/HCV-coinfected patients, particularly in individuals with low CD4 counts (≤350 cells/mm3). Data largely from retrospective cohort studies are inconsistent regarding the effect of ART on the natural history of HCV disease; however, some studies suggest that ART may slow the progression of liver disease by preserving or restoring immune function and by reducing HIV-related immune activation and inflammation. Therefore, ART should be initiated in most HIV/HCV-coinfected patients, regardless of CD4 count **(BII)**. However, in HIV treatment-naive patients with CD4 counts >500 cells/mm3, some clinicians may choose to defer ART until HCV treatment is completed to avoid drug-drug interactions **(CIII)**. Compared to patients with CD4 counts>350 cells/mm3, those with CD4 counts <200 had lower HCV treatment response rates and higher rates of toxicity due to PegIFN/RBV. Data regarding HCV treatment response to combination therapy with DAA agents in those with advanced immunosuppression is lacking. For patients with lower CD4 counts (e.g., <200 cells/mm3), ART should be initiated promptly **(AI)** and HCV therapy may be delayed until the patient is stable on HIV treatment **(CIII)**.

Antiretroviral Drugs to Start and Avoid

Initial ARV combination regimens recommended for most HIV treatment-naive patients with HCV are the same as those recommended for patients without HCV infection. Special considerations for ARV selection in HIV/HCV-coinfected patients include the following:

- When both HIV and HCV treatments are indicated, the ARV regimen should be selected with special considerations of potential drug-drug interactions and overlapping toxicities with the HCV treatment regimen.

- Cirrhotic patients should be carefully evaluated by an expert in advanced liver disease for signs of liver decompensation according to the Child-Turcotte-Pugh classification system. This assessment is necessary because hepatically metabolized ARV and HCV DAA drugs may be contraindicated or require dose modification in patients with Child-Pugh class B and C disease

Hepatotoxicity

Drug-induced liver injury (DILI) following the initiation of ART is more common in HIV/HCV-coinfected patients than in those with HIV monoinfection. The greatest risk of DILI may be observed in coinfected individuals with advanced liver disease (e.g., cirrhosis, end-stage liver disease). Eradication of HCV infection with treatment may decrease the likelihood of ARV-associated DILI.

- Given the substantial heterogeneity in patient populations and drug regimens, comparison of DILI incidence rates for individual ARV agents across clinical trials is difficult. The incidence of significant elevations in liver enzyme levels (more than 5 times the upper limit of the normal laboratory reference range) is low with currently recommended ART regimens. Hypersensitivity (or allergic) reactions associated with rash and elevations in liver enzymes can occur with certain ARVs. Alanine aminotransferase (ALT) and aspartate aminotransferase (AST) levels should be monitored 2 to 8 weeks after initiation of ART and every 3 to 6 months thereafter. Mild to moderate fluctuations in ALT and/or AST are typical in individuals with chronic HCV infection. In the absence of signs and/or symptoms of liver disease or increases in bilirubin, these fluctuations do not warrant interruption of ART. Patients with significant ALT and/or AST elevation should be careful evaluated for signs and symptoms of liver insufficiency and for alternative causes of liver injury (e.g., acute HAV or HBV infection, hepatobiliary disease, or alcoholic hepatitis). Short-term interruption of the ART regimen or of the specific drug suspected of causing the DILI may be required.

Concurrent Treatment of HIV and Hepatitis C Virus Infection

Concurrent treatment of HIV and HCV is feasible but may be complicated by pill burden, drug-drug interactions, and toxicities. In this context, the stage of HCV disease should be assessed to determine the medical need for HCV treatment and inform decision making on when to start HCV. If the decision is to treat HCV, the ART regimen may need to be modified before HCV treatment is initiated to reduce the potential for drug-drug interactions and/or toxicities that may develop during the period of concurrent HIV and HCV treatment. In patients with suppressed plasma HIV RNA and modified ART, HIV RNA should be measured within 4 to 8 weeks after changing HIV therapy to confirm the effectiveness of the new regimen. After completion of HCV treatment, the modified ART regimen should be continued for at least 2 weeks before reinitiating the original regimen. Continued use of the modified regimen is necessary because of the prolonged half-life of some HCV drugs and the potential risk of drug-drug interactions if a prior HIV regimen is resumed soon after HCV treatment is completed.

Drug-Drug Interaction

Considerations for the concurrent use of ART and recommended HCV agents are discussed below.

- Sofosbuvir is an HCV NS5B nucleotide polymerase inhibitors that is not metabolized by the cytochrome P450 enzyme system and, therefore, can be used in combination with most ARV drugs. Sofosbuvir is a substrate of p-glycoprotein (P-gp). P-gp inducers, such as tipranavir (TPV), may decrease sofosbuvir plasma concentrations and should not be co-administered with sofosbuvir. No other clinically significant pharmocokinetic interactions between sofosbuvir and ARVs have been identified. Drug-drug interaction studies in healthy volunteers did not find any significant interaction between sofosbuvir and darunavir/ritonavir (DRV/r), efavirenz (EFV), rilpivirine (RPV), raltegravir (RAL), tenofovir disoproxil fumarate (TDF), or emtricitabine (FTC).

- Ledipasvir is an HCV NS5A inhibitor and is part of a fixed-dose drug combination of sofosbuvir and ledipasvir. Similar to sofosbuvir, ledipasvir is not metabolized by the cytochrome P450 system (CYP) of enzymes and is a substrate for P-gp. Ledipasvir is an inhibitor of the drug transporters P-gp and breast cancer resistance protein (BCRP) and may increase intestinal absorption of coadministered substrates for these transporters. The use of P-gp inducers is not recommended with ledipasivir/sofosbuvir. The coadministration of ledipasvir/sofosbuvir and ARV regimens containing TDF is associated with increased exposure to TDF, especially when TDF is taken with an HIV PI boosted with either RTV or cobicistat (COBI) In some patients, alternative HCV or ARV drugs should be considered to avoid increases in TDF exposures. If the drugs are co-administered, the patient should be monitored for potential TDF-associated renal injury by assessing measurements of renal function (i.e., estimated creatinine clearance, serum phosphorus, urine glucose, and urine protein) before HCV treatment initiation and periodically during treatment.

- The fixed-dose drug combination of ombitasvir (a NS5A inhibitor), paritaprevir (an HCV PI), and RTV (a pharmacokinetic enhancer) is co-packaged and used in combination with dasabuvir, an NS5B inhibitor.38Paritaprevir is a substrate and inhibitor of the CYP3A4 enzymes and therefore may have significant interactions with certain ARVs that are metabolized by, or may induce or inhibit the same pathways. Dasabuvir is primarily metabolized by the CYP2C8 enzymes. Furthermore, ombitasvir, paritaprevir, and dasabuvir are inhibitors of UGT1A1 and also substrates of P-gp and BCRP. Paritaprevir is also a substrate and inhibitor of OATP1B1/3. Co-administration with drugs that are substrates or inhibitors of these enzymes and drug transporters may result in increased plasma concentrations of either the co-administered drug or the HCV drugs. Given that several CYP enzymes and drug transporters are involved in the metabolism of dasabuvir, ombitasvir, paritaprevir, and RTV, complex drug-drug interactions are likely. Therefore clinicians need to consider all coadministered drugs for potential drug-drug interactions. No significant drug-drug interactions have been found when dasabuvir, ombitasvir, paritaprevir, and RTV are used in conjunction with ATV or RAL. When either RTV or COBI is used in conjunction with ATV, the boosting agent should be discontinued during HCV therapy and ATV should be taken in the morning at the same time as ombitasvir, paritaprevir/r, and dasabuvir. RTV or COBI should be restarted after completion of HCV treatment.

- Simeprevir is a HCV NS3/4A PI that has been studied in HIV/HCV-coinfected patients. Simeprevir is a substrate and inhibitor of CYP3A4 and P gp enzymes, and therefore may have significant interactions with certain ARVs that are metabolized by the same pathways. Simeprevir is also an inhibitor of the drug transporter OATP1B1/3. On the basis of drug-drug interaction studies in healthy volunteers, simeprevir can be coadministered with RAL, DTG, RPV, and TDF. However, coadministration of simeprevir with EFV, ETR, HIV PIs, COBI, or EVG/c/TDF/FTC **is not recommended**.

Section 19.3

Hepatitis and Substance Abuse

This section includes text excerpted from "Viral Hepatitis—A Very Real Consequence of Substance Use," National Institute on Drug Abuse (NIDA), May 2013.

What Is Hepatitis?

Hepatitis is an inflammation of the liver. It can be caused by a variety of toxins (such as drugs or alcohol), autoimmune conditions, or pathogens (including viruses, bacteria, or parasites). Viral hepatitis is caused by a family of viruses labeled A, B, C, D, and E; each has its own unique route of transmission and prognosis. Hepatitis B (HBV) and hepatitis C (HCV) are the most common viral hepatitis infections transmitted through the risky behaviors that drug users often engage in. Approximately 800,000–1.4 million people are living with HBV and 2.7–3.9 million people are living with HCV in the United States.

Left untreated, hepatitis can lead to cirrhosis (progressive deterioration and malfunction) of the liver and a type of liver cancer called hepatocellular carcinoma (HCC). In fact, HBV and HCV infections are the major risk factors for liver cancer worldwide. An estimated 22,000 people are expected to die from this disease in 2013 in the United States alone, a number that has been steadily increasing over the past several years and now exceeds deaths linked to human immunodeficiency virus. During the next 40–50 years, 1 million people with untreated chronic HCV infection will likely die from complications related to their HCV.

What Is the Relationship between Drug Use and Viral Hepatitis?

Drug and alcohol use places individuals at particular risk for contracting viral hepatitis. Engaging in risky sexual behavior that often accompanies drug use places individuals at risk for contracting HBV, and less frequently HCV. Injection drug users (IDUs) are at high risk for contracting HBV and HCV from shared needles and other drug preparation equipment, which exposes them to bodily fluids from other infected people. Because of the compulsive nature of addiction, IDUs repeatedly engage in these unsafe behaviors, which can make them "super-spreaders" of the virus. A recent study reported that each IDU infected with HCV is likely to infect about 20 others and that this rapid transmission of the disease occurs within the first three years of initial infection. Drug and alcohol use can also directly damage the liver, increasing risk for chronic liver disease and cancer among those infected with hepatitis. This underscores that early detection and treatment of hepatitis infections in IDUs and other drug users is paramount to protecting both the health of the individual and that of the community.

What Other Health Challenges Do IDUs with Hepatitis Have?

Injection drug users (IDUs) with hepatitis often suffer from several other health conditions at the same time, including mental illness and HIV/AIDS thus requiring care from multiple healthcare providers. Drug abuse treatment is critical for IDUs, as it can reduce risky behaviors that increase the chance of transmitting hepatitis. Research has shown that patients with hepatitis receiving medication-assisted therapy for their opioid addiction can be safely treated with antiviral medications. To enhance HCV care, NIDA is examining coordinated care models that utilize case managers to integrate HCV specialty care with primary care, substance abuse treatment, and mental health services so that these patients get treatment regimens that address all of their health care needs.

What Treatments Are Available for Viral Hepatitis?

Medications are available for the treatment of chronic HBV and HCV infection. For chronic HBV infection, there are several antiviral drugs (adefovir dipivoxil, interferon alfa-2b, pegylated interferon alfa-2a, lamivudine, entecavir, and telbivudine). People who are chronically infected with HBV require consistent medical monitoring to ensure that the medications are keeping the virus in check and that the disease is not progressing to liver damage or cancer.

There are also antiviral medications available for HCV treatment; however, not everyone needs or can benefit from treatment. Until recently, only two antiviral medications (pegylated interferon and ribavirin) were available to treat HCV infection. Although both are effective, serious side effects including depression and suicidal thoughts are experienced by some patients. Now, there are two new safer, direct-acting antiviral (DAA) medications available (bociprevir and telaprevir), which are administered by injection with pegylated interferon. This new treatment lasts between 12–48 weeks depending on the individual and cures HCV infection, unlike treatment for HIV which lasts a lifetime and does not rid the body of HIV. Research on HCV antivirals continues, and several new promising medications that avoid the adverse events associated with pegylated interferon and can be administered orally (not injected) are in development.

Some people are able to clear the HCV virus (that is, rid it from their bodies) without medications. Recently, NIDA researchers have identified genes that are associated with spontaneous clearance of HCV. These genes also enable people who are unable to clear HCV on their own to respond more favorably to treatment medications. This new information can be used to determine which patients can benefit most from HCV treatment. More studies must be done, but this is a first step to personalized medicine for the treatment of HCV.

How Do I Know If I Am Infected with Viral Hepatitis?

The number of new HBV and HCV infections has been declining in recent years, but the number of people living with chronic hepatitis infections is considerable, and deaths associated with untreated, chronic hepatitis infections have been on the rise. This is because most people don't know they are infected until the disease has begun to damage their liver, highlighting why screening for viral hepatitis is so important.

Initial screening for HBV or HCV involves antibody tests, which show whether you have been exposed to the hepatitis virus, although not necessarily whether you are still infected. A positive antibody test should then be followed up with a test that measures the amount of virus in your blood. If this follow-up test is positive, then you should seek advice from a physician that specializes in viral hepatitis treatment. Because screening for hepatitis is so critical for linking people who test positive to the care they need, NIDA is studying new rapid HCV antibody tests that can be used in drug treatment settings.

Section 19.4

Treating Hepatitis

This section contains text excerpted from the following sources: Text under the heading "What Should Be Done for a Patient with Confirmed HCV Infection?" is excerpted from "Hepatitis C FAQs for Health Professionals," Centers for Disease Control and Prevention (CDC), March 11, 2016; Text under the heading "Zepatier for Treatment of Chronic Hepatitis C Genotypes 1 and 4" is excerpted from "FDA Approves Zepatier for Treatment of Chronic Hepatitis C Genotypes 1 and 4," U.S. Food and Drug Administration (FDA), January 28, 2016.

What Should Be Done for a Patient with Confirmed HCV Infection?

HCV-positive persons should be evaluated (by referral or consultation, if appropriate) for presence of chronic liver disease, including assessment of liver function tests, evaluation for severity of liver disease and possible treatment, and determination of the need for Hepatitis A and Hepatitis B vaccination.

When Might a Specialist Be Consulted in the Management of HCV-Infected Persons?

Any physician who manages a person with hepatitis C should be knowledgeable and current on all aspects of the care of a person with hepatitis C; this can include some internal medicine and family practice physicians as well as specialists such as infectious disease physicians, gastroenterologists, or hepatologists.

What Is the Treatment for Acute Hepatitis C?

Treatment for acute hepatitis C is similar to treatment for chronic hepatitis C.

What Is the Treatment for Chronic Hepatitis C?

Until recently, the mainstay of treatment for chronic hepatitis C virus (HCV) infection has been pegylated interferon and ribavirin, with possible addition of boceprevir (Victrelis™) and telaprevir (Incivek™) (both protease inhibitors) for HCV genotype 1 infection. After given for 24–48 weeks, this treatment resulted in a sustained virologic response (a marker for cure), defined as undetectable HCV RNA in the patient's blood 24 weeks after the end of treatment in 50%–80% of patients (with higher SVR among persons with HCV genotypes 2 or 3 infections versus infections with HCV genotype 1, the most common genotype found in the United States).

In late 2013, The U.S. Food and Drug Administration (FDA) approved two new direct acting antiviral drugs, Sofosbuvir (Sovaldi™) and Simeprevir (Olysio™) to treat chronic HCV infection. Both medications have proven efficacy when used as a component of a combination antiviral regimen to treat HCV-infected adults with compensated liver disease, cirrhosis, HIV co-infection, and hepatocellular carcinoma awaiting liver transplant. Clinical trials have shown that these new medications achieve SVR in 80%–95% of patients after 12–24 weeks of treatment.

Sofosbuvir (Sovaldi™) is a nucleotide analogue inhibitor of the hepatitis C virus (HCV) NS5B polymerase enzyme, which plays an important role in HCV replication. It is taken orally once a day at a 400-mg dose. The drug is approved for two chronic hepatitis C indications: In combination with pegylated interferon and ribavirin for treatment-naive adults with HCV genotype 1 and 4 infections, and in combination with ribavirin for adults with HCV genotypes 2 and 3 infection. The second indication is the first approval of an interferon-free regimen for the treatment of chronic HCV infection.

Simeprevir (Olysio™) is a protease inhibitor that blocks a specific protein needed by the hepatitis C virus to replicate. It is to be used as a component of a combination antiviral treatment regimen of peginterferon-alfa and ribavirin for genotype 1 infections only. It is taken orally once a day at a 150-mg dose. The treatment duration is 24–48 weeks depending on prior treatment history and response to treatment. Because the efficacy of simeprevir is substantially reduced in patients infected with HCV genotype 1a with an NS3 Q80K polymorphism, screening for this mutation is strongly recommended by the manufacturer before treatment initiation.

Zepatier for Treatment of Chronic Hepatitis C Genotypes 1 and 4

The U.S. Food and Drug Administration (FDA) approved Zepatier (elbasvir and grazoprevir) with or without ribavirin for the treatment of chronic hepatitis C virus (HCV) genotypes 1 and 4 infections in adult patients.

Hepatitis C is a viral disease that causes inflammation of the liver that can lead to diminished liver function or liver failure. Most people infected with HCV have no symptoms of the disease until liver damage becomes apparent, which may take several years. Some people with chronic HCV infection develop cirrhosis over many years, which can lead to complications such as bleeding, jaundice (yellowish eyes or skin), fluid accumulation in the abdomen, infections or liver cancer. According to the Centers for Disease Control and Prevention, approximately 3 million Americans are infected with HCV, of which genotype 1 is the most common and genotype 4 is one of the least common.

The safety and efficacy of Zepatier with or without ribavirin was evaluated in clinical trials of 1,373 participants with chronic HCV genotype 1 or 4 infections with and without cirrhosis. The participants received Zepatier with or without ribavirin once daily for 12 or 16 weeks. The studies were designed to measure whether a participant's hepatitis C virus was no longer detected in the blood 12 weeks after finishing treatment (sustained virologic response or SVR), suggesting a participant's infection had been cured.

The overall SVR rates ranged from 94–97 percent in genotype 1-infected subjects and from 97–100 percent in genotype 4-infected subjects across trials for the approved treatment regimens. In order to maximize SVR rates for patients, the product label provides recommendations regarding length of treatment with or without ribavirin specifically tailored to the characteristics of the patient and their virus. It is recommended that healthcare professionals screen genotype 1a-infected patients for certain viral genetic variations prior to starting treatment with Zepatier to determine dosage regimen and duration.

The most common side effects of Zepatier without ribavirin were fatigue, headache and nausea. The most common side effects of Zepatier with ribavirin were anemia and headache.

Zepatier carries a warning alerting patients and health care providers that elevations of liver enzymes to greater than five times the upper limit of normal occurred in approximately 1 percent of clinical trial participants, generally at or after treatment week eight. Liver-related blood tests should be performed prior to starting therapy and at certain times during treatment. Zepatier should not be given to patients with moderate or severe liver impairment.

Chapter 20

HIV/AIDS

Chapter Contents

Section 20.1

HIV and AIDS

This section includes text excerpted from "About HIV/AIDS," Centers for Disease Control and Prevention (CDC), December 6, 2015.

About HIV/AIDS

HIV is a virus spread through certain body fluids that attacks the body's immune system, specifically the CD4 cells, often called T cells. Over time, HIV can destroy so many of these cells that the body can't fight off infections and disease. These special cells help the immune system fight off infections. Untreated, HIV reduces the number of CD4 cells (T cells) in the body. This damage to the immune system makes it harder and harder for the body to fight off infections and some other diseases. Opportunistic infections or cancers take advantage of a very weak immune system and signal that the person has AIDS.

What Is HIV?

HIV stands for human immunodeficiency virus. It is the virus that can lead to acquired immunodeficiency syndrome, or AIDS. Unlike some other viruses, the human body cannot get rid of HIV. That means that once you have HIV, you have it for life.

No safe and effective cure currently exists, but scientists are working hard to find one, and remain hopeful. Meanwhile, with proper medical care, HIV can be controlled. Treatment for HIV is often called antiretroviral therapy or ART. It can dramatically prolong the lives of many people infected with HIV and lower their chance of infecting others. Before the introduction of ART in the mid-1990s, people with HIV could progress to AIDS in just a few years. Today, someone diagnosed with HIV and treated before the disease is far advanced can have a nearly normal life expectancy.

HIV affects specific cells of the immune system, called CD4 cells, or T cells. Over time, HIV can destroy so many of these cells that the body can't fight off infections and disease. When this happens, HIV infection leads to AIDS.

HIV attacks the body's immune system, specifically the CD4 cells (T cells), which help the immune system fight off infections. Untreated, HIV reduces the number of CD4 cells (T cells) in the body, making the person more likely to get other infections or infection-related cancers. Over time, HIV can destroy so many of these cells that the body can't fight off infections and disease. These opportunistic infections or cancers take advantage of a very weak immune system and signal that the person has AIDS, the last stage of HIV infection.

No effective cure currently exists, but with proper medical care, HIV can be controlled. The medicine used to treat HIV is called antiretroviral therapy or ART. If taken the right way, every day, this medicine can dramatically prolong the lives of many people infected with HIV, keep them healthy, and greatly lower their chance of infecting others. Before the introduction of ART in the mid-1990s, people with HIV could progress to AIDS in just a few years. Today, someone diagnosed with HIV and treated before the disease is far advanced can live nearly as long as someone who does not have HIV.

Where Did HIV Come From?

Scientists identified a type of chimpanzee in Central Africa as the source of HIV infection in humans. They believe that the chimpanzee version of the immunodeficiency virus (called simian immunodeficiency virus, or SIV) most likely was transmitted to humans and mutated into HIV when humans hunted these chimpanzees for meat and came into contact with their infected blood. Studies show that HIV may have jumped from apes to humans as far back as the late 1800s. Over decades, the virus slowly spread across Africa and later into other parts of the world. We know that the virus has existed in the United States since at least the mid to late 1970s.

What Are the Stages of HIV?

When people get HIV and don't receive treatment, they will typically progress through three stages of disease. Medicine to treat HIV, known as antiretroviral therapy (ART), helps people at all stages of the disease if taken the right way, every day. Treatment can slow or prevent progression from one stage to the next. It can also dramatically reduce the chance of transmitting HIV to someone else.

Stage 1: Acute HIV Infection

Within 2 to 4 weeks after infection with HIV, people may experience a flu-like illness, which may last for a few weeks. This is the body's natural response to infection. When people have acute HIV infection, they have a large amount of virus in their blood and are very contagious. But people with acute infection are often unaware that they're infected because they may not feel sick right away or at all. To know whether someone has acute infection, either a fourth-generation antibody/antigen test or a nucleic acid (NAT) test is necessary. If you think you have been exposed to HIV through sex or drug use and you have flu-like symptoms, seek medical care and ask for a test to diagnose acute infection.

Stage 2: Clinical Latency (HIV Inactivity or Dormancy)

This period is sometimes called *asymptomatic HIV infection* or *chronic HIV infection*. During this phase, HIV is still active but reproduces at very low levels. People may not have any symptoms or get sick during this time. For people who aren't taking medicine to treat HIV, this period can last a decade or longer, but some may progress through this phase faster. People who are taking medicine to treat HIV (ART) the right way, every day may be in this stage for several decades. It's important to remember that people can still transmit HIV to others during this phase, although people who are on ART and stay virally suppressed (having a very low level of virus in their blood) are much less likely to transmit HIV than those who are not virally suppressed. At the end of this phase, a person's viral load starts to go up and the CD4 cell count begins to go down. As this happens, the person may begin to have symptoms as the virus levels increase in the body, and the person moves into Stage 3.

Stage 3: Acquired Immunodeficiency Syndrome (AIDS)

AIDS is the most severe phase of HIV infection. People with AIDS have such badly damaged immune systems that they get an increasing number of severe illnesses, called opportunistic illnesses.

Without treatment, people with AIDS typically survive about 3 years. Common symptoms of AIDS include chills, fever, sweats, swollen lymph glands, weakness, and weight loss. People are diagnosed with AIDS when their CD4 cell count drops below 200 cells/mm or if they develop certain opportunistic illnesses. People with AIDS can have a high viral load and be very infectious.

How Do I Know If I Have HIV?

The only way to know for sure whether you have HIV is to get tested. Knowing your status is important because it helps you make healthy decisions to prevent getting or transmitting HIV.

Some people may experience a flu-like illness within 2 to 4 weeks after infection (Stage 1 HIV infection). But some people may not feel sick during this stage. Flu-like symptoms include fever, chills, rash, night sweats, muscle aches, sore throat, fatigue, swollen lymph nodes, or mouth ulcers. These symptoms can last anywhere from a few days to several weeks. During this time, HIV infection may not show up on an HIV test, but people who have it are highly infectious and can spread the infection to others.

If you have these symptoms, that doesn't mean you have HIV. Each of these symptoms can be caused by other illnesses. But if you have these symptoms after a potential exposure to HIV, see a health care provider and tell them about your risk. The only way to determine whether you are infected is to be tested for HIV infection.

Is There a Cure for HIV?

No effective cure currently exists for HIV. But with proper medical care, HIV can be controlled. Treatment for HIV is called antiretroviral therapy or ART. If taken the right way, every day, ART can dramatically prolong the lives of many people infected with HIV, keep them healthy, and greatly lower their chance of infecting others. Before the introduction of ART in the mid-1990s, people with HIV could progress to AIDS (the last stage of HIV infection) in a few years. Today, someone diagnosed with HIV and treated before the disease is far advanced can live nearly as long as someone who does not have HIV.

Section 20.2

STDs and HIV

This section includes text excerpted from "STDs and HIV–CDC Fact Sheet," Centers for Disease Control and Prevention (CDC), December 16, 2014.

Are STDs Related to HIV?

Yes. In the United States, people who get syphilis, gonorrhea, and herpes often also have HIV or are more likely to get HIV in the future. One reason is the behaviors that put someone at risk for one infection (not using condoms, multiple partners, anonymous partners) often put them at risk for other infections. Also, because STD and HIV tend to be linked, when someone gets an STD it suggests they got it from someone who may be at risk for other STD and HIV. Finally, a sore or inflammation from an STD may allow infection with HIV that would have been stopped by intact skin.

STDs Can Increase the Risk of Spreading HIV

HIV-infected persons are more likely to shed HIV when they have urethritis or a genital ulcer. When HIV-infected persons get another STD such as gonorrhea or syphilis, it suggests that they were having sex without using condoms. If so, they may have spread HIV to their partners.

Some STDs Are More Closely Linked to HIV than Others

In the United States, both syphilis and HIV are highly concentrated epidemics among men who have sex with men. In 2014, MSM accounted for 83% of all primary and secondary syphilis cases among males in which sex of sex partner was known. In Florida, in 2010, among all persons diagnosed with infectious syphilis 42% were also HIV infected. Men who get syphilis are at very high risk of being diagnosed with HIV in the future; among HIV-uninfected men who got syphilis in Florida in 2003, 22% were newly diagnosed with HIV by 2011. HIV is more closely linked to gonorrhea than chlamydia (which is particularly common among young women). Herpes is also commonly associated with HIV; a meta-analysis found persons infected with HSV-2 are at 3-fold increased risk for acquiring HIV infection.

Some Activities Can Put People at Increased Risk for Both STDs and HIV

- Having anal, vaginal, or oral sex without a condom;

- Having multiple sex partners;

- Having anonymous sex partners;

- Having sex while under the influence of drugs or alcohol can lower inhibitions and result in greater sexual risk taking.

Does Treating STDs Prevent HIV?

Not by itself. Given the close link between STD and HIV in many studies, it seems obvious that treating STDs should reduce the risk of HIV. However, studies that have lowered the risk of STD in communities have not necessarily lowered the risk of HIV. Risk of HIV was lowered in one community trial, but not in 3 others.

In Mwanza (Tanzania), improved STD treatment lowered 2-year HIV incidence by 40% in the intervention towns (1.2%) compared to other towns (1.9%).

- In Rakai (Uganda), a more intensive intervention (mass treatment and improved STD control) was done, leading to lower rates of syphilis and trichomoniasis, but the incidence of HIV was the same in intervention and comparison towns (1.5% per year).

- A third community trial found no difference in HIV incidence when behavioral plus STD control interventions were compared to usual services (Incidence rate ratio = 1.00), despite lower rates of syphilis (rate ratio 0.52) and gonorrhea (rate ratio 0.25).

- A fourth community trial found HIV incidence was slightly higher in communities that received a combination of interventions including improved STD treatment when compared to control communities (incidence rate ratio 1.27, not statistically significant).

Treating individuals for STDs has also not necessarily lowered their risk of acquiring HIV.

- One study found there was slightly lower risk of HIV seroconversion among female sex workers who had monthly exams for STD (5.3%) compared to sex workers who were examined when they had symptoms (7.6%, P=0.5); their rates of infection were lower for trichomonas (14% vs 7% P=0.07) but not for gonorrhea, chlamydia, or genital ulcers.

- A second trial in female sex workers found a slightly higher incidence of HIV among women who received monthly treatment with azithromycin (4%) compared to women who did not (3.2%, P=0.5) despite major differences in the incidence of infection with gonorrhea (relative risk RR 0.46), chlamydia (RR 0.38), and trichomoniasis (RR 0.56).

Three placebo-controlled trials have assessed the benefit to individuals from treatment with acyclovir to suppress genital herpes ulcers:

- One enrolled female sex workers who were infected with HSV but not HIV; it found no impact on HIV incidence in the acyclovir group (4.29%) compared to the placebo group (4.25%), though it also found no difference in reported episodes of genital ulceration or in measured HSV shedding.

- A second study of HIV acquisition among persons infected with HSV-2 included women and men who have sex with men; HIV incidence was similar in the acyclovir group (3.9%) and the placebo group (3.3%) despite a 47% reduction in observed genital ulcers in the acyclovir group.

- The third study looked at the effect of acyclovir on HIV transmission from heterosexuals infected with both HIV and HSV-2 to their HIV-uninfected partners; after removing 29% of new infections that were apparently acquired from an outside partner, the incidence was similar in the acyclovir group (1.8%) and the placebo group (1.9%, P=0.69) despite major reductions in genital ulcer disease (risk ratio 0.39).

Screening for STDs can help assess a person's risk for getting HIV. Treatment of STDs is important to prevent the complications of those infections, and to prevent transmission to partners, but it should not be expected to prevent spread of HIV.

What Can People Do to Reduce Their Risk of Getting STDs and HIV?

The only way to avoid STDs is to not have vaginal, anal, or oral sex. If people are sexually active, they can do the following things to lower their chances of getting STDs and HIV:

- Choose less risky sexual behaviors;
- Use condoms consistently and correctly;
- Reduce the number of people with whom they have sex;
- Limit or eliminate drug and alcohol use before and during sex;
- Have an honest and open talk with their healthcare provider and ask whether they should be tested for STDs and HIV;
- Talk with their healthcare provider and find out if pre-exposure prophylaxis, or PrEP, is a good option for them to prevent HIV infection.

If Someone Already Has HIV, and Subsequently Gets an STD, Does That Put Their Sex Partner(s) at an Increased Risk for Getting HIV?

It can. HIV-negative sex partners are at greater risk of getting HIV from someone who is HIV-positive and acquires another STD. The HIV-negative sex partners of persons who are HIV-positive are less likely to get HIV if:

- HIV-positive persons use antiretroviral therapy (ART). ART reduces the amount of virus (viral load) in blood and body fluids. ART can keep HIV-positive persons healthy for many years, and greatly reduce the chance of transmitting HIV to sex partners if taken consistently.
- Sex partners take pre-exposure prophylaxis (PrEP) after discussing this option with his/her healthcare provider and determining whether it is appropriate.

- Choose less risky sexual behaviors.

- Use condoms consistently and correctly.

Will Treating Someone for STDs Prevent Them from Getting HIV?

No. It's not enough. Screening for STDs can help assess a person's risk for getting HIV. Treatment of STDs is important to prevent the complications of those infections, and to prevent transmission to partners, but it should not be expected to prevent spread of HIV.

If someone HIV-positive is diagnosed with an STD, they should receive counseling about risk reduction and how to protect their sex partner(s) from getting re-infected with the same STD or getting HIV.

Section 20.3

Questions and Answers about HIV Transmission

This section includes text excerpted from "HIV Transmission," Centers for Disease Control and Prevention (CDC), December 14, 2015.

How Is HIV Passed from One Person to Another?

You can get or transmit HIV only through specific activities. Most commonly, people get or transmit HIV through sexual behaviors and needle or syringe use.

Only certain body fluids—blood, semen (*cum*), pre-seminal fluid (*pre-cum*), rectal fluids, vaginal fluids, and breast milk—from a person who has HIV can transmit HIV. These fluids must come in contact with a mucous membrane or damaged tissue or be directly injected into the bloodstream (from a needle or syringe) for transmission to occur. Mucous membranes are found inside the rectum, vagina, penis, and mouth.

In the United States, HIV is spread mainly by

- Having anal or vaginal sex with someone who has HIV without using a condom or taking medicines to prevent or treat HIV.

- Anal sex is the highest-risk sexual behavior. For the HIV-negative partner, receptive anal sex (bottoming) is riskier than insertive anal sex (topping).

- Vaginal sex is the second-highest-risk sexual behavior.

- Sharing needles or syringes, rinse water, or other equipment (works) used to prepare drugs for injection with someone who has HIV. HIV can live in a used needle up to 42 days depending on temperature and other factors.

Less commonly, HIV may be spread

- From mother to child during pregnancy, birth, or breastfeeding. Although the risk can be high if a mother is living with HIV and not taking medicine, recommendations to test all pregnant women for HIV and start HIV treatment immediately have lowered the number of babies who are born with HIV.

- By being stuck with an HIV-contaminated needle or other sharp object. This is a risk mainly for health care workers.

In extremely rare cases, HIV has been transmitted by

- Oral sex—putting the mouth on the penis (fellatio), vagina (cunnilingus), or anus (rimming). In general, there's little to no risk of getting HIV from oral sex. But transmission of HIV, though extremely rare, is theoretically possible if an HIV-positive man ejaculates in his partner's mouth during oral sex.

- Receiving blood transfusions, blood products, or organ/tissue transplants that are contaminated with HIV. This was more common in the early years of HIV, but now the risk is extremely small because of rigorous testing of the US blood supply and donated organs and tissues.

- Eating food that has been pre-chewed by an HIV-infected person. The contamination occurs when infected blood from a caregiver's mouth mixes with food while chewing. The only known cases are among infants.

- Being bitten by a person with HIV. Each of the very small number of documented cases has involved severe trauma with extensive tissue damage and the presence of blood. There is no risk of transmission if the skin is not broken.

- Contact between broken skin, wounds, or mucous membranes and HIV-infected blood or blood-contaminated body fluids.

- Deep, open-mouth kissing if both partners have sores or bleeding gums and blood from the HIV-positive partner gets into the bloodstream of the HIV-negative partner. HIV is not spread through saliva.

How Well Does HIV Survive Outside the Body?

HIV does not survive long outside the human body (such as on surfaces), and it cannot reproduce outside a human host. It **is not** spread by

- Mosquitoes, ticks, or other insects.

- Saliva, tears, or sweat that is not mixed with the blood of an HIV-positive person.

- Hugging, shaking hands, sharing toilets, sharing dishes, or closed-mouth or "social" kissing with someone who is HIV-positive.

- Other sexual activities that don't involve the exchange of body fluids (for example, touching).

Can I Get HIV from Anal Sex?

Yes. In fact, having anal sex is the riskiest type of sex for getting or spreading HIV.

HIV can be found in the blood, semen (*cum*), preseminal fluid (*precum*), or rectal fluid of a person infected with the virus. The *bottom* is at greater risk of getting HIV because the lining of the rectum is thin and may allow HIV to enter the body during anal sex, but the top is also at risk because HIV can enter through the opening of the penis or through small cuts, abrasions, or open sores on the penis.

Can I Get HIV from Vaginal Sex?

Yes. Vaginal sex is the sexual behavior with the second-highest risk for getting or transmitting HIV.

It is possible for either partner to get HIV from vaginal sex.

When a woman has vaginal sex with a partner who's HIV-positive, HIV can enter her body through the mucous membranes that line the vagina and cervix. Most women who get HIV get it from vaginal sex.

Men can also get HIV from having vaginal sex with a woman who's HIV-positive. This is because vaginal fluid and blood can carry HIV. Men get HIV through the opening at the tip of the penis (or urethra); the foreskin if they're not circumcised; or small cuts, scratches, or open sores anywhere on the penis.

Can I Get HIV from Oral Sex?

The chance that an HIV-negative person will get HIV from oral sex with an HIV-positive partner is extremely low.

Oral sex involves putting the mouth on the penis (fellatio), vagina (cunnilingus), or anus (anilingus). In general, there's little to no risk of getting or transmitting HIV through oral sex.

Factors that may increase the risk of transmitting HIV through oral sex are ejaculation in the mouth with oral ulcers, bleeding gums, genital sores, and the presence of other sexually transmitted diseases (STDs), which may or may not be visible.

You can get other STDs from oral sex. And, if you get feces in your mouth during anilingus, you can get hepatitis A and B, parasites like *Giardia*, and bacteria like *Shigella*, *Salmonella*, *Campylobacter*, and *E. coli*.

Is There a Connection between HIV and Other Sexually Transmitted Infections?

Yes. Having another sexually transmitted disease (STD) can increase the risk of getting or transmitting HIV.

If you have another STD, you're more likely to get or transmit HIV to others. Some of the most common STDs include gonorrhea, chlamydia, syphilis, trichomoniasis, human papillomavirus (HPV), genital herpes, and hepatitis. The only way to know for sure if you have an STD is to get tested. If you're sexually active, you and your partners should get tested for STDs (including HIV if you're HIV-negative) regularly, even if you don't have symptoms.

If you are HIV-negative but have an STD, you are about 3 times as likely to get HIV if you have unprotected sex with someone who has HIV. There are two ways that having an STD can increase the likelihood of getting HIV. If the STD causes irritation of the skin (for example, from syphilis, herpes, or human papillomavirus), breaks or sores may make it easier for HIV to enter the body during sexual contact. Even STDs that cause no breaks or open sores (for example, chlamydia, gonorrhea, trichomoniasis) can increase your risk by causing inflammation that increases the number of cells that can serve as targets for HIV.

If you are HIV-positive and also infected with another STD, you are about 3 times as likely as other HIV-infected people to spread HIV through sexual contact. This appears to happen because there is an increased concentration of HIV in the semen and genital fluids of HIV-positive people who also are infected with another STD.

Does My HIV-Positive Partner's Viral Load Affect My Risk of Getting HIV?

Yes, as an HIV-positive person's viral load goes down, the chance of transmitting HIV goes down.

Viral load is the amount of HIV in the blood of someone who is HIV-positive. When the viral load is very low, it is called viral suppression. Undetectable viral load is when the amount of HIV in the blood is so low that it can't be measured.

In general, the higher someone's viral load, the more likely that person is to transmit HIV. People who have HIV but are in care, taking HIV medicines, and have a very low or undetectable viral load are much less likely to transmit HIV than people who have HIV and do not have a low viral load.

However, a person with HIV can still potentially transmit HIV to a partner even if they have an undetectable viral load, because

- HIV may still be found in genital fluids (semen, vaginal fluids). The viral load test only measures virus in blood.

- A person's viral load may go up between tests. When this happens, they may be more likely to transmit HIV to partners.

- Sexually transmitted diseases increase viral load in genital fluids.

If you're HIV-positive, getting into care and taking HIV medicines (called antiretroviral therapy or ART) the right way, every day will give you the greatest chance to get and stay virally suppressed, live a longer, healthier life, and reduce the chance of transmitting HIV to your partners.

If you're HIV-negative and have an HIV-positive partner, encourage your partner to get into care and take HIV treatment medicines.

Taking other actions, like using a condom the right way every time you have sex or taking daily medicine to prevent HIV (called pre-exposure prophylaxis or PrEP) if you're HIV-negative, can lower your chances of transmitting or getting HIV even more.

Can I Get HIV from Injecting Drugs?

Yes. Your risk for getting HIV is very high if you use needles or works (such as cookers, cotton, or water) after someone with HIV has used them.

People who inject drugs, hormones, steroids, or silicone can get HIV by sharing needles or syringes and other injection equipment. The needles and equipment may have someone else's blood in them, and blood can transmit HIV. Likewise, you're at risk for getting hepatitis B and C if you share needles and works because these infections are also transmitted through blood.

Another reason people who inject drugs can get HIV (and other sexually transmitted diseases) is that when people are high, they're more likely to have risky sex.

Stopping injection and other drug use can lower your chances of getting HIV a lot. You may need help to stop or cut down using drugs, but many resources are available. To find a substance abuse treatment center near you, check out the locator tools on SAMHSA.gov or AIDS. gov, or call 1-800-662-HELP (4357).

If you keep injecting drugs, you can lower your risk for getting HIV by using only new, sterile needles and works each time you inject. Never share needles or works.

Can I Get HIV from Using Other Kinds of Drugs?

When you're drunk or high, you're more likely to make decisions that put you at risk for HIV, such as having sex without a condom.

Drinking alcohol, particularly binge drinking, and using "club drugs" like Ecstasy, ketamine, GHB, and poppers can alter your judgment, lower your inhibitions, and impair your decisions about sex or other drug use. You may be more likely to have unplanned and unprotected sex, have a harder time using a condom the right way every time you have sex, have more sexual partners, or use other drugs, including injection drugs or meth. Those behaviors can increase your risk of exposure to HIV. If you have HIV, they can also increase your risk of spreading HIV to others. Being drunk or high affects your ability to make safe choices.

If you're going to a party or another place where you know you'll be drinking or using drugs, you can bring a condom so that you can reduce your risk if you have vaginal or anal sex.

Therapy, medicines, and other methods are available to help you stop or cut down on drinking or using drugs. Talk with a counselor, doctor, or other health care provider about options that might be right for you.

If I Already Have HIV, Can I Get Another Kind of HIV?

Yes. Your risk for getting HIV is very high if you use needles or works (such as cookers, cotton, or water) after someone with HIV has used them.

People who inject drugs, hormones, steroids, or silicone can get HIV by sharing needles or syringes and other injection equipment. The needles and equipment may have someone else's blood in them, and blood can transmit HIV. Likewise, you're at risk for getting hepatitis B and C if you share needles and works because these infections are also transmitted through blood.

Another reason people who inject drugs can get HIV (and other sexually transmitted diseases) is that when people are high, they're more likely to have risky sex.

Stopping injection and other drug use can lower your chances of getting HIV a lot. You may need help to stop or cut down using drugs, but many resources are available.

If you keep injecting drugs, you can lower your risk for getting HIV by using only new, sterile needles and works each time you inject. Never share needles or works.

Are Health Care Workers at Risk of Getting HIV on the Job?

When you're drunk or high, you're more likely to make decisions that put you at risk for HIV, such as having sex without a condom.

Drinking alcohol, particularly binge drinking, and using "club drugs" like Ecstasy, ketamine, GHB, and poppers can alter your judgment, lower your inhibitions, and impair your decisions about sex or other drug use. You may be more likely to have unplanned and unprotected sex, have a harder time using a condom the right way every time you have sex, have more sexual partners, or use other drugs, including injection drugs or meth. Those behaviors can increase your risk of exposure to HIV. If you have HIV, they can also increase your risk of spreading HIV to others. Being drunk or high affects your ability to make safe choices.

If you're going to a party or another place where you know you'll be drinking or using drugs, you can bring a condom so that you can reduce your risk if you have vaginal or anal sex.

Therapy, medicines, and other methods are available to help you stop or cut down on drinking or using drugs. Talk with a counselor, doctor, or other health care provider about options that might be right for you.

Can I Get HIV from Receiving Medical Care?

Yes. This is called HIV superinfection.

HIV superinfection is when a person with HIV gets infected with another strain of the virus. The new strain of HIV can replace the original strain or remain along with the original strain.

The effects of superinfection differ from person to person. Superinfection may cause some people to get sicker faster because they become infected with a new strain of the virus that is resistant to the medicine (antiretroviral therapy or ART) they're taking to treat their original infection.

Research suggests that a hard-to-treat superinfection is rare. Taking medicine to treat HIV (ART) may reduce someone's chance of getting a superinfection.

Can I Get HIV from Casual Contact ("Social Kissing," Shaking Hands, Hugging, Using a Toilet, Drinking from the Same Glass, or the Sneezing and Coughing of an Infected Person)?

No. HIV isn't transmitted

- by hugging, shaking hands, sharing toilets, sharing dishes, or closed-mouth or "social" kissing with someone who is HIV-positive.

- through saliva, tears, or sweat that is not mixed with the blood of an HIV-positive person.

- by mosquitoes, ticks or other blood-sucking insects.

- through the air.

Only certain body fluids—blood, semen (*cum*), pre-seminal fluid (*pre-cum*), rectal fluids, vaginal fluids, and breast milk—from an HIV-infected person can transmit HIV. Most commonly, people get or transmit HIV through sexual behaviors and needle or syringe use. Babies can also get HIV from an HIV-positive mother during pregnancy, birth, or breastfeeding.

Can I Get HIV from a Tattoo or a Body Piercing?

There are no known cases in the United States of anyone getting HIV this way. However, it is possible to get HIV from a reused or not properly sterilized tattoo or piercing needle or other equipment, or from contaminated ink.

It's possible to get HIV from tattooing or body piercing if the equipment used for these procedures has someone else's blood in it or if the ink is shared. The risk of getting HIV this way is very low, but the risk increases when the person doing the procedure is unlicensed, because of the potential for unsanitary practices such as sharing needles or ink. If you get a tattoo or a body piercing, be sure that the person doing the procedure is properly licensed and that they use only new or sterilized needles, ink, and other supplies.

Can I Get HIV from Being Spit on or Scratched by an HIV-Infected Person?

No. HIV isn't spread through saliva, and there is no risk of transmission from scratching because no body fluids are transferred between people.

Can I Get HIV from Mosquitoes?

No. HIV is not transmitted by mosquitoes, ticks, or any other insects.

Can I Get HIV from Food?

You can't get HIV from consuming food handled by an HIV-infected person. Even if the food contained small amounts of HIV-infected blood or semen, exposure to the air, heat from cooking, and stomach acid would destroy the virus.

Though it is very rare, HIV can be spread by eating food that has been pre-chewed by an HIV-infected person. The contamination occurs when infected blood from a caregiver's mouth mixes with food while chewing. The only known cases are among infants.

Are Lesbians or Other Women Who Have Sex with Women at Risk for HIV?

Case reports of female-to-female transmission of HIV are rare. The well-documented risk of female-to-male transmission shows that vaginal fluids and menstrual blood may contain the virus and that exposure to these fluids through mucous membranes (in the vagina or mouth) could potentially lead to HIV infection.

Is the Risk of HIV Different for Different People?

Some groups of people in the United States are more likely to get HIV than others because of many factors, including the status of their sex partners, their risk behaviors, and where they live.

When you live in a community where many people have HIV infection, the chances of having sex or sharing needles or other injection equipment with someone who has HIV are higher.

Gay and bisexual men have the largest number of new diagnoses in the United States. Blacks/African Americans and Hispanics/Latinos are disproportionately affected by HIV compared to other racial and ethnic groups. Also, transgender women who have sex with men are among the groups at highest risk for HIV infection, and injection drug users remain at significant risk for getting HIV.

Risky behaviors, like having anal or vaginal sex without using a condom or taking medicines to prevent or treat HIV, and sharing needles or syringes play a big role in HIV transmission. Anal sex is the highest-risk sexual behavior. If you don't have HIV, being a receptive partner (or bottom) for anal sex is the highest-risk sexual activity for getting HIV. If you do have HIV, being the insertive partner (or top) for anal sex is the highest-risk sexual activity for transmitting HIV.

But there are more tools available today to prevent HIV than ever before. Choosing less risky sexual behaviors, taking medicines to prevent and treat HIV, and using condoms with lubricants are all highly effective ways to reduce the risk of getting or transmitting HIV.

Section 20.4

Stages of HIV Infection

This section contains text excerpted from the following sources:
Text under the heading "How Does HIV Progress in Your Body?"
is excerpted from "Stages of HIV Infection," U.S. Department of
Health and Human Services (HHS), August 27, 2015; Text under
the heading "Progression to AIDS" is excerpted from "Symptoms
of HIV," U.S. Department of Health and Human Services (HHS),
December 31, 2015; Text under the heading "AIDS" is excerpted
from "Stages of HIV Infection," U.S. Department of Health and
Human Services (HHS), August 27, 2015.

How Does HIV Progress in Your Body?

Without treatment, HIV advances in stages, overwhelming your
immune system and getting worse over time. The three stages of HIV
infection are: (1) acute HIV infection, (2) clinical latency, and (3) AIDS
(acquired immunodeficiency syndrome).

However, there's good news: by using HIV medicines (called antiretroviral therapy or ART) consistently, you can prevent HIV from progressing to AIDS. ART helps control the virus so that you can live a
longer, healthier life and reduce the risk of transmitting HIV to others.

These are the three stages of HIV infection:

Acute HIV Infection Stage

Within 2–4 weeks after HIV infection, many, but not all, people
develop flu-like symptoms, often described as "the worst flu ever."
Symptoms can include fever, swollen glands, sore throat, rash, muscle
and joint aches and pains, and headache. This is called "acute retro-
viral syndrome" (ARS) or "primary HIV infection," and it's the body's
natural response to the HIV infection.

During this early period of infection, large amounts of virus are
being produced in your body. The virus uses CD4 count to replicate
and destroys them in the process. Because of this, your CD4 cells can
fall rapidly. Eventually your immune response will begin to bring the
level of virus in your body back down to a level called a viral set point,

which is a relatively stable level of virus in your body. At this point, your CD4 count begins to increase, but it may not return to pre-infection levels. It may be particularly beneficial to your health to begin ART during this stage.

During the acute HIV infection stage, you are at high risk of transmitting HIV to your sexual or drug using partners because the levels of HIV in your blood stream are very high. For this reason, it is very important to take steps to reduce your risk of transmission.

Clinical Latency Stage

After the acute stage of HIV infection, the disease moves into a stage called the "clinical latency" stage. "Latency" means a period where a virus is living or developing in a person without producing symptoms. During the clinical latency stage, people who are infected with HIV experience no symptoms, or only mild ones. (This stage is sometimes called "asymptomatic HIV infection" or "chronic HIV infection.")

During the clinical latency stage, the HIV virus continues to reproduce at very low levels, although it is still active. If you take ART, you may live with clinical latency for several decades because treatment helps keep the virus in check. For people who are not on ART, the clinical latency stage lasts an average of 10 years, but some people may progress through this stage faster.

People in this symptom-free stage are still able to transmit HIV to others, even if they are on ART, although ART greatly reduces the risk of transmission.

If you have HIV and you are not on ART, then eventually your viral load will begin to rise and your CD4 count will begin to decline. As this happens, you may begin to have constitutional symptoms of HIV as the virus levels increase in your body.

Progression to AIDS

If you have HIV and you are not on ART, eventually the virus will weaken your body's immune system and you will progress to AIDS (acquired immunodeficiency syndrome), the late stage of HIV infection.

Symptoms can include:

- Rapid weight loss

- Recurring fever or profuse night sweats

- Extreme and unexplained tiredness

- Prolonged swelling of the lymph glands in the armpits, groin, or neck

- Diarrhea that lasts for more than a week

- Sores of the mouth, anus, or genitals

- Pneumonia

- Red, brown, pink, or purplish blotches on or under the skin or inside the mouth, nose, or eyelids

- Memory loss, depression, and other neurologic disorders.

Each of these symptoms can also be related to other illnesses. So the only way to know for sure if you have HIV is to get tested. Many of the severe symptoms and illnesses of HIV disease come from the opportunistic infections that occur because your body's immune system has been damaged.

AIDS

This is the stage of HIV infection that occurs when your immune system is badly damaged and you become vulnerable to opportunistic infections. When the number of your CD4 cells falls below 200 cells per cubic millimeter of blood (200 cells/mm3), you are considered to have progressed to AIDS. (In someone with a healthy immune system, CD4 counts are between 500 and 1,600 cells/mm3.) You are also considered to have progressed to AIDS if you develop one or more opportunistic illnesses, regardless of your CD4 count.

Without treatment, people who progress to AIDS typically survive about 3 years. Once you have a dangerous opportunistic illness, life-expectancy without treatment falls to about 1 year. However, if you are taking ART and maintain a low viral load, then you may enjoy a near normal life span. You will most likely never progress to AIDS.

Factors Affecting Disease Progression

People living with HIV may progress through these stages at different rates, depending on a variety of factors, including their genetic makeup, how healthy they were before they were infected, how soon after infection they are diagnosed and linked to care and treatment, whether they see their healthcare provider regularly and take their HIV medications as directed, and different health-related choices they make, such as decisions to eat a healthful diet, exercise, and not smoke.

Time between HIV Infection and AIDS

Factors that may shorten the time between HIV and AIDS:

- Older age
- HIV subtype
- Co-infection with other viruses (like tuberculosis or hepatitis C)
- Poor nutrition
- Severe stress
- Your genetic background

Factors that may delay the time between HIV and AIDS:

- Taking antiretroviral therapy consistently
- Staying in regular HIV care
- Closely adhering to your doctor's recommendations
- Eating healthful foods
- Taking care of yourself
- Your genetic background

By making healthy choices, you have some control over the progression of HIV infection.

Not everyone is diagnosed early. Some people are diagnosed with HIV and AIDS concurrently, meaning that they have been living with HIV for a long time and the virus has already done damage to their body by the time they find out they are infected. These individuals need to seek a healthcare provider immediately and be linked to care so that they can stay as healthy as possible, as long as possible.

Section 20.5

HIV Signs and Symptoms

This section includes text excerpted from "Symptoms of HIV," U.S. Department of Health and Human Services (HHS), December 31, 2015.

How Can I Tell If I Have HIV?

You cannot rely on symptoms to tell whether you have HIV. **The only way to know for sure if you have HIV is to get tested**. Knowing your status is important because it helps you make healthy decisions to prevent getting or transmitting HIV.

The symptoms of HIV vary, depending on the individual and what stage of the disease you are in: the early stage, the clinical latency stage, or AIDS (the late stage of HIV infection). Below are the symptoms that some individuals may experience in these three stages. Not all individuals will experience these symptoms.

Early Stage of HIV

Some people may experience a flu-like illness within 2–4 weeks after HIV infection. But some people may not feel sick during this stage.

Flu-like symptoms can include:

- Fever
- Chills
- Rash
- Night sweats
- Muscle aches
- Sore throat
- Fatigue
- Swollen lymph nodes
- Mouth ulcers

These symptoms can last anywhere from a few days to several weeks. During this time, HIV infection may not show up on an HIV test, but people who have it are highly infectious and can spread the infection to others.

You should not assume you have HIV just because you have any of these symptoms. Each of these symptoms can be caused by other illnesses. And some people who have HIV do not show any symptoms at all for 10 years or more.

If you think you may have been exposed to HIV, get an HIV test. Most HIV tests detect antibodies (proteins your body makes as a reaction against the presence of HIV), not HIV itself. But it takes a few weeks for your body to produce these antibodies, so if you test too early, you might not get an accurate test result. A new HIV test is available that can detect HIV directly during this early stage of infection. So be sure to let your testing site know if you think you may have been recently infected with HIV.

After you get tested, it's important to find out the result of your test so you can talk to your health care provider about treatment options if you're HIV-positive or learn ways to prevent getting HIV if you're HIV-negative.

You are at high risk of transmitting HIV to others during the early stage of HIV infection, even if you have no symptoms. For this reason, it is very important to take steps to reduce your risk of transmission.

Section 20.6

Testing for HIV

This section includes text excerpted from "Testing," Centers for Disease Control and Prevention (CDC), December 6, 2015.

The only way to know for sure whether you have HIV is to get tested. This section answers some of the most common questions related to HIV testing, including the types of tests available, where to get one, and what to expect when you get tested.

Should I Get Tested for HIV?

CDC recommends that everyone between the ages of 13 and 64 get tested for HIV at least once as part of routine health care. About 1 in 8 people in the United States who have HIV don't know they have it.

People with certain risk factors should get tested more often. If you were HIV-negative the last time you were tested and answer yes to any of the following questions, you should get an HIV test because these things increase your chances of getting HIV:

- Are you a man who has had sex with another man?

- Have you had sex—anal or vaginal—with an HIV-positive partner?

- Have you had more than one sex partner since your last HIV test?

- Have you injected drugs and shared needles or works (for example, water or cotton) with others?

- Have you exchanged sex for drugs or money?

- Have you been diagnosed with or sought treatment for another sexually transmitted disease?

- Have you been diagnosed with or treated for hepatitis or tuberculosis (TB)?

- Have you had sex with someone who could answer yes to any of the above questions or someone whose sexual history you don't know?

You should be tested at least once a year if you keep doing any of these things. Sexually active gay and bisexual men may benefit from more frequent testing (for example, every 3 to 6 months).

If you're pregnant, talk to your health care provider about getting tested for HIV and other ways to protect you and your child from getting HIV. Also, anyone who has been sexually assaulted should get an HIV test as soon as possible after the assault and should consider post-exposure prophylaxis (PEP), taking antiretroviral medicines after being potentially exposed to HIV to prevent becoming infected.

Before having sex for the first time with a new partner, you and your partner should talk about your sexual and drug-use history, disclose your HIV status, and consider getting tested for HIV and learning the results.

How Can Testing Help Me?

The only way to know for sure whether you have HIV is to get tested.

Knowing your HIV status gives you powerful information to help you take steps to keep you and your partner healthy.

- If you test positive, you can take medicine to treat HIV to stay healthy for many years and greatly reduce the chance of transmitting HIV to your sex partner.

- If you test negative, you have more prevention tools available today to prevent HIV than ever before.

- If you are pregnant, you should be tested for HIV so that you can begin treatment if you're HIV-positive. If an HIV-positive woman is treated for HIV early in her pregnancy, the risk of transmitting HIV to her baby can be very low.

I Don't Believe I Am at High Risk. Why Should I Get Tested?

Some people who test positive for HIV were not aware of their risk. That's why CDC recommends that everyone between the ages of 13 and 64 get tested for HIV at least once as part of routine health care.

Even if you are in a monogamous relationship (both you and your partner are having sex only with each other), you should find out for sure whether you or your partner has HIV.

I Am Pregnant. Why Should I Get Tested?

All pregnant women should be tested for HIV so that they can begin treatment if they're HIV-positive. If a woman is treated for HIV early in her pregnancy, the risk of transmitting HIV to her baby can be very low. Testing pregnant women for HIV infection and treating those who are infected have led to a big decline in the number of children infected with HIV from their mothers.

The treatment is most effective for preventing HIV transmission to babies when started as early as possible during pregnancy. However, there are still great health benefits to beginning preventive treatment even during labor or shortly after the baby is born.

What Kinds of Tests Are Available, and How Do They Work?

There are three broad types of tests available: antibody tests, combination or fourth-generation tests, and nucleic acid

tests (NAT). HIV tests may be performed on blood, oral fluid, or urine.

1. Most HIV tests, including most rapid tests and home tests, are **antibody tests**. Antibodies are produced by your immune system when you're exposed to viruses like HIV or bacteria. HIV antibody tests look for these antibodies to HIV in your blood or oral fluid. In general, antibody tests that use blood can detect HIV slightly sooner after infection than tests done with oral fluid.

It can take 3 to 12 weeks (21–84 days) for an HIV-positive person's body to make enough antibodies for an antibody test to detect HIV infection. This is called the window period. Approximately 97% of people will develop detectable antibodies during this window period. If you get a negative HIV antibody test result during the window period, you should be re-tested 3 months after your possible exposure to HIV.

- With a **rapid antibody screening test**, results are ready in 30 minutes or less.

- The **OraQuick HIV Test**, which involves taking an oral swab, provides fast results. You have to swab your mouth for an oral fluid sample and use a kit to test it. Results are available in 20 minutes. The manufacturer provides confidential counseling and referral to follow-up testing sites. Because the level of antibody in oral fluid is lower than it is in blood, blood tests find infection sooner after exposure than oral fluid tests. These tests are available for purchase in stores and online. They may be used at home, or they may be used for testing in some community and clinic testing programs.

- The **Home Access HIV-1 Test System** is a home collection kit, which involves pricking your finger to collect a blood sample, sending the sample by mail to a licensed laboratory, and then calling in for results as early as the next business day. This test is anonymous. The manufacturer provides confidential counseling and referral to treatment.ess.

If you use any type of antibody test and have a positive result, you will need to take a follow-up test to confirm your results. If your first test is a rapid home test and it's positive, you will be sent to a health care provider to get follow-up testing. If your first test is done in a testing lab and it's positive, the lab will conduct the follow-up testing, usually on the same blood sample as the first test.

A **combination, or fourth-generation, test** looks for both HIV antibodies and antigens. Antigens are foreign substances that cause your immune system to activate. The antigen is part of the virus itself and is present during acute HIV infection (the phase of infection right after people are infected but before they develop antibodies to HIV). If you're infected with HIV, an antigen called p24 is produced even before antibodies develop. Combination screening tests are now recommended for testing done in labs and are becoming more common in the United States. There is now a rapid combination test available.

It can take 2 to 6 weeks (13 to 42 days) for a person's body to make enough antigens and antibodies for a combination, or fourth-generation, test to detect HIV. This is called the window period. If you get a negative combination test result during the window period, you should be retested 3 months after your possible exposure.

A **nucleic acid test** (NAT) looks for HIV in the blood. It looks for the virus and not the antibodies to the virus. The test can give either a positive/negative result or an actual amount of virus present in the blood (known as a viral load test). This test is very expensive and not routinely used for screening individuals unless they recently had a high-risk exposure or a possible exposure with early symptoms of HIV infection.

It can take 7 to 28 days for a NAT to detect HIV. Nucleic acid testing is usually considered accurate during the early stages of infection. However, it is best to get an antibody or combination test at the same time to help the doctor interpret the negative NAT. This is because a small number of people naturally decrease the amount of virus in their blood over time, which can lead to an inaccurate negative NAT result. Taking pre-exposure prophylaxis (PrEP) or post-exposure prophylaxis (PEP) may also reduce the accuracy of NAT if you have HIV.

Talk to your health care provider to see what type of HIV test is right for you. After you get tested, it's important for you to find out the result of your test so that you can talk to your health care provider about treatment options if you're HIV-positive. If you're HIV-negative, continue to take actions to prevent HIV, like using condoms the right way every time you have sex and taking medicines to prevent HIV if you're at high risk.

How Soon after an Exposure to HIV Can an HIV Test Detect If I Am Infected?

No HIV test can detect HIV immediately after infection. If you think you've been exposed to HIV, talk to your health care provider as soon as possible.

The time between when a person gets HIV and when a test can accurately detect it is called the *window period*. The window period varies from person to person and also depends upon the type of HIV test.

- Most HIV tests are **antibody tests**. Antibodies are produced by your immune system when you're exposed to viruses like HIV or bacteria. HIV antibody tests look for these antibodies to HIV in your blood or oral fluid.

- The soonest an antibody test will detect infection is 3 weeks. Most (approximately 97%), but not all, people will develop detectable antibodies within 3 to 12 weeks (21 to 84 days) of infection.

- A **combination, or fourth-generation, test** looks for both HIV antibodies and antigens. Antigens are foreign substances that cause your immune system to activate. The antigen is part of the virus itself and is present during acute HIV infection (the phase of infection right after people are infected but before they develop antibodies to HIV).

- Most, but not all people, will make enough antigens and antibodies for fourth-generation or combination tests to accurately detect infection 2 to 6 weeks (13 to 42 days) after infection.

- A **nucleic acid test** (NAT) looks for HIV in the blood. It looks for the virus and not the antibodies to the virus. This test is very expensive and not routinely used for screening individuals unless they recently had a high-risk exposure or a possible exposure with early symptoms of HIV infection.

Most, but not all people, will have enough HIV in their blood for a nucleic acid test to detect infection 1 to 4 weeks (7 to 28 days) after infection.

Ask your health care provider about the window period for the test you're taking. If you're using a home test, you can get that information from the materials included in the test's package. If you get an HIV test within 3 months after a potential HIV exposure and the result is negative, get tested again in 3 more months to be sure.

If you learned you were HIV-negative the last time you were tested, you can only be sure you're still negative if you haven't had a potential HIV exposure since your last test. If you're sexually active, continue to take actions to prevent HIV, like using condoms the right way every time you have sex and taking medicines to prevent HIV if you're at high risk.

Where can I get tested?

You can ask your health care provider for an HIV test. Many medical clinics, substance abuse programs, community health centers, and hospitals offer them too. You can also find a testing site near you by

- calling 1-800-CDC-INFO (232-4636),
- visiting gettested.cdc.gov, or
- texting your ZIP code to KNOW IT (566948).

You can also buy a home testing kit at a pharmacy or online.

What Should I Expect When I Go in for an HIV Test?

If you take a test in a health care setting, when it's time to take the test, a health care provider will take your sample (blood or oral fluid), and you may be able to wait for the results if it's a rapid HIV test. If the test comes back negative, and you haven't had an exposure for 3 months, you can be confident you're not infected with HIV.

If your HIV test result is positive, you may need to get a follow-up test to be sure you have HIV.

Your health care provider or counselor may talk with you about your risk factors, answer questions about your general health, and discuss next steps with you, especially if your result is positive.

What Does a Negative Test Result Mean?

A negative result doesn't necessarily mean that you don't have HIV. That's because of the window period—the time between when a person gets HIV and when a test can accurately detect it. The window period varies from person to person and is also different depending upon the type of HIV test.

Ask your health care provider about the window period for the test you're taking. If you're using a home test, you can get that information from the materials included in the test's package. If you get an HIV test within 3 months after a potential HIV exposure and the result is negative, get tested again in 3 more months to be sure.

If you learned you were HIV-negative the last time you were tested, you can only be sure you're still negative if you haven't had a potential HIV exposure since your last test. If you're sexually active, continue to take actions to prevent HIV, like using condoms the right way every time you have sex and taking medicines to prevent HIV if you're at high risk.

If I Have a Negative Result, Does That Mean That My Partner Is HIV-Negative Also?

No. Your HIV test result reveals only your HIV status.

HIV is not necessarily transmitted every time you have sex. Therefore, taking an HIV test is not a way to find out if your partner is infected.

It's important to be open with your partners and ask them to tell you their HIV status. But keep in mind that your partners may not know or may be wrong about their status, and some may not tell you if they have HIV even if they know they're infected. Consider getting tested together so you can both know your HIV status and take steps to keep yourselves healthy.

What Does a Positive Result Mean?

A follow-up test will be conducted. If the follow-up test is also positive, it means you are HIV-positive.

If you had a rapid screening test, the testing site will arrange a follow-up test to make sure the screening test result was correct. If your blood was tested in a lab, the lab will conduct a follow-up test on the same sample.

It is important that you start medical care and begin HIV treatment as soon as you are diagnosed with HIV. Anti-retroviral therapy or ART (taking medicines to treat HIV infection) is recommended for all people with HIV, regardless of how long they've had the virus or how healthy they are. It slows the progression of HIV and helps protect your immune system. ART can keep you healthy for many years and greatly reduces your chance of transmitting HIV to sex partners if taken the right way, every day.

If you have health insurance, your insurer is required to cover some medicines used to treat HIV. If you don't have health insurance, or you're unable to afford your co-pay or co-insurance amount, you may be eligible for government programs that can help through Medicaid, Medicare, the Ryan White HIV/AIDS Program, and community health centers. Your health care provider or local public health department can tell you where to get HIV treatment.

To lower your risk of transmitting HIV,

- Take medicines to treat HIV (antiretroviral therapy or ART) the right way every day.

- Use condoms the right way every time you have sex.

- If your partner is HIV-negative, encourage them to talk to their health care provider to see if taking daily medicine to prevent HIV (called pre-exposure prophylaxis, or PrEP) is right for them.

- If you think your partner might have been recently exposed to HIV—for example, if the condom breaks during sex and you aren't virally suppressed—they should talk to a health care provider right away (within 3 days) about taking medicines (called post-exposure prophylaxis, or PEP) to prevent getting HIV.

- Get tested and treated for STDs and encourage your partner to do the same.

Receiving a diagnosis of HIV can be a life-changing event. People can feel many emotions—sadness, hopelessness, and even anger. Allied health care providers and social service providers, often available at your health care provider's office, will have the tools to help you work through the early stages of your diagnosis and begin to manage your HIV.

Talking to others who have HIV may also be helpful. Find a local HIV support group. Learn about how other people living with HIV have handled their diagnosis.

If I Test Positive for HIV, Does That Mean I Have AIDS?

No. Being HIV-positive does not mean you have AIDS. AIDS is the most advanced stage of HIV disease. HIV can lead to AIDS if not treated.

Will Other People Know My Test Result?

If you take an anonymous test, no one but you will know the result. If you take a confidential test, your test result will be part of your medical record, but it is still protected by state and federal privacy laws.

- **Anonymous testing** means that nothing ties your test results to you. When you take an anonymous HIV test, you get a unique identifier that allows you to get your test results.

- **Confidential testing** means that your name and other identifying information will be attached to your test results. The results will go in your medical record and may be shared with your health care providers and your health insurance company. Otherwise, the results are protected by state and federal privacy laws, and they can be released only with your permission.

With confidential testing, if you test positive for HIV, the test result and your name will be reported to the state or local health department to help public health officials get better estimates of the rates of HIV in the state. The state health department will then **remove all personal information** about you (name, address, etc.) and share the remaining non-identifying information with CDC. CDC does not share this information with anyone else, including insurance companies.

Should I Share My Positive Test Result with Others?

It's important to share your status with your sex partners. Whether you disclose your status to others is your decision.

Partners

It's important to disclose your HIV status to your sex partners even if you're uncomfortable doing it. Communicating with each other about your HIV status means you can take steps to keep both of you healthy. The more practice you have disclosing your HIV status, the easier it will become.

If you're nervous about disclosing your test result, or you have been threatened or injured by your partner, you can ask your doctor or the local health department to tell them that they might have been exposed to HIV. This is called partner notification services. Health departments do not reveal your name to your partners. They will only tell your partners that they have been exposed to HIV and should get tested.

Many states have laws that require you to tell your sexual partners if you're HIV-positive before you have sex (anal, vaginal, or oral) or tell your drug-using partners before you share drugs or needles to inject drugs. In some states, you can be charged with a crime if you don't tell your partner your HIV status, even if your partner doesn't become infected.

Family and friends

In most cases, your family and friends will not know your test results or HIV status unless you tell them yourself. While telling your family that you have HIV may seem hard, you should know that disclosure actually has many benefits—studies have shown that people who disclose their HIV status respond better to treatment than those who don't.

If you are under 18, however, some states allow your health care provider to tell your parent(s) that you received services for HIV if they think doing so is in your best interest. For more information, see the Guttmacher Institute's State Policies in Brief: Minors' Access to STI Services.

Employers

In most cases, your employer will not know your HIV status unless you tell them. But your employer does have a right to ask if you have any health conditions that would affect your ability to do your job or pose a serious risk to others. (An example might be a health care professional, like a surgeon, who does procedures where there is a risk of blood or other body fluids being exchanged.)

If you have health insurance through your employer, the insurance company cannot **legally** tell your employer that you have HIV. But it is possible that your employer could find out if the insurance company provides detailed information to your employer about the benefits it pays or the costs of insurance.

Who Will Pay for My HIV Test?

HIV screening is covered by health insurance without a co-pay, as required by the Affordable Care Act. If you do not have medical insurance, some testing sites may offer free tests.

Who Will Pay for My Treatment If I Am HIV-Positive?

If you have health insurance, your insurer is required to cover some medicines used to treat HIV. If you don't have health insurance, or you're unable to afford your co-pay or co-insurance amount, you may be eligible for government programs that can help through Medicaid, Medicare, the Ryan White HIV/AIDS Program, and community health centers. Your health care provider or local public health department can tell you where to get HIV treatment.

Section 20.7

HIV and Its Treatment

This section includes text excerpted from "HIV Treatment," Centers for Disease Control and Prevention (CDC), January 12, 2016.

HIV treatment involves taking medicines that slow the progression of the virus in your body. HIV is a type of virus called a retrovirus, and the drugs used to treat it is called antiretrovirals (ARV). These drugs are always given in combination with other ARVs; this combination therapy is called antiretroviral therapy (ART). Many ART drugs have been used since the mid-1990s and are the reason why the annual number of deaths related to AIDS has dropped over the past two decades.

Although a cure for HIV does not yet exist, ART can keep you healthy for many years, and greatly reduces your chance of transmitting HIV to your partner(s) if taken consistently and correctly. ART reduces the amount of virus (or viral load) in your blood and body fluids. ART is recommended for all people living with HIV, regardless of how long they've had the virus or how healthy they are.

Why Is Treatment Important?

To protect your health, it is important to get on and stay on HIV treatment. HIV treatment is important because it helps your body fight HIV. You may hear the phrase "treatment adherence," which means staying on your treatment plan. Most people living with HIV who don't get treatment eventually develop AIDS.

If left untreated, HIV attacks your immune system and can allow different types of life-threatening infections and cancers to develop. If your CD4 cell count falls below a certain level, you are at risk of getting an opportunistic infection. These are infections that don't normally affect people with healthy immune systems but that can infect people with immune systems weakened by HIV infection. Your health care provider may prescribe medicines to prevent certain infections.

HIV treatment is most likely to be successful when you know what to expect and are committed to taking your medicines exactly as prescribed. Working with your health care provider to develop a treatment plan will help you learn more about HIV, manage it effectively, and make decisions that help you live a longer, healthier life. HIV treatment will also greatly reduce your chance of transmitting HIV to sex partners and injection drug-use if taken consistently and correctly.

When Should I Start Treatment?

Treatment guidelines from the United States Department of Health and Human Services recommend that a person living with HIV begin antiretroviral therapy (ART) as soon as possible after diagnosis. Starting ART slows the progression of HIV and can keep you healthy for many years.

If you delay treatment, the virus will continue to harm your immune system and put you at higher risk for developing opportunistic infections that can be life threatening.

How Does ART Work?

Antiretroviral therapy (ART) is the use of HIV medicines to treat HIV infection. There are five different types of HIV medicines. Each medicine helps stop HIV at different points in the virus' life cycle.

When taken consistently and correctly ART helps:

Reduce your viral load (the level of HIV in your body). When you reduce your viral load, you reduce HIV's ability to infect new CD4 cells.

Keep your immune system healthy by increasing your CD4 count. CD4 cells help protect you from developing infections. The right dose and type of ART medicines can help to keep your viral load low and your CD4 cell levels high.

Prevent opportunistic infections and other illnesses.

Reduce, but not eliminate, the chances that you will transmit HIV to others.

Reduce, but not eliminate, the chances that you will transmit the virus to your baby if you are pregnant or plan on becoming pregnant.

Follow your treatment plan exactly as your health care provider has prescribed. Medicines should be taken at specific times of the day, with or without certain kinds of food. If you have questions about when and how to take your medicines, talk to your health care provider or pharmacist.

ART is usually taken as a combination of 3 or more drugs to have the greatest chance of lowering the amount of HIV in your body. Ask your health care provider about the availability of multiple drugs combined into 1 pill. Your health care provider and pharmacist will help you find a treatment combination that works best for you. If the HIV medicines you are taking are not working as well as they should, your health care provider may change your prescription. A change is not unusual because the same treatment does not affect everyone in the same way.

Let your health care provider and pharmacist know about any medical conditions you may have and any other medicines you are taking. Medicines you are taking for other health conditions may interact with your HIV treatment. These conversations will help you receive the best treatment possible. Additionally, if you or your partner is pregnant or considering getting pregnant, talk to your health care provider to determine the right type of ART that can greatly reduce the risk of transmitting HIV to your baby.

Does ART Cause Side Effects?

Like most medicines, antiretroviral therapy (ART) can cause side effects. However, not everyone experiences side effects from ART.

Some common side effects of ART that you may experience can include:

- Nausea and vomiting
- Diarrhea
- Difficulty sleeping
- Dry mouth
- Headache
- Rash
- Dizziness
- Fatigue
- Pain

Side effects can differ for each person and each type of ART medicine. Some side effects can occur once you start a medicine and may only last a few days or weeks. Other side effects can start later and last longer.

Contact your health care provider or pharmacist immediately if you begin to experience problems or if your treatment makes you sick. Medicines are available to help reduce or eliminate side effects or you can change medicines to find a treatment plan that works for you. Your health care provider may prescribe medicines to help manage the side effects or may decide to change your treatment plan.

What Should I Do If I Miss a Dose?

Taking your HIV medicines exactly the way your health care provider tells you to will help keep your viral load low and your CD4 cell count high. If you skip your medicines, even now and then, you are giving HIV the chance to multiply rapidly. This could weaken your immune system, and you could become sick.

Talk to your health care provider if you miss a dose. In most cases, if you realize you missed a dose, take the medicines as soon as you can, then take the next dose at your usual scheduled time (unless your pharmacist or health care provider has told you something different).

If you find you miss a lot of doses, talk to your health care provider or pharmacist about ways to help you remember your medicines. You and your health care provider may even decide to change your treatment regimen to fit your health care needs and life situation, which may change over time.

Do I Have To Take My HIV Medicines If My Viral Load Is Undetectable?

Yes, antiretroviral therapy (ART) reduces viral load, ideally to an undetectable level. If your viral load goes down after starting ART, then the treatment is working, and you should always take your medicine as prescribed by your health care provider. Even when your viral load is undetectable, HIV can still exist in semen, vaginal and rectal fluids, breast milk, and other parts of your body, so you should continue to take steps to prevent HIV transmission. Taking your HIV medications on schedule will help keep your viral load very low and help you maintain your health. It will also make it more difficult for you to pass HIV on to others.

Why Is It Important for Me to Stick to My Treatment Plan?

Sticking to your HIV treatment provides many benefits. Among them, it:

- Allows HIV medications to reduce the amount of HIV in your body. If you skip your medications, even now and then, you are giving HIV the chance to multiply rapidly. Keeping the amount of virus in your blood as low as possible is the best way to protect your health.

- Helps keep your immune system stronger and better able to fight infections.

Reduces the risk of passing HIV to others. Staying on your treatment plan and keeping the amount of HIV in your body as low as possible means that it is less likely that you can pass the virus to others.

Helps prevent drug resistance. Drug resistance develops when the virus changes form and no longer responds to certain HIV medications. This is a problem because that drug no longer works on your HIV. Skipping your medicines makes it easier for drug resistance to develop. Also, HIV can become resistant to the medications you are taking or to similar ones that you have not yet taken. This limits the options for successful HIV treatment. Drug-resistant strains of HIV can be transmitted to others, too.

What Are Some Challenges I Might Expect to Staying on My HIV Treatment?

Staying on an HIV treatment plan can be difficult. That is why it is important to understand some challenges you may face and to think through how you might address them before they happen. For example, remembering when to take your medicines can be complicated. Some treatment plans involve taking several pills every day—with or without food—or before or after other medications. Making a schedule of when and how to take your medicines can be helpful. Or ask your health care provider about the availability of multiple drugs combined into one pill.

Other factors can make sticking to your treatment plan difficult:

Problems taking medications, such as trouble swallowing pills, can make staying on treatment challenging. Your health care provider can offer tips and ideas for addressing these problems.

Side effects from medications, for example, nausea or diarrhea, can make a person not want to take them. Talk to your health care provider. There are medicines or other support, like nutritional counseling to make sure you are getting important nutrients, which can help with the most common side effects. But don't give up. Work with your health care provider to find a treatment that works for you.

A busy schedule. Work or travel away from home can make it easy to forget to take pills. Planning ahead can help. Or, it may be possible to keep extra medicines at work or in your car for the times that you forget to take them at home. But make sure you talk to your health care provider—some medications are affected by extreme temperatures, and it is not always possible to keep medications at work.

Being sick or depressed. How you feel mentally and physically can affect your willingness to stick to your treatment plan. Again, your health care provider is an important source of information to help.

Alcohol or drug use. If substance use is interfering with your ability to keep yourself healthy, it may be time to seek help to quit or better manage it.

Treatment fatigue. Some people find that sticking to their treatment plan becomes harder over time. Every time you see your health care provider, make it a point to talk about staying on your treatment plan.

Your health care provider will help you identify barriers to staying on your plan and ways to address those barriers. Understanding issues that can make staying on your treatment plan difficult will help you and your health care provider select the best treatment for you.

Tell your health care provider right away if you're having difficulty sticking to your plan. Together you can identify the reasons why you're skipping medications and make a plan to address those reasons. Joining a support group, or enlisting the support of family and friends, can also help you stick to your treatment plan.

How Can I Prepare for Sticking to My Treatment Plan before I Start HIV Treatment?

Preparing to stay on your treatment plan before you start taking antiretroviral therapy (ART) is the first step to treatment success. Planning ahead will help you follow your treatment plan once you start treatment.

Begin by talking to your health care provider. Make sure you understand why you're starting HIV treatment and why sticking to your treatment plan is important. Discuss these important details about your treatment plan:

- Each HIV medication that you will take.

- The dose (amount) of each HIV medication in your plan.

- How many pills in each dose.

- When to take each medication.

- How to take each medication—with or without food.

- Possible side effects from each medication, including serious side effects to watch out for.

- How to store your medications.

- Other medications you are taking and how they may interact with your HIV medications.

- Any personal issues such as depression, alcohol or drug abuse, lack of secure housing, or additional medical issues.

- Lack of health insurance to pay for anti-HIV medications.

Tell your health care provider if you have any personal issues, such as depression or alcohol or drug use, that can make staying on your treatment plan difficult. If needed, your health care provider can recommend resources to help you address these issues before you start treatment.

What Are Some Tips to Help Me Stay on My Treatment Plan?

Some tips that may help you stick with your treatment plan are:

- Take your medicine at the same time each day.

- Match your medicine schedule to your life. Add taking your medicines to things you already do each day, like brushing your teeth or eating a meal.

- Try a weekly or monthly pill tray with compartments for each day of the week to help you remember whether you took your medicine that day.

- Set an alarm on your clock, watch, or phone for the time you take your medicines.

- Use a calendar to check off the days you have taken your medicines.

- Download a free app from the Internet to your computer or on your smartphone that can help remind you when it's time to take your medicines. Search for "reminder apps," and you will find many choices.

- Ask a family member or friend to help you remember to take your medicine.

Section 20.8

Living with HIV

This section includes text excerpted from "Living with HIV," Centers
for Disease Control and Prevention (CDC), February 23, 2016.

An estimated 1.2 million people are living with HIV in the United
States. Thanks to better treatments, people with HIV are now living
longer—and with a better quality of life—than ever before. If you are
living with HIV, it's important to make choices that keep you healthy
and protect others.

Stay Healthy

You should start medical care and begin IIIV treatment as soon
as you are diagnosed with HIV. Taking medicine to treat HIV, called
antiretroviral therapy or ART, is recommended for all people with HIV.
Taking medicine to treat HIV slows the progression of HIV and helps
protect your immune system. The medicine can keep you healthy for
many years and greatly reduces your chance of transmitting HIV to
sex partners if taken the right way, every day.

If you're taking medicine to treat HIV, visit your health care provider regularly and always take your medicine as directed to keep
your viral load (the amount of HIV in the blood and elsewhere in the
body) as low as possible.

Do Tell

It's important to disclose your HIV status to your sex and needle-sharing partners even if you are uncomfortable doing it. Communicating with each other about your HIV status allows you and your
partner to take steps to keep both of you healthy.

Many resources can help you learn ways to disclose your status
to your partners. For tips on how to start the conversation with your
partner,

Also, ask your health department about free partner notification services. Health department staff can help find your sex or needle-sharing

partners to let them know they may have been exposed to HIV and provide them with testing, counseling, and referrals for other services. These partner notification services will not reveal your name unless you want to work with them to tell your partners.

Many states have laws that require you to tell your sexual partners if you're HIV-positive before you have sex (anal, vaginal, or oral) or tell your needle-sharing partners before you share drugs or needles to inject drugs. In some states, you can be charged with a crime if you don't tell your partner your HIV status, even if your partner doesn't become infected.

Get Support

Receiving a diagnosis of HIV can be a life-changing event. People can feel many emotions—sadness, hopelessness, and even anger. Allied health care providers and social service providers, often available at your health care provider's office, will have the tools to help you work through the early stages of your diagnosis and begin to manage your HIV.

Talking to others who have HIV may also be helpful. Find a local HIV support group.

Reduce the Risk to Others

Photo of a smiling pregnant woman looking at herself in the mirrorHIV is spread through certain body fluids from an HIV-infected person: blood, semen (cum), pre-seminal fluid (pre-cum), rectal fluids, vaginal fluids, and breast milk. In the United States, HIV is most often transmitted by having anal or vaginal sex with someone who has HIV without using a condom or taking medicines to prevent or treat HIV. In addition, a mother can pass HIV to her baby during pregnancy, during labor, through breastfeeding, or by pre-chewing her baby's food.

The higher your viral load, the more likely you are to transmit HIV to others. When your viral load is very low (called viral suppression, with less than 200 copies per milliliter of blood) or undetectable (about 40 copies per milliliter of blood), your chance of transmitting HIV is greatly reduced. However, this is true only if you can stay virally suppressed. One thing that can increase viral load is not taking HIV medicines the right way, every day.

You can also protect your partners by getting tested and treated for other STDs. If you have both HIV and some other STD with sores, like syphilis, your risk of transmitting HIV can be about 3 times as high as if you didn't have any STD with sores.

Taking other actions, like using a condom the right way every time you have sex or having your partners take daily medicine to prevent HIV (called pre-exposure prophylaxis or PrEP) can lower your chances of transmitting HIV even more.

Section 20.9

How Can I Pay for HIV Care?

This section includes text excerpted from "Cost of HIV Treatment," Centers for Disease Control and Prevention (CDC), February 8, 2016.

Living with HIV can bring up a lot of questions and concerns, especially about how to pay for treatment. Fortunately, resources and programs are available that may help.

Health Insurance

Understanding your health insurance options is key to maintaining good health.

Will My Health Insurance Cover My HIV Treatments?

There is no simple answer to this question. Getting health insurance to help pay for HIV care and treatment can be a challenge for some people living with HIV.

If you are already covered by a private group health insurance plan, such as insurance you have through your employer or a private individual plan, it will typically cover your HIV care, just as it covers care for other medical conditions. Most group health plans require that you pay a portion of your medical costs through:

- Regular payments (sometimes called "premiums"), which are usually subtracted from your paychecks, and/or

- Co-pays, payments made at the time you receive health care services or medications.

If you are covered by a private health insurance policy, review your policy to find out what HIV care and treatment your insurance provider covers. If your policy does not cover portions of your HIV care, some government and private programs may be able to help pay for or provide these services.

What If I Don't Have Health Insurance?

A number of programs may help pay for your care and treatment if you do not have health insurance or if your health insurance doesn't cover the care you need. A social worker or your case manager can help you determine if you are eligible and apply for these programs.

These programs include:

- **Ryan White HIV/AIDS Program:** The Ryan White HIV/AIDS Program provides HIV-related services (like medical care and medications) in the United States for people who do not have enough health care coverage or financial resources to pay for care. The program fills gaps in care not met by other payers. Persons need to meet certain eligibility requirements to access this program. You can call your State HIV/AIDS Hotline and ask them to refer you to the nearest Ryan White provider, or talk to your social worker or case manager to find out more.

- **Medicaid:** The federal-state health insurance program pays for medical care for people with low incomes, older people, and people with disabilities. States manage the Medicaid program, and each state decides who is eligible and what the program covers. Medicaid is currently the biggest source of insurance coverage for people living with HIV. The Affordable Care Act (ACA) expands Medicaid so that, in participating states, more people with HIV who did not qualify in the past can get coverage.

- **Medicare:** The federal health insurance program is for people who are 65 and older or are disabled. All Medicare drug plans cover all HIV medications.

Ask for help. Working with your social worker, case manager, or patient navigator will help you get the care, treatment, and support you need.

How Will the Affordable Care Act Help Me Get Coverage for or Pay for HIV Care and Treatment?

The Affordable Care Act (ACA) is a law that was passed to help ensure that Americans have secure, stable, and affordable health insurance. The ACA created several changes that expand access to coverage for people living with HIV. Because coverage varies by state, talk to your health care provider or social worker to get information about the coverage available where you live.

Can I Get Care and Treatment from a Government Community Health Center?

More than 8,000 Community Health Centers are operated by the U.S. Department of Health and Human Services, Health Resources and Services Administration (HRSA). They help more than 20 million people with limited access to health care. HRSA Community Health Centers provide HIV testing and some offer other services to people with HIV, including medical care. Fees are based on a person's ability to pay. Some patients receive care services at the center itself, while others are referred to an HIV specialist if the Community Health Center does not provide HIV care. Talk to your case manager or social worker for more information on Community Health Centers and whether you are eligible to receive HIV care and treatment from a center near you.

Paying for Medication

Paying for your HIV medication can be a challenge. Fortunately, there are government and private programs that can help pay for medication if you are eligible. Some of these programs include:

- **Ryan White AIDS Drug Assistance Program:** The Ryan White AIDS Drug Assistance Program (ADAP) provides HIV- and AIDS-related prescription drugs to uninsured and underinsured individuals living with HIV and AIDS. ADAP funds are used by states to provide medications to treat HIV, or to prevent the serious deterioration of health, including measures for the prevention and treatment of opportunistic infections. As a payer of last resort, ADAP only helps individuals who have neither public nor private insurance or cannot get all of their medication needs met through their insurance payer. The medication provided by this drug program varies by state. Call your state's HIV and AIDS hotline to ask about the ADAP program in your state or speak to your case manager or social worker.

- **Medicare Prescription Drug Coverage Plans:** Medicare Prescription Drug Coverage Plans are required to provide coverage for common medications that people living with HIV use. Talk to your case manager or social worker to learn more about these plans.

- **Private Prescription Assistance Programs:** Some major drug companies offer patient co-pay savings programs to people living with HIV. In addition, other assistance is available to help qualifying patients with no prescription coverage to obtain free medication. These programs can help you get the medicines you need at low or no cost. Ask your medical provider, case manager, or social worker for more information.

Your case manager, social worker, or patient navigator can help you determine your eligibility and help you apply for these types of assistance. They can also help identify other assistance programs available in your community.

Section 20.10

The Affordable Care Act and People Living with HIV/AIDS

This section includes text excerpted from "The Affordable Care Act and HIV/AIDS," U.S. Department of Health and Human Services (HHS), February 4, 2016.

Improving Access to Instant Coverage

The Affordable Care Act (ACA) provides Americans—including those at risk for and living with HIV/AIDS—better access to healthcare coverage and more health insurance options.

Coverage for people with pre-existing conditions. Thanks to the ACA, no American can ever again be dropped or denied coverage because of a pre-existing health condition, like asthma, cancer, or HIV. Insurers also are prohibited from cancelling or rescinding coverage because of mistakes made on an application, and can no longer impose lifetime caps on insurance benefits. These changes are significant because prior to the ACA, many people living with HIV or other chronic health conditions experienced obstacles in getting health coverage, were dropped from coverage, or avoided seeking coverage for fear of being denied. Now they can get covered and get the care they need. The Ryan White Affordable Care Enrollment (ACE) Technical Assistance Center Exit Disclaimer provides tools and resources to support the enrollment of people living with HIV in health care coverage.

Broader Medicaid eligibility. Under the ACA, states have the option, which is fully Federally funded for the first three years, to expand Medicaid to generally include those with incomes at or below 138% of the Federal poverty line, including single adults without children who were previously not generally eligible for Medicaid. Medicaid is the largest payer for HIV care in the United States, and the expansion of Medicaid to low-income childless adults is particularly important for many gay, bisexual, and other men who have sex with men (MSM) who were previously ineligible for Medicaid, and yet remain the population most affected by the HIV epidemic. Further, in states that opt for Medicaid expansion, people living with HIV who meet the income threshold will no longer have to wait for an AIDS diagnosis in order to become eligible for Medicaid. That means they can get into life-extending care and treatment before the disease has significantly damaged their immune system.

More affordable coverage. The ACA requires most Americans to have qualifying health insurance. To help people access quality, affordable coverage, the ACA created Health Insurance Marketplaces (sometimes called "exchanges") in every state that help consumers compare different health plans and determine what savings they may qualify for. The ACA also provides financial assistance for people with low and middle incomes in the form of tax credits that lower the cost of their monthly premiums and lower their out-of-pocket costs. These tax credits depend on a family's household size and income. The open enrollment period for 2016 coverage is over. However, you may still be able to get coverage if you have a qualifying live event. Also, you can apply for free or low-cost coverage through Medicaid and CHIP at any time, all year.

Lower prescription drug costs for Medicare recipients. In the past, as many as one in four seniors went without a prescription every year because they couldn't afford it. The ACA closes, over time, the Medicare Part D prescription drug benefit "donut hole," giving Medicare enrollees living with HIV and AIDS the peace of mind that they will be better able to afford their medications. Beneficiaries receive a 50% discount on covered brand-name drugs while they are in the "donut hole," a considerable savings for people taking costly HIV/AIDS drugs. And in the years to come, they can expect additional savings on their prescription drugs while they are in the coverage gap until it is closed in 2020. In addition, as a result of the health care law, AIDS Drug Assistance Program (ADAP) benefits are now considered as contributions toward Medicare Part D's True Out of Pocket Spending Limit ("TrOOP"). This is a huge relief for ADAP clients who are Medicare Part D enrollees, since they will now be able to move through the donut hole more quickly, which was difficult, if not impossible, for ADAP clients to do before this change.

Ensuring Quality Coverage

The Affordable Care Act also helps all Americans, including those at risk for or living with HIV, have access to the best quality coverage and care. This includes:

Preventive services. Under the ACA, most new health insurance plans must cover certain recommended preventive services—including HIV testing for everyone ages 15 to 65, and for people of other ages at increased risk—without additional cost-sharing, such as copays or deductibles. Since one in eight people living with HIV in the U.S. are unaware of their infection, improving access to HIV testing will help more people learn their status so they can be connected to care and treatment.

Comprehensive coverage. The law establishes a minimum set of benefits (called "essential health benefits") that must be covered under health plans offered in the individual and small group markets, both inside and outside of the Health Insurance Marketplace. These include many health services that are important for people living with HIV/AIDS, including prescription drug services, hospital inpatient care, lab tests, services and devices to help you manage a chronic disease, and mental health and substance use disorder services.

Coordinated care for those with chronic health conditions. The law recognizes the value of patient-centered medical homes as an effective way to strengthen the quality of care, especially for people with complex chronic conditions such as HIV/AIDS. The patient-centered medical home model of care can foster greater patient retention and higher quality HIV care because of its focus on treating the many needs of the patient at once and better coordination across medical specialties and support services. The Ryan White HIV/AIDS Program has been a pioneer in the development of this model in the HIV health care system. The ACA also authorized an optional Medicaid State Plan benefit for states to establish Health Homes to coordinate care for Medicaid beneficiaries with certain chronic health conditions. HIV/AIDS is one of the chronic health conditions that states may request approval to cover.

Enhancing the Capacity of the Healthcare Delivery System

The ACA expands the capacity of the healthcare delivery system to better serve all Americans, including those at risk for and living with HIV/AIDS.

Expansion of community health centers. The ACA has made a major investment in expanding the network of community health centers that provide preventive and primary care services to more than 20 million Americans every year. These health centers are important partners in implementing the National HIV/AIDS Strategy and expand the opportunities for integrating HIV testing, prevention, care, and treatment services into primary care.

Delivering culturally competent care. The ACA expands initiatives to strengthen cultural competency training for all healthcare providers and ensure all populations are treated equitably. It also bolsters the Federal commitment to reducing health disparities. One effort underway to expand the capacity of health centers to deliver culturally competent care to populations heavily impacted by HIV is the National LGBT Health Education Center, Exit Disclaimer funded by HRSA. This center helps healthcare organizations better address the needs of lesbian, gay, bisexual and transgender individuals, including needs for HIV prevention, testing, and treatment.

Increasing the healthcare workforce for underserved communities. Thanks to the ACA, the National Health Service Corps is providing loans and scholarships to more doctors, nurses, and other health care providers, a critical healthcare workforce expansion to better serve vulnerable populations. This is in line with a key recommendation of the National HIV/AIDS Strategy to increase the number and diversity of available providers of clinical care and related services for people living with HIV, many of whom live in underserved communities.

Section 20.11

Legal Rights in the Workplace under the Americans with Disabilities Act (ADA)

This section includes text excerpted from "Living with HIV Infection: Your Legal Rights in the Workplace Under the ADA," U.S. Equal Employment Opportunity Commission (EEOC), December 1, 2015.

If you have HIV infection or AIDS, you have workplace privacy rights, you are protected against discrimination and harassment at work because of your condition, and you may have a legal right to reasonable accommodations that can help you to do your job. This section briefly explains these rights, which are provided under the Americans with Disabilities Act (ADA). You may also have additional rights under other laws, such as the Family and Medical Leave Act (FMLA) and various medical insurance laws, not discussed here.

Am I Allowed to Keep My Condition Private?

In most situations, you can keep your condition private. Generally, employers cannot ask you whether you are HIV-positive, or whether you have any other medical condition, before making a job offer. An employer is allowed to ask medical questions in four situations:

- When it is engaging in affirmative action for people with disabilities, in which case you may choose whether to respond.

- When you ask for a reasonable accommodation.

- After it has made you a job offer, but before employment begins, as long as everyone entering the same job category is asked the same questions.

- On the job, when there is objective evidence that you may be unable to do your job or that you may pose a safety risk because of your condition. Your employer cannot rely on myths or stereotypes about your condition to conclude that you are unable to do your job or pose a safety risk.

244

If you need to talk about your condition in order to answer a non-medical question (for example, if you are asked why there are gaps on your resume), you may choose whether to respond. However, you should know that the employer could reject you for not answering the question, or for lying. If you do talk about your condition, the employer cannot discriminate against you, and it must keep the information confidential, even from co-workers. (If you wish to discuss your condition with coworkers, you may choose to do so.)

What if My Condition Could Affect My Job Performance?

If your job performance could be affected by HIV infection, the side effects of HIV medication, or another medical condition that has developed because of HIV, you may be entitled to reasonable accommodation that will help to solve the problem.

A reasonable accommodation is some type of change in the way things are done that you need because of a disability. Possible reasonable accommodations include altered break and work schedules (e.g., frequent breaks to rest or use the restroom or modified schedules to accommodate medical appointments), changes in supervisory methods (e.g., written instructions from a supervisor who usually does not provide them), accommodations for visual impairments (e.g., magnifiers, screen reading software, and qualified readers), ergonomic office furniture, unpaid time off (e.g., for treatment or recuperation), permission to work from home, and reassignment to a vacant position if you can no longer do your job because of your condition. These are only examples you are free to request any change that you need because of your condition. However, your employer does not have to remove the essential functions (fundamental duties) of your job, let you do less work for the same amount of pay, or let you do lower-quality work.

Because an employer does not have to excuse poor job performance, even if it was caused by a medical condition or the side effects of medication, it may be better to ask for accommodation before any problems occur or become worse.

How Can I Get Reasonable Accommodation?

Ask for one. Tell a supervisor, HR manager, or other appropriate person that you need a change to the way things are normally done because of a medical condition. You may ask for accommodation at any time. (However, many people choose to wait at least until they receive a job offer, because it's very hard to prove illegal discrimination that takes place before a job offer.)

What Will Happen After I Ask for Reasonable Accommodation?

Your employer may ask you to put your request in writing, and to describe your condition and how it affects your work. You may also be asked to submit a letter from your doctor documenting that you have a medical condition and that you need accommodation. If you do not want the employer to know your specific diagnosis, it may be enough to provide documentation that describes your condition more generally (by stating, for example, that you have an "immune disorder"). The doctor may also be asked whether particular reasonable accommodations would meet your needs.

If a reasonable accommodation would help you do your job, the employer must give you one unless it involves significant difficulty or expense. The employer cannot legally fire you, or refuse to hire or promote you, because you asked for a reasonable accommodation, or because you need one. The employer also cannot charge you for the costs of accommodation. However, if more than one accommodation would work, your employer can choose which one to give you.

If My Employer Knows that I Have HIV Infection, Could I Get Fired?

Employers are not allowed to discriminate against you simply because you have HIV infection. This includes firing you, rejecting you for a job or promotion, and forcing you to take leave.

Although employers do not have to keep employees who are unable to do the job, or who pose a "direct threat" to safety (a significant risk of substantial harm to yourself or others), they cannot rely on myths or stereotypes about HIV infection when deciding what you can safely or effectively do. Before an employer can reject you based on your condition, it must have objective evidence that you are unable to perform your job duties, or that you would create a significant safety risk, even with reasonable accommodation.

What if I Am Being Harassed Because of My Condition?

Harassment based on a disability is not allowed under the ADA. You should tell your employer about any harassment if you want the employer to stop the problem. Follow your employer's reporting procedures if there are any. If you report the harassment, your employer is legally required to take action to prevent it from occurring in the future.

What Should I Do if I Think that My Rights Have Been Violated?

The Equal Employment Opportunity Commission (EEOC) will help you to decide what to do next, and conduct an investigation if you decide to file a charge of discrimination. Because you must file a charge within 180 days of the alleged violation in order to take further legal action (or 300 days if the employer is also covered by a state or local employment discrimination law), it is best to begin the process early. It is illegal for your employer to retaliate against you for contacting the EEOC or filing a charge

Chapter 21

Human Papillomavirus (HPV)

Chapter Contents

Section 21.1

What Is Genital HPV Infection?

This section includes text excerpted from "Genital HPV
Infection—Fact Sheet," Centers for Disease Control
and Prevention (CDC), January 23, 2014.

Human papillomavirus (HPV) is the most common sexually transmitted infection in the United States. Some health effects caused by
HPV can be prevented with vaccines.

What Is HPV?

HPV is the most common sexually transmitted infection (STI). HPV
is a different virus than HIV and HSV (herpes). HPV is so common
that nearly all sexually active men and women get it at some point in
their lives. There are many different types of HPV. Some types can
cause health problems including genital warts and cancers. But there
are vaccines that can stop these health problems from happening.

How Is HPV Spread?

You can get HPV by having vaginal, anal, or oral sex with someone
who has the virus. It is most commonly spread during vaginal or anal
sex. HPV can be passed even when an infected person has no signs
or symptoms.

Anyone who is sexually active can get HPV, even if you have had
sex with only one person. You also can develop symptoms years after
you have sex with someone who is infected making it hard to know
when you first became infected.

Does HPV Cause Health Problems?

In most cases, HPV goes away on its own and does not cause any
health problems. But when HPV does not go away, it can cause health
problems like genital warts and cancer.

Genital warts usually appear as a small bump or group of bumps in
the genital area. They can be small or large, raised or flat, or shaped

like a cauliflower. A healthcare provider can usually diagnose warts by looking at the genital area.

Does HPV Cause Cancer?

HPV can cause cervical and other cancers including cancer of the vulva, vagina, penis, or anus. It can also cause cancer in the back of the throat, including the base of the tongue and tonsils (called oropharyngeal cancer).

Cancer often takes years, even decades, to develop after a person gets HPV. The types of HPV that can cause genital warts are not the same as the types of HPV that can cause cancers.

There is no way to know which people who have HPV will develop cancer or other health problems. People with weak immune systems (including individuals with HIV/AIDS) may be less able to fight off HPV and more likely to develop health problems from it.

How Can I Avoid HPV and the Health Problems It Can Cause?

You can do several things to lower your chances of getting HPV.

Get vaccinated. HPV vaccines are safe and effective. They can protect males and females against diseases (including cancers) caused by HPV when given in the recommended age groups. HPV vaccines are given in three shots over six months; it is important to get all three doses.

Get screened for cervical cancer. Routine screening for women aged 21 to 65 years old can prevent cervical cancer.

If you are sexually active

- Use latex condoms the right way every time you have sex. This can lower your chances of getting HPV. But HPV can infect areas that are not covered by a condom-so condoms may not give full protection against getting HPV;

- Be in a mutually monogamous relationship—or have sex only with someone who only has sex with you.

Who Should Get Vaccinated?

All boys and girls ages 11 or 12 years should get vaccinated.

251

Catch-up vaccines are recommended for males through age 21 and for females through age 26, if they did not get vaccinated when they were younger.

The vaccine is also recommended for gay and bisexual men (or any man who has sex with a man) through age 26. It is also recommended for men and women with compromised immune systems (including people living with HIV/AIDS) through age 26, if they did not get fully vaccinated when they were younger.

How Do I Know If I Have HPV?

There is no test to find out a person's "HPV status." Also, there is no approved HPV test to find HPV in the mouth or throat.

There are HPV tests that can be used to screen for cervical cancer. These tests are recommended for screening only in women aged 30 years and older. They are not recommended to screen men, adolescents, or women under the age of 30 years.

Most people with HPV do not know they are infected and never develop symptoms or health problems from it. Some people find out they have HPV when they get genital warts. Women may find out they have HPV when they get an abnormal Pap test result (during cervical cancer screening). Others may only find out once they've developed more serious problems from HPV, such as cancers.

How Common Is HPV and the Health Problems Caused by HPV?

About 79 million Americans are currently infected with HPV. About 14 million people become newly infected each year. HPV is so common that most sexually-active men and women will get at least one type of HPV at some point in their lives.

Health problems related to HPV include genital warts and cervical cancer.

- **Genital warts:** About 360,000 people in the United States get genital warts each year.

- **Cervical cancer:** More than 11,000 women in the United States get cervical cancer each year.

There are other conditions and cancers caused by HPV that occur in persons living in the United States.

I'm Pregnant. Will Having HPV Affect My Pregnancy?

If you are pregnant and have HPV, you can get genital warts or develop abnormal cell changes on your cervix. Abnormal cell changes can be found with routine cervical cancer screening. You should get routine cervical cancer screening even when you are pregnant.

Can I Be Treated for HPV or Health Problems Caused by HPV?

There is no treatment for the virus itself. However, there are treatments for the health problems that HPV can cause:

1. Genital warts can be treated by you or your physician. If left untreated, genital warts may go away, stay the same, or grow in size or number.

2. Cervical precancer can be treated. Women who get routine Pap tests and follow up as needed can identify problems *before* cancer develops. Prevention is always better than treatment.

3. Other HPV-related cancers are also more treatable when diagnosed and treated early.

Section 21.2

HPV and Men

This section includes text excerpted from "HPV and Men—Fact Sheet," Centers for Disease Control and Prevention (CDC), February 16, 2015.

Nearly all sexually active people will get human papillomavirus (HPV) at some time in their life. Although most HPV infections go away on their own without causing problems, HPV can cause men to develop genital warts, or some kinds of cancer. Getting vaccinated against HPV can help prevent these health problems.

What Is HPV?

HPV is the most common sexually transmitted infection. HPV is a viral infection that can be spread from one person to another person through anal, vaginal, or oral sex, or through other close skin-to-skin touching during sexual activity. If you are sexually active you can get HPV, and nearly all sexually active people get infected with HPV at some point in their lives. It is important to understand that getting HPV is not the same thing as getting HIV or HSV (herpes).

How Do Men Get HPV?

You can get HPV by having sex with someone who is infected with HPV. This disease is spread easily during anal or vaginal sex, and it can also be spread through oral sex or other close skin-to-skin touching during sex. HPV can be spread even when an infected person has no visible signs or symptoms.

Will HPV Cause Health Problems for Me?

Most of the time HPV infections completely go away and don't cause any health problems. However, if an infection does not go away on its own, it is possible to develop HPV symptoms months or years after getting infected. This makes it hard to know exactly when you became infected. Lasting HPV infection can cause genital warts or certain kinds of cancer. It is not known why some people develop health problems from HPV and others do not.

What Are the Symptoms of HPV?

Most men who get HPV never develop symptoms and the infection usually goes away completely by itself. However, if HPV does not go away, it can cause genital warts or certain kinds of cancer.

See your healthcare provider if you have questions about anything new or unusual such as warts, or unusual growths, lumps, or sores on your penis, scrotum, anus, mouth, or throat.

What Are the Symptoms of Genital Warts?

Genital warts usually appear as a small bump or group of bumps in the genital area around the penis or the anus. These warts might be small or large, raised or flat, or shaped like a cauliflower. The warts may go away, or stay the same, or grow in size or number. Usually, a healthcare provider can diagnose genital warts simply by looking at them. Genital warts can come back, even after treatment. The types of HPV that cause warts do not cause cancer.

Can HPV Cause Cancer?

Yes. HPV infection isn't cancer but can cause changes in the body that lead to cancer. HPV infections usually go away by themselves but having an HPV infection can cause certain kinds of cancer to develop. These include cervical cancer in women, penile cancer in men, and anal cancer in both women and men. HPV can also cause cancer in the back of the throat, including the base of the tongue and tonsils (called oropharyngeal cancer). All of these cancers are caused by HPV infections that did not go away. Cancer develops very slowly and may not be diagnosed until years, or even decades, after a person initially gets infected with HPV. Currently, there is no way to know who will have only a temporary HPV infection, and who will develop cancer after getting HPV.

How Common Are HPV-Related Cancers in Men?

Although HPV is the most common sexually transmitted infection, HPV-related cancers are not common in men.

Certain men are more likely to develop HPV-related cancers:

- Men with weak immune systems (including those with HIV) who get infected with HPV are more likely to develop HPV-related health problems.

- Men who receive anal sex are more likely to get anal HPV and develop anal cancer.

Can I Get Tested for HPV?

No, there is currently no approved test for HPV in men.

Routine testing (also called 'screening') to check for HPV or HPV-related disease before there are signs or symptom, is not recommended by the CDC for anal, penile, or throat cancers in men in the United States. However, some healthcare providers do offer anal Pap tests to men who may be at increased risk for anal cancer, including men with HIV or men who receive anal sex. If you have symptoms and are concerned about cancer, please see a healthcare provider.

Can I Get Treated for HPV or Health Problems Caused by HPV?

There is no specific treatment for HPV, but there are treatments for health problems caused by HPV. Genital warts can be treated by your healthcare provider, or with prescription medication. HPV-related cancers are more treatable when diagnosed and treated promptly.

How Can I Lower My Chance of Getting HPV?

There are two steps you can take to lower your chances of getting HPV and HPV-related diseases:

- **Get vaccinated.** HPV vaccines are safe and effective. They can protect men against warts and certain cancers caused by HPV. Ideally, you should get vaccinated before ever having sex. HPV vaccines are given in a series of three shots over a period of about six months.

- **Use condoms the correct way every time you have sex.** This can lower your chances of getting all STIs, including HPV. However, HPV can infect areas that are not covered by a condom, so condoms may not give full protection against getting HPV.

Can I Get an HPV Vaccine?

In the United States, HPV vaccines are recommended for the following men:

- All boys at age 11 or 12 years (or as young as 9 years)

- Older boys through age 21 years, if they did not get vaccinated when they were younger

- Gay, bisexual, and other men who have sex with men through age 26 years, if they did not get vaccinated when they were younger

- Men with HIV or weakened immune systems through age 26 years, if they did not get vaccinated when they were younger

What Does Having HPV Mean for Me or My Sex Partner's Health?

See a healthcare provider if you have questions about anything new or unusual (such as warts, growths, lumps, or sores) on your own or your partner's penis, scrotum, anus, mouth or throat. Even if you are healthy, you and your sex partner(s) may also want to get checked by a healthcare provider for other STIs.

If you or your partner have genital warts, you should avoid having sex until the warts are gone or removed. However, it is not known how long a person is able to spread HPV after warts are gone.

What Does HPV Mean for My Relationship?

HPV infections are usually temporary. A person may have had HPV for many years before it causes health problems. If you or your partner are diagnosed with an HPV-related disease, there is no way to know how long you have had HPV, whether your partner gave you HPV, or whether you gave HPV to your partner. HPV is not necessarily a sign that one of you is having sex outside of your relationship. It is important that sex partners discuss their sexual health, and risk for all STIs, with each other.

Section 21.3

HPV and Women

This section includes text excerpted from "HPV—Women's Health Guide," Centers for Disease Control and Prevention (CDC), June 3, 2015.

Human papillomavirus or HPV is the most common viral sexually transmitted disease (STD) in the United States. According to the Centers for Disease Control and Prevention (CDC), at least one out of every two sexually active people will have HPV at some point in their life.

The Number of Known HPV Types Are over 100

About 40 types can infect female and male genital areas. Genital HPV are grouped into two types:

- Low-risk types of HPV can cause genital warts or may be completely harmless.

- High-risk types of HPV increase the chances for some types of cancer, like cervical cancer.

How Is It Spread?

HPV is spread by skin-to-skin contact. Women get HPV from sexual contact with someone who has it. HPV can be spread by vaginal, anal, oral or hand-genital sexual contact. Someone who is infected but has no visible signs can still spread HPV to others. People can be infected with more than one type of HPV. Long-term sexual partners with HPV often have the same HPV types.

Most sexually active men and women get genital HPV at some time in their lives.

There is an increased risk of genital HPV infection if you:

- Become sexually active at an earlier age
- Have multiple sexual partners
- Smoke
- Have an immune system that does not work well due to a medical condition (e.g., cancer, HIV/AIDS) or from a medicine that weakens the immune system

What Are Signs of HPV in Women?

Most HPV infections have no signs that can been seen or felt. You can have HPV even if years have passed since you had sexual contact with an infected person. You may never know which sexual partner gave you HPV. HPV infection may cause:

- Genital warts (infection with low-risk viruses)
- Cancer (infection with high-risk viruses)
- Cervical cancer (more common)
- Cancers of the vagina, vulva, anus, throat, tongue or tonsils (less common)

How Do You Know If You Have HPV?

Most women with HPV have no signs of infection. Since most HPV infections go away on their own within two years, many women never know they had an infection. Some HPV infections cause genital warts that can be seen or felt. The only way to know if you have HPV is to ask your health care provider to do an HPV test. Your health care provider may also examine you for other infections.

High-risk types of HPV infection can cause cervical cancer. To detect changes in the cervix caused by HPV, all women should get regular Pap tests. You should talk to your health care provider about when to start, how often, and when to stop having Pap tests.

Pap tests:

- Screen for cervical cancer and changes in the cervix that might turn into cancer

- Are done by a health care provider who collects a cell sample from the cervix with a small brush

- Can find abnormal cells on the cervix caused by HPV

- Can be done with an HPV test if:

  - You are age 30 or older.

  - You have had an abnormal Pap test result. This will show if HPV caused the changes.

- Should be done within three years of first sexual contact or starting at age 21

- Are important, as treating pre-cancer changes on the cervix can prevent cervical cancer

All women, aged 21 and older, should have regular Pap tests.

How Is It Treated?

Although genital HPV infections are very common, most show no signs and go away without treatment within a few years. If HPV does not go away, treatments are different for low risk HPV and high-risk HPV:

- **Low-Risk HPV** (Genital warts)–Even when genital warts are treated, HPV infection may remain. Warts can also come back after treatment. Over-the-counter treatments for other types of warts should not be used. Treatments for genital warts include:

  - Watch and wait to see if the warts stay the same, get bigger, or go away

  - Medicines put directly on the warts

  - Burning off the warts

- Freezing off the warts

- Cutting the warts out

- Using special lights or lasers to destroy the warts

- **High-Risk HPV**–Pap tests can find pre-cancer changes in the cervix and other abnormal cells. Removing the abnormal cells is the best way to prevent cervical cancer.

- Abnormal cells can be surgically removed without removing the uterus or damaging the cervix. After, women can still have normal pregnancies.

What Can Happen If You Have HPV for a Long Time?

Certain types of low-risk HPV can cause genital warts. Without treatment genital warts may:

- Go away

- Remain unchanged

- Increase in size or number

High-risk HPV can cause abnormal cells in the cervix and cancer if not treated. Almost all cervical cancers are thought to be caused by HPV infections. While there are often no signs of early cervical cancer, some signs may include:

- Increased vaginal discharge, which may be pale, watery, pink, brown, bloody, or foul-smelling

- Abnormal vaginal bleeding between menstrual periods, after sex, douching or a pelvic exam

- Longer or heavier menstrual periods

- Bleeding after menopause

- Pelvic pain

- Pain during sex

If you have high-risk HPV the risk of cervical cancer is further increased if you:

- Smoke

- Have had more than three children

- Have used a birth control pill for more than five years
- Have a family history of cervical cancer
- Have limited access to medical testing and care
- Have a suppressed immune system

Almost all cervical cancers are caused by high-risk HPV infection.

If You Have HPV

- Get regular Pap tests.
- Discuss treatment and follow-up care with your health care provider.
- Know that partners that have been together for a while often share the same HPV types, even if both have no symptoms

How Can You Avoid HPV?

- Get vaccinated against HPV.
  - HPV vaccines can protect against 70% of cervical cancers.
  - One type of HPV vaccine can protect against the low-risk HPV that causes 90% of genital warts.
  - HPV vaccine is recommended for all females 9 to 26 years old.
  - The Centers for Disease Control and Prevention (CDC) recommends all 11–12 year old girls and boys get the HPV vaccine.
- Avoid sexual contact.
- Have safer sex:
  - Reduce the number of sexual partners.
  - Condoms, when used correctly, can reduce the risk of getting HPV. But, condoms may not cover all infected areas. Each time you have sex use a condom (male or female type):
    - Before vaginal sex
    - Before anal sex
    - Before oral sex

- Have sex with only one partner who does not have sex with others and does not have HPV.

- Know that other forms of birth control do not protect against HPV.

Condoms may not fully protect against HPV since HPV can infect areas not covered by a condom.

What about Pregnancy?

Genital warts rarely cause problems during pregnancy and birth. Most women who no longer have visible genital warts do not have problems with pregnancy or birth. If you are pregnant, you should discuss treatment options with your health care provider as the warts may:

- Grow larger and bleed

- Make it difficult to urinate if growing in the urinary tract (rare)

- Make the vagina less elastic during birth if the warts are in the vagina (rare)

- Cause a need for a cesarean section (C-section) birth if the warts block the birth canal (rare)

- Be passed on to the baby during birth (rare)

If you are pregnant and have a HPV infection and an abnormal Pap test, you should discuss your pregnancy with your health care provider.

Section 21.4

Recurrent Respiratory Papillomatosis

This section includes text excerpted from "Recurrent
Respiratory Papillomatosis or Laryngeal Papillomatosis," National
Institute on Deafness and Other Communication
Disorders (NIDCD), April 1, 2011. Reviewed April 2016.

What Is Recurrent Respiratory Papillomatosis?

Recurrent respiratory papillomatosis (RRP) is a disease in which tumors grow in the air passages leading from the nose and mouth into the lungs (respiratory tract). Although the tumors can grow anywhere in the respiratory tract, their presence in the larynx (voice box) causes the most frequent problems, a condition called laryngeal papillomatosis. The tumors may vary in size and grow very quickly. They often grow back even when removed.

What Is the Cause of RRP?

RRP is caused by two types of human papilloma virus (HPV), called HPV 6 and HPV 11. There are more than 150 types of HPV and they do not all have the same symptoms.

Most people who encounter HPV never develop any illness. However, many HPVs can cause small wart-like, non-cancerous tumors called papillomas. The most common illness caused by HPV 6 and HPV 11 is genital warts. Although scientists are uncertain how people are infected with HPV 6 or HPV 11, the virus is thought to be spread through sexual contact or when a mother with genital warts passes it to her baby during childbirth. HPV 6 and HPV 11 can also cause disease of the uterine cervix and, in rare cases, cervical cancer.

According to the Centers for Disease Control and Prevention, the incidence of RRP is rare. Fewer than 2,000 children get RRP each year.

Who Is Affected by RRP?

RRP affects adults as well as infants and small children who may have contracted the virus during childbirth. According to the RRP

Foundation, there are roughly 20,000 cases in the United States. Among children, the incidence of RRP is approximately 4.3 per 100,000; among adults, it's about 1.8 per 100,000.

What Are the Symptoms of RRP?

Normally, voice is produced when air from the lungs is pushed past two side-by-side elastic muscles—called vocal folds or vocal cords—with sufficient pressure to cause them to vibrate. When the tumors interfere with the normal vibrations of the vocal folds, it causes hoarseness, which is the most common symptom of RRP. Eventually, the tumors may block the airway passage and cause difficulty breathing.

Because the tumors grow quickly, young children with the disease may find it difficult to breathe when sleeping, or they may experience difficulty swallowing. Adults and children may experience hoarseness, chronic coughing, or breathing problems. The symptoms tend to be more severe in children than in adults; however, some children experience some relief or remission of the disease when they begin puberty. Because of the similarity of the symptoms, RRP is sometimes misdiagnosed as asthma or chronic bronchitis.

How Is RRP Diagnosed?

Two routine tests for RRP are indirect and direct laryngoscopy. In an indirect laryngoscopy, an otolaryngologist—a doctor who specializes in diseases of the ear, nose, throat, head, and neck—or speech-language pathologist will typically insert a flexible fiberoptic telescope, called an endoscope, into a patient's nose or mouth and then view the larynx on a monitor. Some medical professionals use a video camera attached to a flexible tube to examine the larynx. An older, less common method is for the otolaryngologist to place a small mirror in the back of the throat and angle the mirror down toward the larynx to inspect it for tumors.

- A direct laryngoscopy is conducted in the operating room with the use of general anesthesia. This method allows the otolaryngologist to view the vocal folds and other parts of the larynx under high magnification. This procedure is usually used to minimize discomfort, especially with children, or to enable the doctor to collect tissue samples from the larynx or other parts of the throat to examine them for abnormalities.

How Is RRP Treated?

There is no cure for RRP. Surgery is the primary method for removing tumors from the larynx or airway. Because traditional surgery can result in problems due to scarring of the larynx tissue, many surgeons are now using laser surgery, which uses an intense laser light as the surgical tool. Carbon dioxide lasers—which pass electricity through a tube containing carbon dioxide and other gases to generate light—are currently the most popular type used for this purpose. In the past 10 years, surgeons have begun using a device called a microdebrider, which uses suction to hold the tumor while a small internal rotary blade removes the growth.

Once the tumors have been removed, they have a tendency to return unpredictably. It is common for patients to require repeat surgery. With some patients, surgery may be required every few weeks in order to keep the breathing passage open, while others may require surgery only once a year. In the most extreme cases where tumor growth is aggressive, a tracheotomy may be performed.

A tracheotomy is a surgical procedure in which an incision is made in the front of the patient's neck and a breathing tube (trach tube) is inserted through an opening, called a stoma, into the trachea (windpipe). Rather than breathing through the nose and mouth, the patient will now breathe through the trach tube. Although the trach tube keeps the breathing passage open, doctors try to remove it as soon as it is feasible.

Some patients may be required to keep a trach tube indefinitely in order to keep the breathing passage open. In addition, because the trach tube re-routes all or some of the exhaled air away from the vocal folds, the patient may find it difficult to speak. With the help of a voice specialist or speech-language pathologist who specializes in voice, the patient can learn how to use his or her voice.

Adjuvant therapies—therapies that are used in addition to surgery—have been used to treat more severe cases of RRP. Drug treatments may include antivirals such as interferon and cidofovir, which block the virus from making copies of itself, and indole-3-carbinol, a cancer-fighting compound found in cruciferous vegetables, such as broccoli and Brussels sprouts. To date, the results of these and other adjuvant therapies have been mixed or not yet fully proven.

Section 21.5

Pap Tests and Cervical Cancer Screening to Check for HPV

This section includes text excerpted from "Pap and HPV Testing,"
National Institutes of Health (NIH), September 9, 2014.

What Causes Cervical Cancer?

Nearly all cases of cervical cancer are caused by infection with oncogenic, or high-risk, types of human papillomavirus, or HPV. There are about 12 high-risk HPV types. Infections with these sexually transmitted viruses also cause most anal cancers; many vaginal, vulvar, and penile cancers; and some oropharyngeal cancers.

Although HPV infection is very common, most infections will be suppressed by the immune system within 1 to 2 years without causing cancer. These transient infections may cause temporary changes in cervical cells. If a cervical infection with a high-risk HPV type persists, the cellular changes can eventually develop into more severe precancerous lesions. If precancerous lesions are not treated, they can progress to cancer. It can take 10 to 20 years or more for a persistent infection with a high-risk HPV type to develop into cancer.

What Is Cervical Cancer Screening?

Cervical cancer screening is an essential part of a woman's routine health care. It is a way to detect abnormal cervical cells, including precancerous cervical lesions, as well as early cervical cancers. Both precancerous lesions and early cervical cancers can be treated very successfully. Routine cervical screening has been shown to greatly reduce both the number of new cervical cancers diagnosed each year and deaths from the disease.

Cervical cancer screening includes two types of screening tests: cytology-based screening, known as the Pap test or Pap smear, and HPV testing. The main purpose of screening with the Pap test is to detect abnormal cells that may develop into cancer if left untreated. The Pap test can also find noncancerous conditions, such as infections

266

and inflammation. It can also find cancer cells. In regularly screened populations, however, the Pap test identifies most abnormal cells before they become cancer.

HPV testing is used to look for the presence of high-risk HPV types in cervical cells. These tests can detect HPV infections that cause cell abnormalities, sometimes even before cell abnormalities are evident. Several different HPV tests have been approved for screening. Most tests detect the DNA of high-risk HPV, although one test detects the RNA of high-risk HPV. Some tests detect any high-risk HPV and do not identify the specific type or types that are present. Other tests specifically detect infection with HPV types 16 and 18, the two types that cause most HPV-associated cancers.

How Is Cervical Cancer Screening Done?

Cervical cancer screening can be done in a medical office, a clinic, or a community health center. It is often done during a pelvic examination.

While a woman lies on an exam table, a health care professional inserts an instrument called a speculum into her vagina to widen it so that the upper portion of the vagina and the cervix can be seen. This procedure also allows the health care professional to take a sample of cervical cells. The cells are taken with a wooden or plastic scraper and/ or a cervical brush and are then prepared for Pap analysis in one of two ways. In a conventional Pap test, the specimen (or smear) is placed on a glass microscope slide and a fixative is added. In an automated liquid-based Pap cytology test, cervical cells collected with a brush or other instrument are placed in a vial of liquid preservative. The slide or vial is then sent to a laboratory for analysis.

In the United States, automated liquid-based Pap cytology testing has largely replaced conventional Pap tests. One advantage of liquid-based testing is that the same cell sample can also be tested for the presence of high-risk types of HPV, a process known as "Pap and HPV cotesting." In addition, liquid-based cytology appears to reduce the likelihood of an unsatisfactory specimen. However, conventional and liquid-based Pap tests appear to have a similar ability to detect cellular abnormalities.

When Should a Woman Begin Cervical Cancer Screening, and How Often Should She Be Screened?

Women should talk with their doctor about when to start screening and how often to be screened. In March 2012, updated screening guidelines were released by the United States Preventive Services Task Force and jointly by the American Cancer Society, the American Society for Colposcopy and Cervical Pathology, and the American Society for Clinical Pathology. These guidelines recommend that women have their first Pap test at age 21. Although previous guidelines recommended that women have their first Pap test 3 years after they start having sexual intercourse, waiting until age 21 is now recommended because adolescents have a very low risk of cervical cancer and a high likelihood that cervical cell abnormalities will go away on their own.

According to the updated guidelines, women ages 21 through 29 should be screened with a Pap test every 3 years. Women ages 30 through 65 can then be screened every 5 years with Pap and HPV cotesting or every 3 years with a Pap test alone.

The guidelines also note that women with certain risk factors may need to have more frequent screening or to continue screening beyond age 65. These risk factors include being infected with the human immunodeficiency virus (HIV), being immunosuppressed, having been exposed to diethylstilbestrol before birth, and having been treated for a precancerous cervical lesion or cervical cancer.

Women who have had a hysterectomy (surgery to remove the uterus and cervix) do not need to have cervical screening, unless the hysterectomy was done to treat a precancerous cervical lesion or cervical cancer.

What Are the Benefits of Pap and HPV Cotesting?

For women age 30 and older, Pap and HPV cotesting is less likely to miss an abnormality (i.e., has a lower false-negative rate) than Pap testing alone. Therefore, a woman with a negative HPV test and normal Pap test has very little risk of a serious abnormality developing over the next several years. In fact, researchers have found that, when Pap and HPV cotesting is used, lengthening the screening interval to 5 years still allows abnormalities to be detected in time to treat them while also reducing the detection of HPV infections that would have gone away on their own.

Adding HPV testing to Pap testing may also improve the detection of glandular cell abnormalities, including adenocarcinoma of the cervix (cancer of the glandular cells of the cervix). Glandular cells are mucus-producing cells found in the endocervical canal (the opening in the center of the cervix) or in the lining of the uterus. Glandular cell abnormalities and adenocarcinoma of the cervix are much less common than squamous cell abnormalities and squamous cell carcinoma.

There is some evidence that Pap testing is not as good at detecting adenocarcinoma and glandular cell abnormalities as it is at detecting squamous cell abnormalities and cancers.

Can HPV Testing Be Used Alone for Cervical Cancer Screening?

On April 24, 2014, the U.S. Food and Drug Administration (FDA) approved the use of one HPV DNA test (cobas HPV test, Roche Molecular Systems, Inc.) as a first-line primary screening test for use alone for women age 25 and older. This test detects each of HPV types 16 and 18 and gives pooled results for 12 additional high-risk HPV types.

The new approval was based on long-term findings from the ATHENA trial, a clinical trial that included more than 47,000 women. The results showed that the HPV test used in the study performed better than the Pap test at identifying women at risk of developing severe cervical cell abnormalities.

The greater assurance against future cervical cancer risk with HPV testing has also been demonstrated by a cohort study of more than a million women, which found that, after 3 years, women who tested negative on the HPV test had an extremely low risk of developing cervical cancer—about half the already low risk of women who tested negative on the Pap test.

First-line HPV testing has not yet been incorporated into the current professional cervical cancer screening guidelines. Professional societies are developing interim guidance documents, and some medical practices might incorporate primary HPV screening.

How Are the Results of Cervical Cancer Screening Tests Reported?

A doctor may simply describe Pap test results to a patient as "normal" or "abnormal." Likewise, HPV test results can either be "positive," meaning that a patient's cervical cells are infected with high-risk HPV, or "negative," indicating that high-risk HPV types were not found. A woman may want to ask her doctor for specific information about her Pap and HPV test results and what these results mean.

Most laboratories in the United States use a standard set of terms, called the Bethesda System, to report Pap test results. Under the Bethesda System, samples that have no cell abnormalities are reported as "negative for intraepithelial lesion or malignancy." A negative Pap test report may also note certain benign (non-neoplastic) findings, such as common infections or inflammation. Pap test results also indicate whether the specimen was satisfactory or unsatisfactory for examination.

The Bethesda System considers abnormalities of squamous cells and glandular cells separately. Squamous cell abnormalities are divided into the following categories, ranging from the mildest to the most severe.

Atypical squamous cells (ASC) are the most common abnormal finding in Pap tests. The Bethesda System divides this category into two groups, ASC-US and ASC-H.

1. **ASC-US**: atypical squamous cells of undetermined significance. The squamous cells do not appear completely normal, but doctors are uncertain about what the cell changes mean. The changes may be related to an HPV infection, but they can also be caused by other factors.

2. **ASC-H**: atypical squamous cells, cannot exclude a high-grade squamous intraepithelial lesion. The cells do not appear normal, but doctors are uncertain about what the cell changes mean. ASC-H lesions may be at higher risk of being precancerous compared with ASC-US lesions.

Low-grade squamous intraepithelial lesions (LSILs) are considered mild abnormalities caused by HPV infection. Low-grade means that there are early changes in the size and shape of cells. Intraepithelial refers to the layer of cells that forms the surface of the cervix. When cells from the abnormal area are removed and examined under a microscope (in a procedure called a biopsy), LSILs are usually found to have mild cell changes that may be classified as mild dysplasia or as cervical intraepithelial neoplasia, grade 1 (CIN-1).

High-grade squamous intraepithelial lesions (HSILs) are more severe abnormalities that have a higher likelihood of progressing to cancer if left untreated. High-grade means that there are more evident changes in the size and shape of the abnormal (precancerous) cells and that the cells look very different from normal cells. When examined under a microscope, the cells from HSILs are often found to have more extensive changes that may be classified as moderate or severe dysplasia or as CIN-2, CIN-2/3, or CIN-3 (in order of increasing severity). Microscopic examination of HSILs may also reveal carcinoma in situ (CIS), which is commonly included in the CIN-3 category.

Squamous cell carcinoma is cervical cancer. The abnormal squamous cells have invaded more deeply into the cervix or into other tissues or organs. In a well-screened population, such as that in the United States, a finding of cancer during cervical screening is extremely rare.

Glandular cell abnormalities describe abnormal changes that occur in the glandular tissues of the cervix. These abnormalities are divided into the following categories:

- **Atypical glandular cells (AGC)**, meaning the glandular cells do not appear normal, but doctors are uncertain about what the cell changes mean.

- **Endocervical adenocarcinoma in situ (AIS)**, meaning that severely abnormal cells are found but have not spread beyond the glandular tissue of the cervix.

- **Adcnocarcinoma** includes not only cancer of the endocervical canal itself but also, in some cases, endometrial, extrauterine, and other cancers.

What Follow-Up Tests Are Done If Cervical Cancer Screening Results Are Abnormal?

For a woman receiving Pap and HPV cotesting:

If a woman is found to have a **normal Pap test result with a positive HPV test** that detects the group of high-risk HPV types, the doctor will usually have her return in a year for repeat screening to see if the HPV infection persists and whether any cell changes have developed that need further follow-up testing. Alternatively, the woman may have another HPV test that looks specifically for HPV-16 and HPV-18, the two HPV types that cause most cervical cancers.

If either of these two HPV types is present, a woman will usually have follow-up testing with colposcopy. Colposcopy is the use of an instrument much like a microscope (called acolposcope) to examine the vagina and the cervix. During a colposcopy, the doctor inserts a speculum into the vagina to widen it and may apply a dilute vinegar solution to the cervix, which causes abnormal areas to turn white. The doctor then uses the colposcope (which remains outside the body) to observe the cervix. When a doctor performs colposcopy, he or she will usually remove cells or tissues from the abnormal area for examination under a microscope, a procedure called a biopsy.

If a woman is found to have an **abnormal Pap test result with a negative (normal) HPV test**, the follow-up tests will depend on the Pap test result. If the Pap test result is ASC-US, the doctor will usually have the woman return in 3 to 5 years for a repeat screen. If the Pap test result is LSIL, the doctor may recommend colposcopy or might have the woman return in a year for repeat screening.

If a woman is found to have an **abnormal Pap test result with a positive HPV test** that detects any high-risk HPV type, the doctor will usually have the woman receive follow-up testing with colposcopy.

For a woman receiving Pap testing alone:

If a woman who is receiving Pap testing alone is found to have an **ASC-US Pap test result**, her doctor may have the sample tested for high-risk HPV types or may repeat the Pap test to determine whether further follow-up is needed. Many times, ASC-US cell changes in the cervix go away without treatment, especially if there is no evidence of infection with high-risk HPV. Doctors may prescribe estrogen cream for women with ASC-US who are near or past menopause. Because ASC-US cell changes can be caused by low hormone levels, applying an estrogen cream to the cervix for a few weeks can usually help to clarify their cause.

Follow-up testing for **all other abnormal Pap results** will typically involve a colposcopy.

For a woman receiving HPV-alone testing:

If a woman who is having HPV-alone testing **tests positive for HPV types 16 or 18**, she should, according to guidance from the FDA, have a colposcopy. A women who tests negative for types 16 and 18 but is positive for one of the 12 other high-risk HPV types should have a Pap test to determine whether a colposcopy is needed.

How Are Cervical Abnormalities Treated?

If biopsy analysis of cells from the affected area of the cervix shows that the cells have CIN-2 or more severe abnormalities, further treatment is probably needed depending on a woman's age, pregnancy status, and future fertility concerns. Without treatment, these cells may turn into cancer. Treatment options include the following:

- LEEP (loop electrosurgical excision procedure), in which an electrical current that is passed through a thin wire loop acts as a knife to remove tissue

- Cryotherapy, in which abnormal tissue is destroyed by freezing it

- Laser therapy, the use of a narrow beam of intense light to destroy or remove abnormal cells

- Conization, the removal of a cone-shaped piece of tissue using a knife, a laser, or the LEEP technique.

The screening guidelines call for women who have been treated for CIN-2 or more severe abnormalities to continue screening for at least 20 years, even if they are over 65.

Do Women Who Have Been Vaccinated against HPV Still Need to Be Screened for Cervical Cancer?

Yes. Because current HPV vaccines do not protect against all HPV types that cause cervical cancer, it is important for vaccinated women to continue to undergo routine cervical cancer screening.

What Are the Limitations of Cervical Cancer Screening?

Although cervical cancer screening tests are highly effective, they are not completely accurate. Sometimes a patient can be told that she has abnormal cells when the cells are actually normal (a false-positive result), or she can be told that her cells are normal when in fact there is an abnormality that was not detected (a false-negative result).

Cervical cancer screening has another limitation, caused by the nature of HPV infections. Because most HPV infections are transient and produce only temporary changes in cervical cells, overly frequent cervical screening could detect HPV infections or cervical cell changes that would never cause cancer. Treating abnormalities that would have gone away on their own can cause needless psychological stress. In addition, follow-up tests and treatments can be uncomfortable, and some treatments that remove cervical tissue, such as LEEP and conization, have the potential to weaken the cervix and may affect fertility or slightly increase the rate of premature delivery, depending on how much tissue is removed.

The screening intervals in the 2012 guidelines are intended to minimize the harms caused by treating abnormalities that would never progress to cancer while also limiting false-negative results that would delay the diagnosis and treatment of a precancerous condition or cancer. With these intervals, if an HPV infection or abnormal cells are missed at one screen, chances are good that abnormal cells will be detected at the next screening exam, when they can still be treated successfully.

Section 21.6

Making Sense of Your HPV Test Results

This section includes text excerpted from
"Making Sense of Your Pap and HPV Test Results,"
Centers for Disease Control and Prevention (CDC),
January 5, 2012. Reviewed April 2016.

What Is Cervical Cancer?

Cancer that starts to grow on a woman's cervix is called "cervical cancer." Cancer can grow on a woman's cervix the same way it can grow on other body parts. Most times, cervical cancer forms slowly. Cervical cancer often does not cause symptoms until it is advanced. When cervical cancer is advanced, it may cause abnormal bleeding, discharge, or pain.

The cervix is the opening of your uterus (womb). It is part of a woman's reproductive system.

What Is HPV?

HPV is a common virus. There are about 40 types of HPV that can infect the genitals or sex organs of men and women. These HPV types can also infect the mouth and throat. HPV is so common that most people get it at some time in their lives. But HPV usually causes no symptoms so you can't tell that you have it.

Cervical Cancer Screening Tests

One important way to prevent cervical cancer is through regular screening with the Pap test. An HPV test can also be used at the same time as the Pap test for women 30 years and older. **Since cervical cancer often does not cause symptoms until it is advanced, it is important to get screened even when you feel healthy.**

274

The Pap and HPV tests can find early problems that could lead to cervical cancer over time. These tests do NOT:

- Check for early signs of other cancers

- Check your fertility (ability to get pregnant)

- Check for all HPV types –The HPV test only checks for specific HPV types that are linked to cervical cancer.

- Check for other sexually transmitted infections (STIs).

What Does My Pap Test Result Mean?

Your Pap test will come back as either "normal," "unclear," or "abnormal."

Normal

A normal result means that no cell changes were found on your cervix. This is good news. But you still need to get Pap tests in the future. New cell changes can still form on your cervix.

Unclear

It is common for test results to come back unclear. Your doctor may use other words to describe this result, like: equivocal, inconclusive, or ASC-US. These all mean the same thing: that your cervical cells look like they could be abnormal. It is not clear if it's related to HPV. It could be related to life changes like pregnancy, menopause, or an infection. The HPV test can help find out if your cell changes are related to HPV.

Abnormal

An abnormal result means that cell changes were found on your cervix. This usually does not mean that you have cervical cancer.

Abnormal changes on your cervix are likely caused by HPV. The changes may be minor (low-grade) or serious (high-grade). Most of the time, minor changes go back to normal on their own. But more serious changes can turn into cancer if they are not removed. The more serious changes are often called "precancer" because they are not yet cancer, but they can turn into cancer over time. It is important to make sure these changes do not get worse.

In rare cases, an abnormal Pap test can show that you may have cancer. You will need other tests to be sure. The earlier you find cervical cancer, the easier it is to treat.

If your Pap test results are unclear or abnormal, you will likely need more tests so your doctor can tell if your cell changes could be related to cancer.

Making Sense of Your Pap and HPV Test Results

If you have an HPV test at the same time as your Pap test, it can be confusing to get both results at the same time.

Your HPV test will come back as either "positive" or "negative":

- A negative HPV test means you do not have an HPV type that is linked to cervical cancer.

- A positive HPV test means you do have an HPV type that has been linked to cervical cancer. This does not mean you have cervical cancer now. But it could be a warning.

HPV test results are only meaningful WITH your Pap test results. To understand what these tests mean together:

- If your HPV test is negative (normal).
- If your HPV test is positive (abnormal).

If your HPV Test is Negative (normal), and your Pap test is...
Pap test is Normal

This means:

- Your cervical cells are normal.
- You do not have HPV.
- You have a very low chance of getting cervical cancer in the next few years.

You should:

- Wait three years before getting your next Pap and HPV test.
- Ask your doctor when to come in for your next visit.

Experts used to suggest yearly Pap tests. But now you can safely wait longer because having two tests gives you extra peace of mind.

Pap test is Unclear (ASC-US)

This means:

- You do not have HPV, but you may have cell changes on your cervix.

- Even if you do have cell changes, it is unlikely that they are caused by HPV (or related to cervical cancer).

You should:

- Get another Pap test in one year.

Pap test is Abnormal

This means:

- Your cervical cells are abnormal.
- You do not have HPV.

It's important to find out why the two tests are showing different things.

For minor cell changes, your doctor will:

- Take a closer look at your cervix to decide next steps.

For major cell changes, your doctor will:

- Take a closer look at your cervix and/or treat you right away.

If your HPV Test is Positive (abnormal), and your Pap test is...
Pap test is Normal

This means:

- Your cervical cells are normal, but you do have HPV.

You may fight off HPV naturally and never get cell changes. Or, you may not fight off HPV, and HPV could cause cell changes in the future.
It is believed that most women fight off HPV within two years. It is not known why some women fight off HPV and others do not.

You should:

- Get another Pap test and HPV test in one year.

Cell changes happen slowly. Some time must pass before your doctor can tell if HPV will go away or cause cell changes.

Pap Test Is Unclear (ASC-US)

This means:

- You have HPV, and you may have cell changes on your cervix.

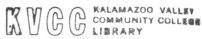

Your doctor will:

- Take a closer look at your cervix to find out if your cells are abnormal.

Your doctor may need to remove the abnormal cells or follow up with you over time to make sure the cells do not get worse.

Pap Test Is Abnormal

This means:

- You have HPV.

- Your cervical cells are abnormal.

This does not usually mean you have cancer.

For minor cell changes, your doctor will:

- Take a closer look at your cervix to decide next steps.

For major cell changes, your doctor will:

- Take a closer look at your cervix and/or treat you right away.

What Else Can I Do to Prevent Cervical Cancer?

- Keep your next doctor's appointment. Mark your calendar or post a note on your fridge, so you remember it.

- Go back for more testing or treatment if your doctor tells you to.

- Keep getting regular Pap tests—at least once every three years.

- Do not smoke. Smoking harms all of your body's cells, including your cervical cells. If you smoke and have HPV, you have higher chances of getting cervical cancer. If you smoke, ask your doctor for help quitting.

- If you are age 26 or younger, you can get vaccinated against HPV. HPV vaccines do not cure existing HPV or related problems (like abnormal cervical cells), but they can protect you from getting new HPV infections in the future.

Questions to Ask Your Doctor

- How do I know if I got an HPV test?

- When and how should I expect to get my test results?

- What do my test results mean?

- What other tests or treatment will I need if my Pap or HPV test is abnormal?

- When do I need to come back for more testing or treatment?

- What should I expect during and after these tests or treatments?

- Are there risks or side effects?

- Will the testing or treatment affect my chance to get or stay pregnant?

- Will the added tests or treatment be covered by my insurance?

- Where can I get help to cover the costs?

Be sure to ask your doctor about anything you don't understand.

How Do I Talk to My Partner about HPV?

You and your partner may benefit from talking openly about HPV. Here are some things to know before talking to your partner.

- HPV is very common. It can infect both men and women. Usually, HPV has no signs or symptoms, and the body fights it off naturally before it causes health problems.

- Most sexually active people get HPV at some time in their lives, though most will never know it. Even people with only one lifetime sex partner can get HPV, if their partner had it when the relationship started.

- HPV testing is not recommended for men, nor is it recommended for finding HPV on the genitals or in the mouth or throat. But the body usually fights off HPV naturally, before HPV causes health problems. So an HPV infection that is found today will most likely not be there a year or two from now.

- Partners who are age 26 or younger should consider HPV vaccination to protect against the types of HPV that most commonly cause health problems in men and women.

- The types of HPV found on a woman's HPV test can cause cervical cancer; they do not cause genital warts.

- Partners who have been together for a while tend to share HPV. This means that your partner likely has HPV already, even though your partner may have no signs or symptoms.

- Having HPV does not mean that you or your partner is having sex outside of your relationship. There is no sure way to know when you got HPV or who gave it to you. A person can have HPV for many years before it is found.

If your sex partner is female, you should talk to her about the link between HPV and cervical cancer, and encourage her to get a Pap test to screen for cervical cancer.

Common Questions about HPV

Is There a Treatment for HPV or Abnormal Cells?

There is no treatment for HPV (a virus). But there are treatments for abnormal cervical cells, which can be killed or removed. Treating abnormal cells will stop them from growing into cancer. But it may not remove the virus (HPV). That's why it's important to go back to your doctor as told, to make sure abnormal cells do not grow back. You may need to get Pap tests more often for a while. But most people do eventually fight the virus off.

Does Having HPV or Abnormal Cervical Cells Affect My Chances of Getting Pregnant or Having Healthy Babies?

Having HPV or cell changes on your cervix does not make it harder to get or stay pregnant. The type of HPV that is linked to cancer should not affect the health of your future babies. But if you need treatment for your cell changes, the treatment could affect your chance of having babies, in rare cases. If you need treatment, ask your doctor if the treatment can affect your ability to get pregnant or have a normal delivery.

Will I Pass HPV to My Current Partner?

If you have been with your partner for a while, your partner likely has HPV too. But your partner likely has no signs or symptoms of HPV. Partners usually share HPV, until your bodies fight it off naturally. There is no way to know if your partner gave you HPV, or if you gave HPV to your partner.

Can I Prevent Passing HPV to a New Partner?

Condoms may lower your chances of passing HPV to your new partner, if used with every sex act, from start to finish. But HPV can infect areas that are not covered by a condom—so condoms may not fully protect against HPV. If your partner is age 26 years or younger, vaccinations are available to prevent the types of HPV that most commonly cause health problems in men and women. But the only sure way to prevent passing HPV to a new partner is to not have sex.

Can My Male Partner Get Tested for HPV?

Right now, there is no HPV test for men. The approved HPV tests on the market are not useful for screening for HPV-related cancers or genital warts in men.

I Heard about an HPV Vaccine. Can It Help Me?

Three vaccines are available to prevent the HPV types that cause most cervical cancers as well as some cancers of the anus, vulva (area around the opening of the vagina), vagina, and oropharynx (back of throat including base of tongue and tonsils). Two of these vaccines also prevent HPV types that cause most genital warts. HPV vaccines are given in 3 shots over 6 months. They do not treat existing HPV, cervical cell changes, or genital warts. The vaccines are recommended at age 11 or 12 because they are most effective when given before a person's first sexual contact. But you can get vaccinated through age 26, if you did not get all three vaccine doses when you were younger. These vaccines may one day become available to women older than 26 years, if they are found to be safe and effective for them.

If I've Had a Hysterectomy, Do I Still Need to Get Screened for Cervical Cancer?

This depends on why you got your hysterectomy, and if you still have your cervix. If you got a total hysterectomy for reasons other than cancer, you may not need cervical cancer screening. Talk to your doctor to find out if you still need to get screened.

Free or Low-Cost Cervical Cancer Screening and Follow-Up Tests

You may be able to get cervical cancer screening and follow-up tests for free or at low cost if you:

- **have health insurance**. If you have questions about coverage, talk to your insurance company.

- **are eligible for Medicaid.** To learn more, call **1-800-MEDI-CARE (1-800-633-4227)** or visit Medicaid.gov.

- **are age 65 or older.** Medicare pays for the Pap test every 2 years, or every year for some women. To learn more about Medicare's Pap test coverage, call 1-800-MEDICARE (1-800- 633-4227). The call is free and you can speak to someone in English or Spanish.

- **have a low income or do not have health insurance.**

To find out if you can get free or low-cost tests and where to go, call or visit:

- **Your state or local health department**

  Find your state health department

- **CDC's National Breast and Cervical Cancer Early Detection Program**

  Find a Local Program

- **Federally Funded Health Centers**

  Find a local clinic

- **National Cancer Institute (NCI)**

  To find out where else you can get free or low-cost screening and follow-up care, call 1-800-4-CANCER (1-800-422-6237). 1-800-332-9615 (TTY).

- **Planned Parenthood**

  1-800-230-PLAN (1-800-230-7526)
  Find a local health center

- **National Family Planning and Reproductive Health Association**

Section 21.7

What You Should Know When You Are Diagnosed with Genital Warts

This section includes text excerpted from "Genital Warts-Women's Health Guide," U.S. Department of Veterans Affairs (VA), June 3, 2015.

Genital warts are caused by low-risk types of human papillomavirus (HPV). These viruses may not cause warts in everyone.

How Are They Spread?

Women can get genital warts from sexual contact with someone who has HPV. Genital warts are spread by skin-to-skin contact, usually from contact with the warts. It can be spread by vaginal, anal, oral, or hand-genital sexual contact. Genital warts will spread HPV while visible, and after recent treatment. Long-term sexual partners usually have the same type of wart-causing HPV.

What Are Signs of Genital Warts in Women?

Genital warts can grow anywhere in the genital area:

- In the vagina
- Around the vaginal opening
- On the cervix (the opening to the womb)
- On the groin
- In or around the anus
- In the mouth or throat (rare)

Genital warts:

- Can be any size—from so small they can't be seen, to big clusters and lumps
- Can be smooth with a "mosaic" pattern or bumpy like a cauliflower

- Are soft, moist and flesh-colored

- Can cause itching, burning or pain

Not all HPV infections cause genital warts. HPV infections often do not have any signs that you can see or feel.

Even if you can't see any genital warts, you could still have an HPV infection.

How Do You Know If You Have Genital Warts?

Genital warts can be detected by:

- Yourself

- A sexual partner

- A health care provider

The only way to confirm HPV infection is if your health care provider does an HPV test

How Is It Treated?

See your health care provider to discuss treatment. Even when genital warts are treated, the HPV infection may remain. Warts may also return after treatment. Over-the-counter treatments for other types of warts should not be used. Treatments for genital warts include:

- Watch and wait to see if the warts stay the same, get bigger, or go away

- Medicines applied directly to the warts. These can include prescribed creams.

- Burning off the warts

- Freezing off the warts

- Cutting the warts out

- Using special lights or lasers to destroy the warts.

What Can Happen If You Have Genital Warts for a Long Time?

The immune system fights HPV infection. The types of HPV that cause genital warts do not cause cancer. Without any treatment, genital warts may:

- Go away

- Remain unchanged
- Increase in size or number

If You Have Genital Warts

- Discuss treatment for genital warts with your health care provider.
- Know that it you may never know when you got HPV or who gave it to you.
- Know that partners that have been together for a while often share the same HPV types, even if both have no symptoms.
- Condoms may not fully protect against HPV since HPV can infect areas not covered by a condom.

How Can You Avoid Genital Warts?

- Get vaccinated against HPV.
  - Certain types of HPV vaccines protect against the low-risk HPV that causes 90% of genital warts.
  - HPV vaccine is safe for all females 9 to 26 years old.
  - The Centers for Disease Control and Prevention (CDC) recommends all 11–12 year old girls get the HPV vaccine.
- Avoid sexual contact.
- Have safer sex:
  - Reduce the number of sexual partners.
  - Condoms, when used correctly, can reduce the risk of getting HPV. But, condoms may not cover all infected areas. Each time you have sex use a condom (male or female type):
    - Before vaginal sex
    - Before anal sex
    - Before oral sex
  - Have sex with only one partner who does not have sex with others and does not have HPV.

- Know that other forms of birth control do not protect against HPV.

What about Pregnancy?

Genital warts rarely cause problems during pregnancy and birth. Most women who no longer have visible genital warts do not have problems with pregnancy or birth. If you are pregnant, you should discuss treatment options with your health care provider as the warts may:

- Grow larger and bleed

- Make it difficult to urinate if growing in the urinary tract (rare)

- Make the vagina less elastic during birth if the warts are in the vagina (rare)

- Cause a need for a cesarean section (C-section) birth if the warts block the birth canal (rare)

- Be passed to the baby during birth (rare)

Section 21.8

Prevention and Treatment for HPV

This section includes text excerpted from "Human Papillomavirus (HPV) Infection," Centers for Disease Control and Prevention (CDC), June 4, 2015.

Human Papillomavirus (HPV) Infection

Approximately 100 types of human papillomavirus infection (HPV) have been identified, at least 40 of which can infect the genital area. Most HPV infections are self-limited and are asymptomatic or unrecognized. Most sexually active persons become infected with HPV at least once in their lifetime. Oncogenic, high-risk HPV infection (e.g., HPV types 16 and 18) causes most cervical, penile, vulvar, vaginal, anal, and oropharyngeal cancers and precancers, whereas nononcogenic, low-risk HPV infection (e.g., HPV types 6 and 11) causes genital warts and recurrent respiratory papillomatosis. Persistent oncogenic HPV infection is the strongest risk factor for development of HPV-associated precancers and cancers. A substantial burden of cancers and anogenital warts are attributable to HPV in the United States: in 2009, an estimated 34,788 new HPV-associated cancers and approximately 355,000 new cases of anogenital warts were associated with HPV infection.

HPV Vaccines

There are several HPV vaccines licensed in the United States: a bivalent vaccine (Cervarix) that prevents infection with HPV types 16 and 18, a quadrivalent vaccine (Gardasil) that prevents infection with HPV types 6, 11, 16, and 18, and a 9-valent vaccine that prevents infection with HPV types 6, 11, 16, and 18, 31, 33, 45, 52, and 58. The bivalent and quadrivalent vaccines offer protection against HPV types 16 and 18, which account for 66% of all cervical cancers, and the 9-valent vaccine protects against five additional types accounting for 15% of cervical cancers. The quadrivalent HPV vaccine also protects against types 6 and 11, which cause 90% of genital warts.

All HPV vaccines are administered as a 3-dose series of IM injections over a 6-month period, with the second and third doses given 1–2 and 6 months after the first dose, respectively. The same vaccine product should be used for the entire 3-dose series. For girls, either vaccine is recommended routinely at ages 11–12 years and can be administered beginning at 9 years of age; girls and women aged 13–26 years who have not started or completed the vaccine series should receive the vaccine.

The quadrivalent or 9-valent HPV vaccine is recommended routinely for boys aged 11–12 years; boys can be vaccinated beginning at 9 years of age. Boys and men aged 13–21 years who have not started or completed the vaccine series should receive the vaccine. For previously unvaccinated, immunocompromised persons (including persons with HIV infection) and MSM, vaccination is recommended through age 26 years.

In the United States, the vaccines are not licensed or recommended for use in men or women aged >26 years. HPV vaccines are not recommended for use in pregnant women. HPV vaccines can be administered regardless of history of anogenital warts, abnormal Pap/HPV tests, or anogenital precancer. Women who have received HPV vaccine should continue routine cervical cancer screening if they are aged ≥21 years. HPV vaccine is available for eligible children and adolescents aged <19 years through the Vaccines for Children (VFC) program. For uninsured persons aged 19–26 years, patient assistance programs are available from the vaccine manufacturers. Prelicensure and postlicensure safety evaluations have found the vaccine to be well tolerated. Impact-monitoring studies in the United States have demonstrated reductions of genital warts, as well as the HPV types contained within the quadrivalent vaccine. Settings that provide STD services should either administer the vaccine to eligible clients who have not started or completed the vaccine series or refer these persons to another facility equipped to provide the vaccine. Clinicians providing services to children, adolescents, and young adults should be knowledgeable about HPV and HPV vaccine. HPV vaccination has not been associated with initiation of sexual activity or sexual risk behaviors or perceptions about sexually transmitted infections.

Abstaining from sexual activity is the most reliable method for preventing genital HPV infection. Persons can decrease their chances of infection by practicing consistent and correct condom use and limiting their number of sex partners. Although these interventions might not fully protect against HPV, they can decrease the chances of HPV acquisition and transmission.

Diagnostic Considerations

HPV tests are available to detect oncogenic types of HPV infection and are used in the context of cervical cancer screening and management or follow-up of abnormal cervical cytology or histology. These tests should not be used for male partners of women with HPV or women aged <25 years, for diagnosis of genital warts, or as a general STD test.

The application of 3%–5% acetic acid, which might cause affected areas to turn white, has been used by some providers to detect genital mucosa infected with HPV. The routine use of this procedure to detect mucosal changes attributed to HPV infection is not recommended because the results do not influence clinical management.

Prevention of HPV

Two HPV vaccines can prevent diseases and cancers caused by HPV. The Cervarix and Gardasil vaccines protect against most cases of cervical cancer; Gardasil also protects against most genital warts. HPV vaccines are recommended routinely for boys and girls aged 11–12 years; either vaccine is recommended for girls/women, whereas only one vaccine (Gardasil) is recommended for boys/men. These vaccines are safe and effective.

Condoms used consistently and correctly can lower the chances of acquiring and transmitting HPV and developing HPV-related diseases (e.g., genital warts and cervical cancer). However, because HPV can infect areas not covered by a condom, condoms might not fully protect against HPV.

Limiting number of sex partners can reduce the risk for HPV. However, even persons with only one lifetime sex partner can get HPV.

Abstaining from sexual activity is the most reliable method for preventing genital HPV infection.

Treatment

Treatment is directed to the macroscopic (e.g., genital warts) or pathologic precancerous lesions caused by HPV. Subclinical genital HPV infection typically clears spontaneously; therefore, specific antiviral therapy is not recommended to eradicate HPV infection. Precancerous lesions are detected through cervical cancer screening; HPV-related precancer should be managed based on existing guidance.

Counseling

Key Messages for Persons with HPV Infection

General

- Anogenital HPV infection is very common. It usually infects the anogenital area but can infect other areas including the mouth and throat. Most sexually active people get HPV at some time in their lives, although most never know it.

- Partners who have been together tend to share HPV, and it is not possible to determine which partner transmitted the original infection. Having HPV does not mean that a person or his/her partner is having sex outside the relationship.

- Most persons who acquire HPV clear the infection spontaneously and have no associated health problems. When the HPV infection does not clear, genital warts, precancers, and cancers of the cervix, anus, penis, vulva, vagina, head, and neck might develop.

- The types of HPV that cause genital warts are different from the types that can cause cancer.

- Many types of HPV are sexually transmitted through anogenital contact, mainly during vaginal and anal sex. HPV also might be transmitted during genital-to-genital contact without penetration and oral sex. In rare cases, a pregnant woman can transmit HPV to an infant during delivery.

- Having HPV does not make it harder for a woman to get pregnant or carry a pregnancy to term. However, some of the precancers or cancers that HPV can cause, and the treatments needed to treat them, might lower a woman's ability to get pregnant or have an uncomplicated delivery. Treatments are available for the conditions caused by HPV, but not for the virus itself.

- No HPV test can determine which HPV infection will clear and which will progress. However, in certain circumstances, HPV tests can determine whether a woman is at increased risk for cervical cancer. These tests are not for detecting other HPV-related problems, nor are they useful in women aged<25 years or men of any age.

Chapter 22

Lymphogranuloma Venereum

What Is Lymphogranuloma Venereum (LGV)?

Lymphogranuloma venereum (LGV) is caused by *C. trachomatis* serovars L1, L2, or L3. The most common clinical manifestation of LGV among heterosexuals is tender inguinal and/or femoral lymphadenopathy that is typically unilateral. A self-limited genital ulcer or papule sometimes occurs at the site of inoculation. However, by the time patients seek care, the lesions have often disappeared. Rectal exposure in women or MSM can result in proctocolitis mimicking inflammatory bowel disease, and clinical findings may include mucoid and/or hemorrhagic rectal discharge, anal pain, constipation, fever, and/or tenesmus.

Outbreaks of LGV protocolitis have been reported among MSM. LGV can be an invasive, systemic infection, and if it is not treated early, LGV proctocolitis can lead to chronic colorectal fistulas and strictures; reactive arthropathy has also been reported. However, reports indicate that rectal LGV can be asymptomatic. Persons with genital and colorectal LGV lesions can also develop secondary bacterial infection or can be coinfected with other sexually and nonsexually transmitted pathogens.

This chapter includes text excerpted from "Lymphogranuloma Venereum (LGV)," Centers for Disease Control and Prevention (CDC), June 4, 2015.

Diagnostic Considerations

Diagnosis is based on clinical suspicion, epidemiologic information, and the exclusion of other etiologies for proctocolitis, inguinal lymphadenopathy, or genital or rectal ulcers. Genital lesions, rectal specimens, and lymph node specimens (i.e., lesion swab or bubo aspirate) can be tested for *C. trachomatis* by culture, direct immunofluorescence, or nucleic acid detection. NAATs for *C. trachomatis* perform well on rectal specimens, but are not FDA-cleared for this purpose. Many laboratories have performed the CLIA validation studies needed to provide results from rectal specimens for clinical management. MSM presenting with protocolitis should be tested for chlamydia; NAAT performed on rectal specimens is the preferred approach to testing.

Additional molecular procedures (e.g., PCR-based genotyping) can be used to differentiate LGV from non-LGV *C. trachomatis* in rectal specimens. However, they are not widely available, and results are not available in a timeframe that would influence clinical management.

Chlamydia serology (complement fixation titers >1:64 or microimmunofluorescence titers >1:256) might support the diagnosis of LGV in the appropriate clinical context. Comparative data between types of serologic tests are lacking, and the diagnostic utility of these older serologic methods has not been established. Serologic test interpretation for LGV is not standardized, tests have not been validated for clinical proctitis presentations, and C. trachomatis serovar-specific serologic tests are not widely available.

Treatment

At the time of the initial visit (before diagnostic tests for chlamydia are available), persons with a clinical syndrome consistent with LGV, including proctocolitis or genital ulcer disease with lymphadenopathy, should be presumptively treated for LGV. As required by state law, these cases should be reported to the health department.

Treatment cures infection and prevents ongoing tissue damage, although tissue reaction to the infection can result in scarring. Buboes might require aspiration through intact skin or incision and drainage to prevent the formation of inguinal/femoral ulcerations.

Although clinical data are lacking, azithromycin 1 g orally once weekly for 3 weeks is probably effective based on its chlamydial antimicrobial activity. Fluoroquinolone-based treatments also might be effective, but the optimal duration of treatment has not been evaluated.

Other Management Considerations

Patients should be followed clinically until signs and symptoms have resolved. Persons who receive an LGV diagnosis should be tested for other STDs, especially HIV, gonorrhea, and syphilis. Those who test positive for another infection should be referred for or provided with appropriate care and treatment.

Follow-Up

Patients should be followed clinically until signs and symptoms resolve.

Special Considerations

Pregnancy

Pregnant and lactating women should be treated with erythromycin. Doxycycline should be avoided in the second and third trimester of pregnancy because of risk for discoloration of teeth and bones, but is compatible with breastfeeding. Azithromycin might prove useful for treatment of LGV in pregnancy, but no published data are available regarding an effective dose and duration of treatment.

HIV Infection

Persons with both LGV and HIV infection should receive the same regimens as those who are HIV negative. Prolonged therapy might be required, and delay in resolution of symptoms might occur.

Chapter 23

Syphilis

Chapter Contents

Section 23.1

What Is Syphilis?

This section includes text excerpted from "Syphilis—CDC Fact Sheet (Detailed)," Centers for Disease Control and Prevention (CDC), September 24, 2015.

Syphilis: The Great Imitator

Syphilis is a sexually transmitted disease (STD) caused by the bacterium Treponema pallidum. Syphilis can cause long-term complications if not adequately treated.

How Common Is Syphilis?

During 2014, there were 63,450 reported new cases of syphilis, compared to 47,352 estimated new diagnoses of HIV infection in 2013 and 350,062 cases of gonorrhea in 2014. Of syphilis cases, 19.999 were of primary and secondary (P and S) syphilis, the earliest and most transmissible stages of syphilis. During the 1990s, syphilis primarily occurred among heterosexual men and women of racial and ethnic minority groups; during the 2000s, however, cases increased among men who have sex with men (MSM). In 2014, MSM accounted for 83% of all P and S syphilis cases among males in which sex of sex partner was known.

Congenital syphilis (syphilis passed from pregnant women to their babies) continues to be a concern in the United States. During 2014, 458 cases of congenital syphilis were reported, compared to an estimated 107 cases of perinatal HIV infection during 2013. Congenital syphilis rates were 10.3 times and 3.3 times higher among infants born to black and Hispanic mothers (38.2 and 12.1 cases per 100,000 live births, respectively) compared to white mothers (3.7 cases per 100,000 live births).

How Do People Get Syphilis?

Syphilis is transmitted from person to person by direct contact with a syphilitic sore, known as a chancre. Chancres occur mainly on the external genitals, vagina, anus, or in the rectum. Chancres also can occur on the lips and in the mouth. Transmission of syphilis occurs during vaginal, anal, or oral sex. Pregnant women with the disease can transmit it to their unborn child.

How Quickly Do Symptoms Appear after Infection?

The average time between infection with syphilis and the start of the first symptom is 21 days, but can range from 10 to 90 days.

What Are the Signs and Symptoms in Adults?

Syphilis has been called "The Great Pretender", as its symptoms can look like many other diseases. However, syphilis typically follows a progression of stages that can last for weeks, months, or even years:

Primary Stage

The appearance of a single chancre marks the primary (first) stage of syphilis symptoms, but there may be multiple sores. The chancre is usually firm, round, and painless. It appears at the location where syphilis entered the body. These painless chancres can occur in locations that make them difficult to find (e.g., the vagina or anus). The chancre lasts 3 to 6 weeks and heals regardless of whether a person is treated or not. However, if the infected person does not receive adequate treatment, the infection progresses to the secondary stage.

Secondary Stage

Skin rashes and/or mucous membrane lesions (sores in the mouth, vagina, or anus) mark the second stage of symptoms. This stage typically starts with the development of a rash on one or more areas of the body. Rashes associated with secondary syphilis can appear when the primary chancre is healing or several weeks after the chancre has healed. The rash usually does not cause itching. The characteristic rash of secondary syphilis may appear as rough, red, or reddish brown spots both on the palms of the hands and the bottoms of the feet.

However, rashes with a different appearance may occur on other parts of the body, sometimes resembling rashes caused by other diseases. Sometimes rashes associated with secondary syphilis are so faint that they are not noticed. Large, raised, gray or white lesions, known as condyloma lata, may develop in warm, moist areas such as the mouth, underarm or groin region. In addition to rashes, symptoms of secondary syphilis may include fever, swollen lymph glands, sore throat, patchy hair loss, headaches, weight loss, muscle aches, and fatigue. The symptoms of secondary syphilis will go away with or without treatment, but without treatment, the infection will progress to the latent and possibly late stages of disease.

Latent and Late Stages

The latent (hidden) stage of syphilis begins when primary and secondary symptoms disappear. Without treatment, the infected person will continue to have syphilis infection in their body even though there are no signs or symptoms. Early latent syphilis is latent syphilis where infection occurred within the past 12 months. Late latent syphilis is latent syphilis where infection occurred more than 12 months ago. Latent syphilis can last for years.

The late stages of syphilis can develop in about 15% of people who have not been treated for syphilis, and can appear 10–20 years after infection was first acquired. In the late stages of syphilis, the disease may damage the internal organs, including the brain, nerves, eyes, heart, blood vessels, liver, bones, and joints. Symptoms of the late stage of syphilis include difficulty coordinating muscle movements, paralysis, numbness, gradual blindness, and dementia. This damage may be serious enough to cause death.

Neurosyphilis

Syphilis can invade the nervous system at any stage of infection, and causes a wide range of symptoms varying from no symptoms at all, to headache, altered behavior, and movement problems that look like other neurologic diseases, such as Parkinson's or Huntington's disease. This invasion of the nervous system is called "neurosyphilis."

Ocular syphilis, a clinical manifestation of neurosyphilis, can involve almost any eye structure, but posterior uveitis and panuveitis are the most common. Ocular syphilis may lead to decreased visual acuity including permanent blindness. Clinicians should be aware of ocular syphilis and screen for visual complaints in any patient at risk for syphilis (e.g., MSM, HIV-infected persons, others with risk factors and persons with multiple or anonymous partners).

HIV Infection and Syphilis Symptoms

Individuals who are HIV-positive can develop symptoms very different from the symptoms described above, including hypopigmented skin rashes. HIV can also increase the chances of developing syphilis with neurological involvement.

How Does Syphilis Affect a Pregnant Woman and Her Baby?

The syphilis bacterium can infect the baby of a woman during her pregnancy. All pregnant women should be tested for syphilis at the first prenatal visit. The syphilis screening test should be repeated during the third trimester (28 to 32 weeks gestation) and at delivery in women who are at high risk for syphilis, live in areas of high syphilis morbidity, are previously untested, or had a positive screening test in the first trimester.

Depending on how long a pregnant woman has been infected, she may have a high risk of having a stillbirth (a baby born dead) or of giving birth to a baby who dies shortly after birth; untreated syphilis in pregnant women results in infant death in up to 40 percent of cases. Any woman who delivers a stillborn infant after 20 week's gestation should also be tested for syphilis.

An infected baby born alive may not have any signs or symptoms of disease. However, if not treated immediately, the baby may develop serious problems within a few weeks. Untreated babies may become developmentally delayed, have seizures, or die. All babies born to mothers who test positive for syphilis during pregnancy should be screened for syphilis and examined thoroughly for evidence of congenital syphilis.

For pregnant women only penicillin therapy can be used to treat syphilis and prevent passing the disease to her baby; treatment with penicillin is extremely effective (success rate of 98%) in preventing mother-to-child transmission. Pregnant women who are allergic to penicillin should be referred to a specialist for desensitization to penicillin.

How Is Syphilis Diagnosed?

The definitive method for diagnosing syphilis is visualizing the spirochete via darkfield microscopy. This technique is rarely performed today because it is a technologically difficult method. Diagnoses are thus more commonly made using blood tests. There are two types of blood tests available for syphilis: nontreponemal tests and treponemal tests.

1. Nontreponemal tests (e.g., VDRL and RPR) are simple, inexpensive, and are often used for screening. However, they are not specific

for syphilis, can produce false-positive results, and, by themselves, are insufficient for diagnosis. VDRL and RPR should each have their antibody titer results reported quantitatively. Persons with a reactive nontreponemal test should receive a treponemal test to confirm a syphilis diagnosis. This sequence of testing (nontreponemal, then treponemal test) is considered the "classical" testing algorithm.

2. Treponemal tests (e.g., FTA-ABS, TP-PA, various EIAs, chemiluminescence immunoassays, immunoblots, and rapid treponemal assays) detect antibodies that are specific for syphilis. Treponemal antibodies appear earlier than nontreponemal antibodies and usually remain detectable for life, even after successful treatment. If a treponemal test is used for screening and the results are positive, a nontreponemal test with titer should be performed to confirm diagnosis and guide patient management decisions. Based on the results, further treponemal testing may be indicated. This sequence of testing (treponemal, then nontreponemal, test) is considered the "reverse" sequence testing algorithm. Reverse sequence testing can be more convenient for laboratories, but its clinical interpretation is problematic, as this testing sequence can identify individuals not previously described (e.g., treponemal test positive, nontreponemal test negative), making optimal management choices difficult.

Special Note: Because untreated syphilis in a pregnant woman can infect and possibly kill her developing baby, every pregnant woman should have a blood test for syphilis. All women should be screened at their first prenatal visit. For patients who belong to communities and populations with high prevalence of syphilis and for patients at high risk, blood tests should also be performed during the third trimester (at 28–32 weeks) and at delivery. All infants born to mothers who have reactive nontreponemal and treponemal test results should be evaluated for congenital syphilis. A quantitative nontreponemal test should be performed on infant serum and, if reactive, the infant should be examined thoroughly for evidence of congenital syphilis. Suspicious lesions, body fluids, or tissues (e.g., umbilical cord, placenta) should be examined by darkfield microscopy, PCR testing, and/or special stains. Other recommended evaluations may include analysis of cerebrospinal fluid by VDRL, cell count and protein, CBC with differential and platelet count, and long-bone radiographs.

What Is the Link between Syphilis and HIV?

Genital sores caused by syphilis make it easier to transmit and acquire HIV infection sexually. There is an estimated 2- to 5-fold increased risk of acquiring HIV if exposed to that infection when syphilis is present.

Ulcerative STDs that cause sores, ulcers, or breaks in the skin or mucous membranes, such as syphilis, disrupt barriers that provide protection against infections. The genital ulcers caused by syphilis can bleed easily, and when they come into contact with oral and rectal mucosa during sex, increase the infectiousness of and susceptibility to HIV. Studies have observed that infection with syphilis was associated with subsequent HIV infection among MSM.

Having other STDs can also indicate increased risk for becoming HIV infected.

What Is the Treatment for Syphilis?

There are no home remedies or over-the-counter drugs that will cure syphilis, but syphilis is easy to cure in its early stages. A single intramuscular injection of long acting Benzathine penicillin G (2.4 million units administered intramuscularly) will cure a person who has primary, secondary or early latent syphilis. Three doses of long acting Benzathine penicillin G (2.4 million units administered intramuscularly) at weekly intervals is recommended for individuals with late latent syphilis or latent syphilis of unknown duration. Treatment will kill the syphilis bacterium and prevent further damage, but it will not repair damage already done.

Selection of the appropriate penicillin preparation is important to properly treat and cure syphilis. Combinations of some penicillin preparations (e.g., Bicillin C-R, a combination of benzathine penicillin and procaine penicillin) are not appropriate treatments for syphilis, as these combinations provide inadequate doses of penicillin.

Although data to support the use of alternatives to penicillin is limited, options for non-pregnant patients who are allergic to penicillin may include doxycycline, tetracycline, and for neurosyphilis, potentially ceftriaxone. These therapies should be used only in conjunction with close clinical and laboratory follow-up to ensure appropriate serological response and cure.

Persons who receive syphilis treatment must abstain from sexual contact with new partners until the syphilis sores are completely healed. Persons with syphilis must notify their sex partners so that they also can be tested and receive treatment if necessary.

Who Should Be Tested for Syphilis?

Any person with signs or symptoms of primary infection, secondary infection, neurologic infection, or tertiary infection should be tested for syphilis.

Providers should routinely test persons who

- are pregnant;

- are members of an at-risk subpopulation (i.e., persons in correctional facilities and MSM);

- have HIV infection;

- are taking PrEP for HIV prevention;

- have partner(s) who have tested positive for syphilis;

- are sexually active and live in areas with high syphilis morbidity.

Will Syphilis Recur?

Syphilis does not recur. However, having syphilis once does not protect a person from becoming infected again. Even following successful treatment, people can be reinfected. Patients with signs or symptoms that persist or recur or who have a sustained fourfold increase in nontreponemal test titer probably failed treatment or were reinfected. These patients should be retreated.

Because chancres can be hidden in the vagina, rectum, or mouth, it may not be obvious that a sex partner has syphilis. Unless a person knows that their sex partners have been tested and treated, they may be at risk of being reinfected by an untreated partner.

How Can Syphilis Be Prevented?

Correct and consistent use of latex condoms can reduce the risk of syphilis only when the infected area or site of potential exposure is protected. However, a syphilis sore outside of the area covered by a latex condom can still allow transmission, so caution should be exercised even when using a condom.

The surest way to avoid transmission of sexually transmitted diseases, including syphilis, is to abstain from sexual contact or to be in a long-term mutually monogamous relationship with a partner who has been tested and is known to be uninfected.

Partner-based interventions include partner notification—a critical component in preventing the spread of syphilis. Sexual partners of infected patients should be considered at risk and provided treatment per the 2015 STD Treatment Guidelines.

Transmission of an STD, including syphilis, cannot be prevented by washing the genitals, urinating, and/or douching after sex. Any unusual discharge, sore, or rash, particularly in the groin area, should be a signal to refrain from having sex and to see a doctor immediately.

Section 23.2

Syphilis and MSM (Men Who Have Sex with Men)

This section includes text excerpted from "Syphilis and MSM (Men Who Have Sex With Men)—CDC Fact Sheet," Centers for Disease Control and Prevention (CDC), November 9, 2015.

Once nearly eliminated in the United States, syphilis is increasing, especially among gay, bisexual, and other men who have sex with men (MSM).

What Is Syphilis?

Syphilis is a sexually-transmitted disease (STD) caused by a specific type of bacteria. If not treated promptly and correctly syphilis can cause long-term complications. Symptoms of syphilis in adults arc divided into stages. The terms used for these stages are primary, secondary, latent, and late syphilis.

Should I Be Concerned about Syphilis?

Syphilis continues to increase among gay, bisexual, and other men who have sex with men. Recent outbreaks among MSM have been marked by high rates of HIV coinfection and high-risk sexual behaviors (such as sex without a condom, new or multiple partners, and substance abuse). Cases of ocular syphilis have also been reported among MSM. Ocular syphilis occurs when syphilis affects the eye and can lead to permanent blindness. While the health problems caused by syphilis in adults are serious, it is also known that the genital sores caused by syphilis in adults also make it easier to get and give HIV infection sexually.

How Could I Get Syphilis?

Any sexually-active person can get syphilis. Syphilis is passed from person to person through direct contact with a syphilis sore. In men, sores occur mainly on the external genitals, the anus, or in the rectum. Sores also can occur on the lips and in the mouth. As a gay or bisexual man, you should know that you can get infected with syphilis during anal or oral sex, as well as vaginal sex. Sometimes sores can occur in areas not covered by a condom, so you could still get syphilis from contact with these sores, even if you are wearing a condom. You cannot get syphilis through casual contact with objects such as toilet seats, doorknobs, swimming pools, hot tubs, bathtubs, shared clothing, or eating utensils.

What Does Syphilis Look Like?

Syphilis has been called 'the great imitator' because it has so many possible symptoms, many of which look like symptoms from other diseases. The painless syphilis sore that you would get after you are first infected can be confused for an ingrown hair, zipper cut, or other seemingly harmless bump. This is a symptom of the primary stage of syphilis. The non-itchy body rash that develops during the secondary stage of syphilis can show up on the palms of your hands and soles of your feet, all over your body, or in just a few places. You could also be infected with syphilis and have very mild symptoms, or no symptoms at all.

How Common Is Syphilis among MSM?

Between 2013 and 2014, the number of reported primary and secondary (P and S) cases increased by 15%. Most cases are among MSM. In 2014, 83% of the reported male P and S syphilis cases where sex of sex partner was known were among gay, bisexual, and other men who have sex with men.

How Can I Reduce My Risk of Getting Syphilis?

The only way to avoid getting syphilis or other STDs is to not have anal, oral, or vaginal sex.

If you are sexually active, doing the following things will lower your chances of getting syphilis:

Being in a long-term mutually monogamous relationship with a partner who has been tested and has negative STD test results.

Using latex condoms the right way every time you have sex. Condoms prevent the spread of syphilis by preventing contact with a sore. Sometimes sores can occur in areas not covered by a condom, so you could still get syphilis from contact with these sores, even if you are wearing a condom.

How Do I Know If I Have Syphilis?

The only way to know is by getting tested. Many men who are infected with syphilis do not have any symptoms for years, yet they remain at risk for health problems later on if they are not treated. Additionally, the painless sores that show up during the early stages of a syphilis infection often go unrecognized by the person who has them. Individuals who are unaware of their infection may be spreading it to their sex partners.

How Will My Doctor Know If I Have Syphilis?

Have an honest and open talk with your healthcare provider about your sexual history and ask whether you should be tested for syphilis or other STDs. Your doctor can do a blood test to determine if you have syphilis. Sometimes, healthcare providers will diagnose syphilis by testing fluid from a syphilis sore. If you are a man who has sex with men, has HIV infection, and/or has partner(s) who have tested positive for HIV, you should get tested regularly for syphilis.

What Is the Link between Syphilis and HIV?

In the United States, people who get syphilis often also have HIV, or are more likely to get HIV in the future. This is because having a sore or break in the skin from an STD such as syphilis may allow HIV to more easily enter your body. You may also be more likely to get HIV because the same behaviors and circumstances that put you at risk for getting other STDs can also put you at greater risk for getting HIV.

Can Syphilis Be Cured?

Yes, syphilis can be cured with the right medicine from your healthcare provider. However, treatment might not undo damage that the infection has already done.

I've Been Treated. Can I Get Syphilis Again?

Having syphilis once does not protect you from getting it again. Even after you've been successfully treated, you can still be reinfected. Only laboratory tests can confirm whether you have syphilis. Follow-up testing by your healthcare provider is recommended to make sure that your treatment was successful.

Because syphilis sores can be hidden in the vagina, anus, under the foreskin of the penis, or in the mouth, it may not be obvious that a sex partner has syphilis. Unless you know that all of your sex partner(s) have been tested and treated, you may be at risk of getting syphilis again from an untreated partner.

Section 23.3

Treatment of Syphilis

This section contains text excerpted from the following
sources: Text under the heading "Treatment," is excerpted
from "Syphilis," National Institute of Allergy and Infectious
Diseases (NIAID), October 27, 2014; Text under the heading
"Syphilis" is excerpted from "Syphilis," Centers for Disease
Control and Prevention (CDC), June 4, 2015.

Syphilis is easy to cure in its early stages. Penicillin, an antibiotic, injected into the muscle, is the best treatment for syphilis. If you are allergic to penicillin, your healthcare provider may give you another antibiotic to take by mouth.

If you have neurosyphilis, you may need to get daily doses of penicillin intravenously (in the vein) and you may need to be treated in the hospital.

If you have late syphilis, damage done to your body organs cannot be reversed.

While you are being treated, you should abstain from sex until any sores are completely healed. You should also notify your sex partners so they can be tested for syphilis and treated if necessary.

Syphilis

Syphilis is a systemic disease caused by Treponema pallidum. The disease has been divided into stages based on clinical findings, helping to guide treatment and follow-up. Persons who have syphilis might seek treatment for signs or symptoms of primary syphilis infection (i.e., ulcers or chancre at the infection site), secondary syphilis (i.e., manifestations that include, but are not limited to, skin rash, mucocutaneous lesions, and lymphadenopathy), or tertiary syphilis (i.e., cardiac, gummatous lesions, tabes dorsalis, and general paresis). Latent infections (i.e., those lacking clinical manifestations) are detected by serologic testing. Latent syphilis acquired within the preceding year is referred to as early latent syphilis; all other cases of latent syphilis are late latent syphilis or syphilis of unknown duration. *T. pallidum* can infect the central nervous system and result in neurosyphilis, which can occur at any stage of syphilis.

Early neurologic clinical manifestations (i.e., cranial nerve dysfunction, meningitis, stroke, acute altered mental status, and auditory or ophthalmic abnormalities) are usually present within the first few months or years of infection. Late neurologic manifestations (i.e., tabes dorsalis and general paresis) occur 10–30 years after infection.

Diagnostic Considerations

Darkfield examinations and tests to detect *T. pallidum* directly from lesion exudate or tissue are the definitive methods for diagnosing early syphilis. Although no *T. pallidum* detection tests are commercially available, some laboratories provide locally developed and validated PCR tests for the detection of *T. pallidum* DNA. A presumptive diagnosis of syphilis requires use of two tests: a nontreponemal test (i.e., Venereal Disease Research Laboratory [VDRL] or Rapid Plasma Reagin [RPR]) and a treponemal test (i.e., fluorescent treponemal antibody absorbed [FTA-ABS] tests, the *T. pallidum* passive particle agglutination [TP-PA] assay, various enzyme immunoassays [EIAs], chemiluminescence immunoassays, immunoblots, or rapid treponemal assays).

Although many treponemal-based tests are commercially available, only a few are approved for use in the United States. Use of only one type of serologic test is insufficient for diagnosis and can result in false-negative results in persons tested during primary syphilis and false-positive results in persons without syphilis. False-positive nontreponemal test results can be associated with various medical conditions and factors unrelated to syphilis, including other infections (e.g., HIV), autoimmune conditions, immunizations, pregnancy, injection-drug use, and older age. Therefore, persons with a reactive nontreponemal test should always receive a treponemal test to confirm the diagnosis of syphilis.

Nontreponemal test antibody titers might correlate with disease activity and are used to follow treatment response. Results should be reported quantitatively. A fourfold change in titer, equivalent to a change of two dilutions (e.g., from 1:16 to 1:4 or from 1:8 to 1:32), is considered necessary to demonstrate a clinically significant difference between two nontreponemal test results obtained using the same serologic test.

Sequential serologic tests in individual patients should be performed using the same testing method (VDRL or RPR), preferably by the same laboratory. The VDRL and RPR are equally valid assays, but quantitative results from the two tests cannot be compared directly because RPR titers frequently are slightly higher than VDRL titers. Nontreponemal test titers usually decline after treatment and might become nonreactive with time; however, in some persons, nontreponemal antibodies can persist for a long period of time, a response referred to as the "serofast reaction."

Most patients who have reactive treponemal tests will have reactive tests for the remainder of their lives, regardless of treatment or disease activity. However, 15%–25% of patients treated during the primary stage revert to being serologically nonreactive after 2–3 years. Treponemal antibody titers do not predict treatment response and therefore should not be used for this purpose.

Some clinical laboratories are screening samples using treponemal tests, typically by EIA or chemiluminescence immunoassays. This reverse screening algorithm for syphilis testing can identify persons previously treated for syphilis, those with untreated or incompletely treated syphilis, and persons with false-positive results that can occur with a low likelihood of infection.

Persons with a positive treponemal screening test should have a standard nontreponemal test with titer performed reflexively by the laboratory to guide patient management decisions. If the nontreponemal test is negative, the laboratory should perform a different treponemal test (preferably one based on different antigens than the original test) to confirm the results of the initial test. If a second treponemal test is positive, persons with a history of previous treatment will require no further management unless sexual history suggests likelihood of re-exposure. In this instance, a repeat nontreponemal test in 2–4 weeks is recommended to evaluate for early infection. Those without a history of treatment for syphilis should be offered treatment. Unless history or results of a physical examination suggest a recent infection, previously untreated persons should be treated for late latent syphilis. If the second treponemal test is negative and the epidemiologic risk and clinical probability for syphilis are low, further evaluation or treatment is not indicated.

Two studies demonstrate that high quantitative index values from treponemal EIA/CIA tests correlate with TPPA positivity; however, the range of optical density values varies among different treponemal immunoassays, and the clinical significance of these findings warrant further investigation.

For most persons with HIV infection, serologic tests are accurate and reliable for diagnosing syphilis and following a patient's response to treatment. However, atypical nontreponemal serologic test results (i.e., unusually high, unusually low, or fluctuating titers) might occur regardless of HIV-infection status. When serologic tests do not correspond with clinical findings suggestive of early syphilis, presumptive treatment is recommended for persons with risk factors for syphilis, and use of other tests (e.g., biopsy and PCR) should be considered.

Further testing is warranted for persons with clinical signs of neurosyphilis (e.g., cranial nerve dysfunction, auditory or ophthalmic abnormalities, meningitis, stroke, acute or chronic altered mental status, and loss of vibration sense). Laboratory testing is helpful in supporting the diagnosis of neurosyphilis; however, no single test can be used to diagnose neurosyphilis in all instances. The diagnosis of neurosyphilis depends on a combination of cerebrospinal fluid (CSF) tests (CSF cell count or protein and a reactive CSF-VDRL) in the presence of reactive serologic test results and neurologic signs and symptoms. CSF laboratory abnormalities are common in persons with early syphilis and are of unknown significance in the absence of neurologic signs or symptoms. CSF-VDRL is highly specific but insensitive.

In a person with neurologic signs or symptoms, a reactive CSF-VDRL (in the absence of blood contamination) is considered diagnostic of neurosyphilis. When CSF-VDRL is negative despite the presence of clinical signs of neurosyphilis, reactive serologic test results, and abnormal CSF cell count and/or protein, neurosyphilis should be considered. In this instance, additional evaluation using FTA-ABS testing on CSF may be warranted. The CSF FTA-ABS test is less specific for neurosyphilis than the CSF-VDRL but is highly sensitive. Neurosyphilis is highly unlikely with a negative CSF FTA-ABS test, especially among persons with nonspecific neurologic signs and symptoms.

Among persons with HIV infection, CSF leukocyte count usually is elevated (>5 white blood cell count [WBC]/mm3). Using a higher cutoff (>20 WBC/ mm3) might improve the specificity of neurosyphilis diagnosis.

Treatment

Penicillin G, administered parenterally, is the preferred drug for treating persons in all stages of syphilis. The preparation used (i.e., benzathine, aqueous procaine, or aqueous crystalline), dosage, and length of treatment depend on the stage and clinical manifestations of the disease. Treatment for late latent syphilis and tertiary syphilis require a longer duration of therapy, because organisms theoretically might be dividing more slowly (the validity of this rationale has not been assessed). Longer treatment duration is required for persons with latent syphilis of unknown duration to ensure that those who did not acquire syphilis within the preceding year are adequately treated.

Selection of the appropriate penicillin preparation is important, because *T. pallidum* can reside in sequestered sites (e.g., the CNS and aqueous humor) that are poorly accessed by some forms of penicillin. Combinations of benzathine penicillin, procaine penicillin, and oral penicillin preparations are not considered appropriate for the treatment of syphilis. Reports have indicated that practitioners have inadvertently prescribed combination benzathine-procaine penicillin (Bicillin C-R) instead of the standard benzathine penicillin product (Bicillin L-A) widely used in the United States. Practitioners, pharmacists, and purchasing agents should be aware of the similar names of these two products to avoid using the inappropriate combination therapy agent for treating syphilis.

The effectiveness of penicillin for the treatment of syphilis was well established through clinical experience even before the value of randomized controlled clinical trials was recognized. Therefore, nearly all recommendations for the treatment of syphilis are based not only on clinical trials and observational studies, but many decades of clinical experience.

Special Considerations

Pregnancy

Parenteral penicillin G is the only therapy with documented efficacy for syphilis during pregnancy. Pregnant women with syphilis in any stage who report penicillin allergy should be desensitized and treated with penicillin.

Jarisch-Herxheimer Reaction

The Jarisch-Herxheimer reaction is an acute febrile reaction frequently accompanied by headache, myalgia, fever, and other symptoms that can occur within the first 24 hours after the initiation of any therapy for syphilis. Patients should be informed about this possible adverse reaction and how to manage it if it occurs. The Jarisch-Herxheimer reaction occurs most frequently among persons who have early syphilis, presumably because bacterial burdens are higher during these stages. Antipyretics can be used to manage symptoms, but they have not been proven to prevent this reaction. The Jarisch-Herxheimer reaction might induce early labor or cause fetal distress in pregnant women, but this should not prevent or delay therapy.

Primary and Secondary Syphilis

Treatment

Parenteral penicillin G has been used effectively to achieve clinical resolution (i.e., the healing of lesions and prevention of sexual transmission) and to prevent late sequelae. However, no comparative trials have been conducted to guide the selection of an optimal penicillin regimen. Substantially fewer data are available for nonpenicillin regimens.

Available data demonstrate that use of additional doses of benzathine penicillin G, amoxicillin, or other antibiotics do not enhance efficacy when used to treat primary and secondary syphilis, regardless of HIV status.

Infants and children aged >1 month who receive a diagnosis of syphilis should have birth and maternal medical records reviewed to assess whether they have congenital or acquired syphilis. Infants and children aged ≥1 month with primary and secondary syphilis should be managed by a pediatric infectious-disease specialist and evaluated for sexual abuse (e.g., through consultation with child-protection services).

Other Management Considerations

All persons who have primary and secondary syphilis should be tested for HIV infection. In geographic areas in which the prevalence of HIV is high, persons who have primary or secondary syphilis should be retested for acute HIV in 3 months if the first HIV test result was negative.

Persons who have syphilis and symptoms or signs suggesting neurologic disease (e.g., cranial nerve dysfunction, meningitis, stroke, and hearing loss) or ophthalmic disease (e.g., uveitis, iritis, neuroretinitis, and optic neuritis) should have an evaluation that includes CSF analysis, ocular slit-lamp ophthalmologic examination, and otologic examination. Treatment should be guided by the results of this evaluation.

Invasion of CSF by *T. pallidum* accompanied by CSF laboratory abnormalities is common among adults who have primary or secondary syphilis. In the absence of clinical neurologic findings, no evidence supports variation from the recommended treatment regimen for primary and secondary syphilis. Symptomatic neurosyphilis develops in only a limited number of persons after treatment with the penicillin regimens recommended for primary and secondary syphilis. Therefore, unless clinical signs or symptoms of neurologic or ophthalmic involvement are present, routine CSF analysis is not recommended for persons who have primary or secondary syphilis.

Follow-Up

Clinical and serologic evaluation should be performed at 6 and 12 months after treatment; more frequent evaluation might be prudent if follow-up is uncertain or if repeat infection is a concern. Serologic response (i.e., titer) should be compared with the titer at the time of treatment. However, assessing serologic response to treatment can be difficult, and definitive criteria for cure or failure have not been well established. In addition, nontreponemal test titers might decline more slowly for persons previously treated for syphilis.

Persons who have signs or symptoms that persist or recur and those with at least a fourfold increase in nontreponemal test titer persisting for >2 weeks likely experienced treatment failure or were re-infected. These persons should be retreated and reevaluated for HIV infection. Because treatment failure usually cannot be reliably distinguished from reinfection with *T. pallidum*, a CSF analysis also should be performed; treatment should be guided by CSF findings.

Failure of nontreponemal test titers to decline fourfold within 6–12 months after therapy for primary or secondary syphilis might be indicative of treatment failure. However, clinical trial data have demonstrated that 15%–20% of persons with primary and secondary syphilis treated with the recommended therapy will not achieve the fourfold decline in nontreponemal titer used to define response at 1 year after treatment. Serologic response to treatment appears to be associated with several factors, including the person's stage of syphilis (earlier stages are more likely to decline fourfold and become negative) and initial nontreponemal antibody titers (lower titers are less likely to decline fourfold than higher titers).

Optimal management of persons who have less than a fourfold decline in titers after treatment of syphilis is unclear. At a minimum, these persons should receive additional clinical and serologic follow-up and be evaluated for HIV infection. If additional follow-up cannot be ensured, retreatment is recommended. Because treatment failure might be the result of unrecognized CNS infection, CSF examination can be considered in such situations.

For retreatment, weekly injections of benzathine penicillin G 2.4 million units IM for 3 weeks is recommended, unless CSF examination indicates that neurosyphilis is present. Serologic titers might not decline despite a negative CSF examination and a repeated course of therapy. In these circumstances, although the need for additional therapy or repeated CSF examinations is unclear, it is not generally recommended.

Chapter 24

Trichomoniasis

Chapter Contents

Section 24.1

What Is Trichomoniasis?

This section includes text excerpted from "Trichomoniasis,"
Office on Women's Health (OWH), March 25, 2014.

Trichomoniasis or "trich" is a sexually transmitted infection (STI) caused by a parasite. The parasite is spread most often through vaginal, oral, or anal sex. It is one of the most common STIs in the United States and affects more women than men. It is treated easily with antibiotics, but many women do not have symptoms. If left untreated, trichomoniasis can raise your risk of getting HIV.

What Is Trichomoniasis?

Trichomoniasis is an STI caused by a parasite. It is one of the most common STIs in the United States.

Who Gets Trichomoniasis?

Trichomoniasis is more common in women than men. It affects more than 2 million women ages 14 to 49 in the United States.

Trichomoniasis affects more African-American women than white and Hispanic women. The risk for African-American women goes up with age and lifetime number of sex partners.

How Do You Get Trichomoniasis?

Trichomoniasis is spread through:

- **Vaginal, oral, or anal sex.** Trichomoniasis can be spread even if there are no symptoms. This means you can get trichomoniasis from someone who has no signs or symptoms.

- **Genital touching.** A man does not need to ejaculate (come) for trichomoniasis to spread. Trichomoniasis can also be passed between women who have sex with women.

What Are the Signs and Symptoms of Trichomoniasis?

Most infected women have no signs or symptoms. If you do get signs or symptoms, they might appear five to 28 days after exposure and can include:

- Irritation and itching in the genital area
- Thin or frothy discharge with an unusual foul odor that can be clear, white, yellowish, or greenish
- Discomfort during sex and when urinating
- Lower abdominal pain (this is rare)

If you think you may have trichomoniasis, you and your sex partner(s) need to see a doctor or nurse as soon as possible.

How Is Trichomoniasis Diagnosed?

To find out whether you have trichomoniasis, your doctor or nurse may:

- Do a pelvic exam
- Use a cotton swab to take a fluid sample from your vagina to look for the parasite under a microscope
- Do a lab test, such as a DNA test or a fluid culture. A culture tests uses urine or a swab from your vagina. The parasite then grows in a lab. It takes up to a week for the parasite to grow enough to be seen.

  A Pap test is not used to detect trichomoniasis.
  If you have trichomoniasis, you need to be tested for other STIs too.

How Is Trichomoniasis Treated?

Trichomoniasis is easily cured with one of two antibiotics:

- Metronidazole
- Tinidazole

These antibiotics are usually a pill you swallow in a single dose.
If you are treated for trichomoniasis, your sex partner(s) needs to be treated too. Do not have sex until you and your sex partner(s) finish taking all of the antibiotics and have no symptoms.

What Can Happen If Trichomoniasis Is Not Treated?

Most people with trichomoniasis have no symptoms and never know they have it. Even without symptoms, it can be passed to others.

If you have trichomoniasis, you are at higher risk of getting HIV (the virus that causes AIDS) if you are exposed to HIV. If you are HIV-positive, having trichomoniasis also raises your risk of passing HIV to your sex partner(s). The Centers for Disease Control and Prevention recommends that women with HIV get screened for trichomoniasis at least once a year.

What Should I Do If I Have Trichomoniasis?

Trichomoniasis is easy to treat. But you need to be tested and treated as soon as possible.

If you have trichomoniasis:

- **See a doctor or nurse as soon as possible.** Antibiotics will treat trichomoniasis.

- **Take all of your medicine.** Even if symptoms go away, you need to finish all of the antibiotics.

- **Tell your sex partner(s)** so they can be tested and treated.

- **Avoid sexual contact until you and your partner(s) have been treated and cured.** Even after you finish your antibiotics, you can get trichomoniasis again if you have sex with someone who has trichomoniasis.

- **See your doctor or nurse again if you have symptoms that don't go away** within a few days after finishing the antibiotics.

How Does Trichomoniasis Affect Pregnancy?

Pregnant women with trichomoniasis are at higher risk of premature birth (babies born before 37 weeks of pregnancy) or a low-birth-weight baby (less than 5 1/2 pounds). Premature birth and a low birth weight raise the risk of health and developmental problems at birth and later in life.

The antibiotic metronidazole can be used to treat trichomoniasis during any stage of pregnancy. Talk to your doctor about the benefits and risks of taking any medicine during pregnancy.

Can I Take Medicine for Trichomoniasis If I Am Breastfeeding?

You can take the antibiotic metronidazole if you are breastfeeding. Your doctor may suggest waiting 12 to 24 hours after taking metronidazole before breastfeeding. Do not take tinidazole if you are breastfeeding.

How Can I Prevent Trichomoniasis?

The best way to prevent trichomoniasis or any STI is to not have vaginal, oral, or anal sex.

If you do have sex, lower your risk of getting an STI with the following steps:

- **Use condoms.** Condoms are the best way to prevent STIs when you have sex. Because a man does not need to ejaculate (come) to give or get trichomoniasis, make sure to put the condom on before the penis touches the vagina, mouth, or anus. Other methods of birth control, like birth control pills, shots, implants, or diaphragms, will not protect you from STIs.

- **Get tested.** Be sure you and your partner are tested for STIs. Talk to each other about the test results before you have sex.

- **Be monogamous.** Having sex with just one partner can lower your risk for STIs. After being tested for STIs, be faithful to each other. That means that you have sex only with each other and no one else.

- **Limit your number of sex partners.** Your risk of getting STIs goes up with the number of partners you have.

- **Do not douche.** Douching removes some of the normal bacteria in the vagina that protects you from infection. This may increase your risk of getting STIs.

- **Do not abuse alcohol or drugs.** Drinking too much alcohol or using drugs increases risky behavior and may put you at risk of sexual assault and possible exposure to STIs.

The steps work best when used together. No single step can protect you from every single type of STI.

Can Women Who Have Sex with Women Get Trichomoniasis?

Yes. It is possible to get trichomoniasis, or any other STI, if you are a woman who has sex only with women.

Talk to your partner about her sexual history before having sex, and ask your doctor about getting tested if you have signs or symptoms of trichomoniasis.

Section 24.2

Treatment of Trichomoniasis

This section includes text excerpted from "Trichomoniasis—2015 STD Treatment Guidelines," Centers for Disease Control and Prevention (CDC), June 4, 2015.

Trichomoniasis

Trichomoniasis is the most prevalent nonviral sexually transmitted infection in the United States, affecting an estimated 3.7 million persons. Health disparities persist in the epidemiology of *T. vaginalis* infection in the United States: 13% of black women are affected compared with 1.8% of non-Hispanic white women. *T. vaginalis* infection affects >11% of women aged ≥40 years, and particularly high prevalence has been detected among STD clinic patients (26% of symptomatic women and 6.5% asymptomatic women tested) and incarcerated persons (9%–32% of incarcerated women and 2%–9% of incarcerated men). The prevalence of trichomoniasis in MSM is low.

Some infected men have symptoms of urethritis, epididymitis, or prostatitis, and some infected women have vaginal discharge that might be diffuse, malodorous, or yellow-green with or without vulvar irritation. However, most infected persons (70%–85%) have minimal or no symptoms, and untreated infections might last for months to years. Although partners might be unaware of their infection, it is readily passed between sex partners during penile-vaginal sex. Among persons who are sexually active, the best way to prevent trichomoniasis is through consistent and correct use of condoms during all penile-vaginal sexual encounters. Partners of men who have been circumcised might have a somewhat reduced risk of *T. vaginalis* infection. Douching is not recommended because it might increase the risk for vaginal infections, including trichomoniasis.

T. vaginalis infection is associated with two- to threefold increased risk for HIV acquisition, preterm birth, and other adverse pregnancy outcomes among pregnant women. Among women with HIV infection, *T. vaginalis* infection is associated with increased risk for PID. Routine screening of asymptomatic women with HIV infection for T. vaginalis is recommended because of the adverse events associated with asymptomatic trichomoniasis and HIV infection.

Diagnostic testing for *T. vaginalis* should be performed in women seeking care for vaginal discharge. Screening might be considered for persons receiving care in high-prevalence settings (e.g., STD clinics and correctional facilities) and for asymptomatic persons at high risk for infection (e.g., persons with multiple sex partners, exchanging sex for payment, illicit drug use, or a history of STD). However, data are lacking on whether screening and treatment for asymptomatic trichomoniasis in high prevalence settings or persons at high risk can reduce any adverse health events and health disparities or reduce community burden of infection. Decisions about screening might be informed by local epidemiology of *T. vaginalis* infection.

Whether the rectum can be a reservoir for *T. vaginalis* infection is unclear; data are needed to clarify whether this occasional finding might reflect recent depositing contamination in up to 5% of persons reporting recent receptive anal sex. Further, the efficacy, benefit, and cost-effectiveness of rectal screening are unknown; therefore, rectal testing for *T. vaginalis* is not recommended. Similarly, oral testing for *T. vaginalis* is not recommended because of a lack of evidence for oral infections. *T. vaginalis* infection is not a nationally notifiable condition in the United States.

Diagnostic Considerations

The use of highly sensitive and specific tests is recommended for detecting *T. vaginalis*. Among women, NAAT is highly sensitive, often detecting three to five times more *T. vaginalis* infections than wet-mount microscopy, a method with poor sensitivity (51%–65%). The APTIMA *T. vaginalis* assay (Hologic Gen-Probe, San Diego, CA) is FDA-cleared for detection of *T. vaginalis* from vaginal, endocervical, or urine specimens from women. This assay detects RNA by transcription-mediated amplification with a clinical sensitivity of 95.3%–100% and specificity of 95.2%–100%. Among women, vaginal swab and urine have up to 100% concordance. As analyte-specific reagents, this assay can be used with urine or urethral swabs from men if validated per CLIA regulations.

The sale, distribution, and use of analyte-specific reagents are allowed under 21 C.F.R. 809.30 pertaining to in vitro diagnostic products for human use. For *T. vaginalis* diagnosis in men, the sensitivity of self-collected penile-meatal swabs was higher than that of urine in one study (80% and 39%, respectively). The BD Probe Tec TV Qx Amplified DNA Assay (Becton Dickinson, Franklin Lakes, New Jersey) is FDA-cleared for detection of *T. vaginalis* from endocervical, vaginal, or urine specimens from women. Although it might be feasible to perform these tests on the same specimen used for chlamydia and gonorrhea screening, the epidemiology of trichomoniasis is distinct and should not be overlooked in older adults.

Other FDA-cleared tests to detect *T. vaginalis* in vaginal secretions include the OSOM Trichomonas Rapid Test (Sekisui Diagnostics, Framingham, MA), an antigen-detection test using immunochromatographic capillary flow dipstick technology that can be performed at the point of care, and the Affirm VP III (Becton Dickinson, Sparks, MD), a DNA hybridization probe test that evaluates for *T. vaginalis*, G. vaginalis, and *Candida albicans*. The results of the OSOM Trichomonas Rapid Test are available in approximately 10 minutes, with sensitivity 82%–95% and specificity 97%–100%. Self-testing might become an option, as a study of 209 young women aged 14–22 years found that >99% could correctly perform and interpret her own self-test using the OSOM assay, with a high correlation with clinician interpretation (96% agreement). The results of the Affirm VP III are available within 45 minutes. Sensitivity and specificity are 63% and 99.9%, respectively, compared with culture and TMA; sensitivity might be higher among women who are symptomatic. Neither the OSOM nor the Affirm VP III test is FDA-cleared for use with specimens obtained from men.

Culture was considered the gold standard method for diagnosing *T. vaginalis* infection before molecular detection methods became available. Culture has a sensitivity of 75%–96% and a specificity of up to 100%. In women, vaginal secretions are the preferred specimen type for culture, as urine culture is less sensitive. In men, culture specimens require a urethral swab, urine sediment, and/or semen. To improve yield, multiple specimens from men can be used to inoculate a single culture.

The most common method for *T. vaginalis* diagnosis might be microscopic evaluation of wet preparations of genital secretions because of convenience and relatively low cost. Unfortunately, the sensitivity of wet mount is low (51%–65%) in vaginal specimens and lower in specimens from men (e.g., urethral specimens, urine sediment, and semen). Clinicians using wet mounts should attempt to evaluate slides immediately because sensitivity declines as evaluation is delayed, decreasing by up to 20% within 1 hour after collection. When highly sensitive (e.g., NAAT) testing on specimens is not feasible, a testing algorithm (e.g., wet mount first, followed by NAAT if negative) can improve diagnostic sensitivity in persons with an initial negative result by wet mount. Although *T. vaginalis* may be an incidental finding on a Pap test, neither conventional nor liquid-based Pap tests are considered diagnostic tests for trichomoniasis, because false negatives and false positives can occur.

Treatment

Treatment reduces symptoms and signs of *T. vaginalis* infection and might reduce transmission. Likelihood of adverse outcomes in women with HIV also is reduced with *T. vaginalis* therapy.

Alcohol consumption should be avoided during treatment with nitroimidazoles. To reduce the possibility of a disulfiram-like reaction, abstinence from alcohol use should continue for 24 hours after completion of metronidazole or 72 hours after completion of tinidazole.

The nitroimidazoles are the only class of antimicrobial medications known to be effective against *T. vaginalis* infections. Of these drugs, metronidazole and tinidazole have been cleared by FDA for the oral or parenteral treatment of trichomoniasis. Tinidazole is generally more expensive, reaches higher levels in serum and the genitourinary tract, has a longer half-life than metronidazole (12.5 hours versus 7.3 hours), and has fewer gastrointestinal side effects. In randomized clinical trials, recommended metronidazole regimens have resulted in cure rates of approximately 84%–98%, and the recommended tinidazole regimen has resulted in cure rates of approximately 92%–100%. Randomized controlled trials comparing single 2 g doses of metronidazole and tinidazole suggest that tinidazole is equivalent or superior to metronidazole in achieving parasitologic cure and resolution of symptoms.

Metronidazole gel does not reach therapeutic levels in the urethra and perivaginal glands. Because it is less efficacious than oral metronidazole, it is not recommended.

Other Management Considerations

Providers should advise persons infected with *T. vaginalis* to abstain from sex until they and their sex partners are treated (i.e., when therapy has been completed and any symptoms have resolved). Testing for other STDs including HIV should be performed in persons infected with T vaginalis.

Follow-Up

Because of the high rate of reinfection among women treated for trichomoniasis (17% within 3 months in one study), retesting for *T. vaginalis* is recommended for all sexually active women within 3 months following initial treatment regardless of whether they believe their sex partners were treated. Testing by nucleic acid amplification can be conducted as soon as 2 weeks after treatment. Data are insufficient to support retesting men.

Persistent or Recurrent Trichomoniasis

Persistent or recurrent infection caused by antimicrobial-resistant *T. vaginalis* or other causes should be distinguished from the possibility of reinfection from an untreated sex partner. Although most recurrent *T. vaginalis* infections are thought to result from reinfection, some infections might be attributed to antimicrobial resistance. Metronidazole resistance occurs in 4%–10% of cases of vaginal trichomoniasis, and tinidazole resistance in 1%.

In general, *T. vaginalis* isolates have lower minimum lethal concentrations to tinidazole than metronidazole. Emerging nitroimidazole-resistant trichomoniasis is concerning, because few alternatives to standard therapy exist. Single-dose therapy should be avoided for treating recurrent trichomoniasis that is not likely a result of reinfection. If treatment failure has occurred with metronidazole 2 g single dose and reinfection is excluded, the patient (and their partner[s]) can be treated with metronidazole 500 mg orally twice daily for 7 days. If this regimen fails, clinicians should consider treatment with metronidazole or tinidazole at 2 g orally for 7 days. If several 1-week regimens have failed in a person who is unlikely to have nonadherence or reinfection, testing of the organism for metronidazole and tinidazole susceptibility is recommended.

CDC has experience with susceptibility testing for nitroimidazole-resistant *T. vaginalis* and treatment management of infected persons and can provide assistance. Higher dose tinidazole at 2–3g for 14 days, often in combination with intravaginal tinidazole, can be considered in cases of nitroimidazole-resistant infections; however, such cases should be managed in consultation with an expert.

Alternative regimens might be effective but have not been systematically evaluated; therefore, consultation with an infectious-disease specialist is recommended. The most anecdotal experience has been with intravaginal paromomycin in combination with high-dose tinidazole; clinical improvement has been reported with other alternative regimens including intravaginal boric acid and nitazoxanide. The following topically applied agents have shown minimal success (<50%) and are not recommended: intravaginal betadine (povidone-iodine), clotrimazole, acetic acid, furazolidone, gentian violet, nonoxynol-9, and potassium permanganate. No other topical microbicide has been shown to be effective against trichomoniasis.

Special Considerations

Allergy, Intolerance, and Adverse Reactions

Metronidazole and tinidazole are both nitroimidazoles. Patients with an IgE mediated-type allergy to a nitroimidazole can be managed by metronidazole desensitization according to a published regimen and in consultation with a specialist.

Pregnancy

T. vaginalis infection in pregnant women is associated with adverse pregnancy outcomes, particularly premature rupture of membranes, preterm delivery, and delivery of a low birthweight infant. Although metronidazole treatment produces parasitologic cure, certain trials have shown no significant difference in perinatal morbidity following metronidazole treatment.

One trial suggested the possibility of increased preterm delivery in women with *T. vaginalis* infection who received metronidazole treatment, yet study limitations prevented definitive conclusions regarding the risks of treatment. More recent, larger studies have shown no positive or negative association between metronidazole use during pregnancy and adverse outcomes of pregnancy. If treatment is considered, the recommended regimen in pregnant women is metronidazole 2 g orally in a single dose. Symptomatic pregnant women, regardless of pregnancy stage, should be tested and considered for treatment.

Treatment of *T. vaginalis* infection can relieve symptoms of vaginal discharge in pregnant women and reduce sexual transmission to partners. Although perinatal transmission of trichomoniasis is uncommon, treatment also might prevent respiratory or genital infection of the newborn. Clinicians should counsel symptomatic pregnant women with trichomoniasis regarding the potential risks for and benefits of treatment and about the importance of partner treatment and condom use in the prevention of sexual transmission.

The benefit of routine screening for *T. vaginalis* in asymptomatic pregnant women has not been established. However, screening at the first prenatal visit and prompt treatment, as appropriate, are recommended for pregnant women with HIV infection, because *T. vaginalis* infection is a risk factor for vertical transmission of HIV. Pregnant women with HIV who are treated for *T. vaginalis* infection should be retested 3 months after treatment.

Although metronidazole crosses the placenta, data suggest that it poses a low risk to pregnant women. No evidence of teratogenicity or mutagenic effects in infants has been found in multiple cross-sectional and cohort studies of pregnant women. Women can be treated with 2 g metronidazole in a single dose at any stage of pregnancy.

Metronidazole is secreted in breast milk. With maternal oral therapy, breastfed infants receive metronidazole in doses that are lower than those used to treat infections in infants, although the active metabolite adds to the total infant exposure. Plasma levels of the drug and metabolite are measurable, but remain less than maternal plasma levels. Although several reported case series found no evidence of adverse effects in infants exposed to metronidazole in breast milk, some clinicians advise deferring breastfeeding for 12–24 hours following maternal treatment with a single 2-g dose of metronidazole. Maternal treatment with metronidazole (400 mg three times daily for 7 days) produced a lower concentration in breast milk and was considered compatible with breastfeeding over longer periods of time.

Data from studies involving human subjects are limited regarding use of tinidazole in pregnancy; however, animal data suggest this drug poses moderate risk. Thus, tinidazole should be avoided in pregnant women, and breastfeeding should be deferred for 72 hours following a single 2-g dose of tinidazole.

HIV Infection

Up to 53% of women with HIV infection also are infected with *T. vaginalis*. *T. vaginalis* infection in these women is significantly associated with PID, and treatment of trichomoniasis is associated with significant decreases in genital-tract HIV viral load and viral shedding. For these reasons, routine screening and prompt treatment are recommended for all women with HIV infection; screening should occur at entry to care and then at least annually thereafter. A randomized clinical trial involving women with HIV infection and *T. vaginalis* infection demonstrated that a single dose of metronidazole 2 g orally was less effective than 500 mg twice daily for 7 days. Thus, to improve cure rates, women with HIV infection who receive a diagnosis of *T. vaginalis* infection should be treated with metronidazole 500 mg orally twice daily for 7 days (rather than with a 2-g single dose of metronidazole). Factors that might interfere with standard single-dose treatment for trichomoniasis in these women include high rates of asymptomatic BV co-infections, use of antiretroviral therapy, changes in vaginal ecology, and impaired immunity.

Treatment

Treatment reduces symptoms and signs of *T. vaginalis* infection and might reduce transmission. Likelihood of adverse outcomes in women with HIV is also reduced with *T. vaginalis* therapy.

In women with HIV infection who receive a diagnosis of *T. vaginalis* infection, retesting is recommended within 3 months following initial treatment; NAAT is encouraged because of higher sensitivity of these tests. Data are insufficient to recommend routine screening, alternative treatment regimens of longer duration, or retesting in men. In women with HIV infection who receive a diagnosis of *T. vaginalis* infection, retesting is recommended within 3 months following initial treatment; NAAT is encouraged because of higher sensitivity of these tests. Data are insufficient to recommend routine screening, alternative treatment regimens of longer duration, or retesting in men.

Part Three

Complications That May Accompany STD Infection

Chapter 25

Infections and Syndromes That Develop after Sexual Contact

Chapter Contents

Section 25.1

Bacterial Vaginosis

This section includes text excerpted from "Bacterial Vaginosis,"
Office on Women's Health (OWH), November 19, 2014.

What Is Bacterial Vaginosis?

Bacterial vaginosis (BV) is an infection in the vagina. BV is caused by changes in the amount of certain types of bacteria in your vagina. BV is common, and any woman can get it. BV is easily treatable with medicine from your doctor or nurse. If left untreated, it can raise your risk for sexually transmitted infections (STIs) and cause problems during pregnancy. Bacterial vaginosis (BV) is an infection in the vagina. BV is caused by changes in the amount of certain types of bacteria in your vagina. BV is common, and any woman can get it. BV is easily treatable with medicine from your doctor or nurse. If left untreated, it can raise your risk for sexually transmitted infections (STIs) and cause problems during pregnancy.

Who Gets BV?

BV is the most common vaginal infection in women ages 15 to 44. But women of any age can get it, even if they have never had sex.
You may be more at risk for BV if you:

- Have a new sex partner

- Have multiple sex partners

- Douche

- Do not use condoms or dental dams

- Are pregnant. BV is common during pregnancy. About 1 in 4 pregnant women get BV. The risk for BV is higher for pregnant women because of the hormonal changes that happen during pregnancy.

- Are African-American. BV is twice as common in African-American women as in white women.

- Have an intrauterine device (IUD), especially if you also have irregular bleeding.

How Do You Get BV?

Researchers are still studying how women get BV. You can get BV without having sex, but BV can also be caused by vaginal, oral, or anal sex. You can get BV from male or female partners.

What Are the Signs and Symptoms of BV?

Many women have no signs or symptoms. If you do have signs or symptoms, they may include:

- Unusual vaginal discharge. The discharge can be white (milky) or gray. It may also be foamy or watery. Some women report a strong fish like odor, especially after sex.

- Burning when urinating

- Itching around the outside of the vagina

- Vaginal irritation

These symptoms may be similar to vaginal yeast infections and other health problems. Only your doctor or nurse can tell you for sure whether you have BV.

How Is BV Diagnosed?

There are tests to find out if you have BV. Your doctor or nurse takes a sample of vaginal discharge. Your doctor or nurse may then look at the sample under a microscope, use an in-office test, or send it to a lab to check for harmful bacteria. Your doctor or nurse may also see signs of BV during an exam.

Before you see a doctor or nurse for a test:

- Don't douche or use vaginal deodorant sprays. They might cover odors that can help your doctor diagnose BV. They can also irritate your vagina.

- Make an appointment for a day when you do not have your period.

How Is BV Treated?

BV is treated with antibiotics prescribed by your doctor.

If you get BV, your male sex partner won't need to be treated. But, BV can be spread to female partners. If your current partner is female, she needs to see her doctor. She may also need treatment.

It is also possible to get BV again.

BV and vaginal yeast infections are treated differently. BV is treated with antibiotics prescribed by your doctor. Yeast infections can be treated with over-the-counter medicines. But you cannot treat BV with over-the-counter yeast infection medicine.

What Can Happen If BV Is Not Treated?

If BV is untreated, possible problems may include:

- **Higher risk of getting STIs, including HIV.** Having BV can raise your risk of getting HIV, genital herpes, chlamydia, pelvic inflammatory disease, and gonorrhea. Women with HIV who get BV are also more likely to pass HIV to a male sexual partner.

- **Pregnancy problems.** BV can lead to premature birth or a low-birth-weight baby (smaller than 5 1/2 pounds at birth). All pregnant women with symptoms of BV should be tested and treated if they have it.

What Should I Do If I Have BV?

BV is easy to treat. If you think you have BV:

- **See a doctor or nurse.** Antibiotics will treat BV.

- **Take all of your medicine.** Even if symptoms go away, you need to finish all of the antibiotic.

- **Tell your sex partner(s) if she is female** so she can be treated.

- **Avoid sexual contact until you finish your treatment.**

- **See your doctor or nurse again if you have symptoms that don't go away** within a few days after finishing the antibiotic.

Is It Safe to Treat Pregnant Women Who Have BV?

Yes. The medicine used to treat BV is safe for pregnant women. All pregnant women with symptoms of BV should be tested and treated if they have it.

If you do have BV, you can be treated safely at any stage of your pregnancy. You will get the same antibiotic given to women who are not pregnant.

How Can I Lower My Risk of BV?

Steps you can take to lower your risk of BV include:

- **Help keep your vaginal bacteria balanced.** Use warm water only to clean the outside of your vagina. You do not need to use soap. Even mild soap can cause infection or irritate your vagina. Always wipe front to back from your vagina to your anus. Keep the area cool by wearing cotton or cotton-lined underpants.

- **Do not douche.** Douching removes some of the normal bacteria in the vagina that protect you from infection. This may raise your risk of BV. It may also make it easier to get BV again after treatment. Doctors do not recommend douching.

- **Practice safe sex.** The best way to prevent the spread of BV through sex is to not have vaginal, oral, or anal sex. If you do have sex, you can lower your risk of getting BV, and any STI, with the following steps. The steps work best when used together. No single step can protect you from BV or every single type of STI. Steps to lower your risk of BV or STIs include:

  - **Use condoms**. Condoms are the best way to prevent BV or STIs when you have sex. Make sure to put on the condom before the penis touches the vagina, mouth, or anus. Other methods of birth control, like birth control pills, shots, implants, or diaphragms, will not protect you from STIs.

  - **Get tested.** Be sure you and your partner are tested for STIs. Talk to each other about your test results before you have sex.

  - **Be monogamous.** Having sex with just one partner can lower your risk for BV or STIs. Be faithful to each other. That means that you only have sex with each other and no one else.

  - **Limit your number of sex partners.** Your risk of getting BV and STIs goes up with the number of partners you have.

  - **Don't abuse alcohol or drugs, which are linked to sexual risk-taking.** Drinking too much alcohol or using drugs also puts you at risk of sexual assault and possible exposure to STIs.

How Can I Protect Myself If My Female Partner Has BV?

If your partner has BV, you can lower your risk by using protection during sex.

- Use a dental dam every time you have sex. A dental dam is a thin piece of latex that is placed over the vagina before oral sex.

- Cover sex toys with condoms before use. Remove the condom and replace it with a new one before sharing the toy with your partner.

Section 25.2

Cytomegalovirus

This section includes text excerpted from "Help Children with Congenital CMV Live Healthy," Centers for Disease Control and Prevention (CDC), June 29, 2015.

CMV (Cytomegalovirus)

CMV is a virus that pregnant women can be infected with and pass to their unborn babies. This is called congenital CMV. About 1 in 150 children is born with congenital CMV infection. Most babies who get congenital CMV will not have signs or symptoms. However, about 20 out of 100 babies born with CMV infection will have symptoms or long-term health issues. These can include developmental disabilities, hearing and vision loss, problems with the liver, spleen or lungs, and seizures.

How CMV Spreads?

CMV is passed from infected people to others through direct contact with body fluids such as blood, urine, saliva, breast milk, or semen. Common ways people become infected with CMV differ by age group:

- Infants usually get infection from breast milk

- Children typically get infection through contact with other children

- Teenagers or adults mostly get infection through contact with saliva or urine of young children or through sexual contact.

Pregnant women can pass CMV to their unborn baby if they were infected before or during pregnancy. It is not known what factors lead to a woman with CMV giving birth to a baby with congenital CMV.

Early Treatment May Help

Babies who have symptoms from CMV when they are born have had moderate benefits for long-term hearing and brain development when they get antiviral medicine beginning in the first month of their lives. But this medicine has side effects, and babies who get it should be closely monitored by their doctor. Antiviral medicine has not been studied in babies with congenital CMV who do not show any symptoms, or only have hearing loss as a symptom.

Get Hearing Checks and Therapies

Symptoms of congenital CMV infection will be different for each child. The symptoms can range from mild to severe.

Parents can help children with congenital CMV infection live a healthy, full life by

- Having your child's hearing checked regularly.

- Hearing loss can affect your child's ability to develop communication, language, and social skills. The earlier your child's hearing loss is diagnosed, the sooner you can get them the services they need.

- Bringing your child to services such as speech, occupational, and physical therapy.

- Access to these services early in life will often help children with congenital CMV infection to develop to their full potential.

Signs of Congenital CMV

Babies may be diagnosed with congenital CMV while they are still in their mother's womb, or after they are born. Signs that a baby might have congenital CMV infection when they are born are:

- jaundice (yellowish coloring of the skin)

- enlarged liver

- enlarged spleen

- petechiae (skin rash resulting from bleeding in the skin)

- pneumonia

- central nervous system damage with small head size, brain abnormalities, eye problems or hearing loss

Blood, urine or saliva tests are done to confirm a diagnosis of congenital CMV. Some babies with congenital CMV infection are identified after they are diagnosed with hearing loss.

Talk with your doctor if you suspect your child might have congenital CMV infection.

Section 25.3

Fungal (Yeast) Infection

This section includes text excerpted from "Vaginal Yeast Infection,"
Office on Women's Health (OWH), December 4, 2014.

Vaginal Yeast Infection

Most women will get a vaginal yeast infection at some point in their life. Symptoms of vaginal yeast infections include burning, itching, and thick, white discharge. Yeast infections are easy to treat, but it is important to see your doctor or nurse if you think you have an infection. Yeast infection symptoms are similar to other vaginal infections and sexually transmitted infections (STIs). If you have a more serious infection, and not a yeast infection, it can lead to major health problems.

Who Gets Vaginal Yeast Infections?

Women and girls of all ages can get vaginal yeast infections. Three out of four women will have a yeast infection at some point in their life. Almost half of women have two or more infections.

Vaginal yeast infections are rare before puberty and after menopause.

Are Some Women More at Risk for Yeast Infections?

Yes. Your risk for yeast infections is higher if:

- You are pregnant
- You have diabetes and your blood sugar is not under control
- You use a type of hormonal birth control that has higher doses of estrogen
- You douche or use vaginal sprays
- You recently took antibiotics such as amoxicillin or steroid medicines
- You have a weakened immune system, such as from HIV

What Are the Signs and Symptoms of a Vaginal Yeast Infection?

The most common symptom of a vaginal yeast infection is extreme itchiness in and around the vagina.

Other signs and symptoms include:

- Burning, redness, and swelling of the vagina and the vulva
- Pain when urinating
- Pain during sex
- Soreness
- A thick, white vaginal discharge that looks like cottage cheese and does not have a bad smell

You may have only a few of these symptoms. They may be mild or severe.

What Causes Yeast Infections?

Yeast infections are caused by overgrowth of the microscopic fungus Candida.

Your vagina may have small amounts of yeast at any given time without causing any symptoms. But when too much yeast grows, you can get an infection.

Can I Get a Yeast Infection from Having Sex?

Yes. A yeast infection is not considered an STI, because you can get a yeast infection without having sex. But you can get a yeast infection from your sexual partner. Condoms and dental dams may help prevent getting or passing yeast infections through vaginal, oral, or anal sex.

Should I Call My Doctor or Nurse If I Think I Have a Yeast Infection?

Yes. Seeing your doctor or nurse is the only way to know for sure if you have a yeast infection and not a more serious type of infection.

The signs and symptoms of a yeast infection are a lot like symptoms of other more serious infections, such as STIs and bacterial vaginosis (BV). If left untreated, STIs and BV raise your risk of getting other STIs, including HIV, and can lead to problems getting pregnant. BV can also lead to problems during pregnancy, such as premature delivery.

How Is a Yeast Infection Diagnosed?

Your doctor will do a pelvic exam to look for swelling and discharge. Your doctor may also use a cotton swab to take a sample of the discharge from your vagina. A lab technician will look at the sample under a microscope to see whether there is an overgrowth of the fungus Candida that causes a yeast infection.

How Is a Yeast Infection Treated?

Yeast infections are usually treated with antifungal medicine. See your doctor or nurse to make sure that you have a vaginal yeast infection and not another type of infection.

You can then buy antifungal medicine for yeast infections at a store, without a prescription. Antifungal medicines come in the form of creams, tablets, ointments, or suppositories that you insert into your vagina. You can apply treatment in one dose or daily for up to seven days, depending on the brand you choose.

Your doctor or nurse can also give you a single dose of antifungal medicine taken by mouth, such as fluconazole. If you get more than four vaginal yeast infections a year, or if your yeast infection doesn't go away after using over-the-counter treatment, you may need to take regular doses of antifungal medicine for up to six months.

Is It Safe to Use Over-the-Counter Medicines for Yeast Infections?

Yes, but always talk with your doctor or nurse before treating yourself for a vaginal yeast infection. This is because:

- **You may be trying to treat an infection that is not a yeast infection.** Studies show that two out of three women who buy yeast infection medicine don't really have a yeast infection. Instead, they may have an STI or bacterial vaginosis (BV). STIs and BV require different treatments than yeast infections and, if left untreated, can cause serious health problems.

- **Using treatment when you do not actually have a yeast infection can cause your body to become resistant to the yeast infection medicine.** This can make actual yeast infections harder to treat in the future.

- **Some yeast infection medicine may weaken condoms and diaphragms, increasing your chance of getting pregnant or an STI when you have sex.** Talk to your doctor or nurse about what is best for you, and always read and follow the directions on the medicine carefully.

How Do I Treat a Yeast Infection If I'm Pregnant?

During pregnancy, it's safe to treat a yeast infection with vaginal creams or suppositories that contain miconazole or clotrimazole.

Do not take the oral fluconazole tablet to treat a yeast infection during pregnancy. It may cause birth defects.

Can I Get a Yeast Infection from Breastfeeding?

Yes. Yeast infections can happen on your nipples or in your breast (commonly called "thrush") from breastfeeding. Yeast thrive on milk and moisture. A yeast infection you get while breastfeeding is different from a vaginal yeast infection. However, it is caused by an overgrowth of the same fungus.

Symptoms of thrush during breastfeeding include:

- Sore nipples that last more than a few days, especially after several weeks of pain-free breastfeeding

- Flaky, shiny, itchy, or cracked nipples

- Deep pink and blistered nipples

- Achy breast

- Shooting pain in the breast during or after feedings

If you have any of these signs or symptoms or think your baby might have thrush in his or her mouth, call your doctor.

If I Have a Yeast Infection, Does My Sexual Partner Need to Be Treated?

Maybe. Yeast infections are not STIs. But it is possible to pass yeast infections to your partner during vaginal, oral, or anal sex.

- **If your partner is a man,** the risk of infection is low. About 15% of men get an itchy rash on the penis if they have unprotected sex with a woman who has a yeast infection. If this happens to your partner, he should see a doctor. Men who haven't been circumcised and men with diabetes are at higher risk.

- **If your partner is a woman,** she may be at risk. She should be tested and treated if she has any symptoms.

How Can I Prevent a Yeast Infection?

You can take steps to lower your risk of getting yeast infections:

- Do not douche. Douching removes some of the normal bacteria in the vagina that protects you from infection.

- Do not use scented feminine products, including bubble bath, sprays, pads, and tampons.

- Change tampons, pads, and panty liners often.

- Do not wear tight underwear, pantyhose, pants, or jeans. These can increase body heat and moisture in your genital area.

- Wear underwear with a cotton crotch. Cotton underwear helps keep you dry and doesn't hold in warmth and moisture.

- Change out of wet swimsuits and workout clothes as soon as you can.

- After using the bathroom, always wipe from front to back.

- Avoid hot tubs and very hot baths.

- If you have diabetes, be sure your blood sugar is under control.

Does Yogurt Prevent or Treat Yeast Infections?

Maybe. Studies suggest that eating eight ounces of yogurt with "live cultures" daily or taking Lactobacillus acidophilus capsules can help prevent infection.

But, more research still needs to be done to say for sure if yogurt with Lactobacillus or other probiotics can prevent or treat vaginal yeast infections. If you think you have a yeast infection, see your doctor or nurse to make sure before taking any over-the-counter medicine.

What Should I Do If I Get Repeat Yeast Infections?

If you get four or more yeast infections in a year, talk to your doctor or nurse.

About 5% of women get four or more vaginal yeast infections in one year. This is called recurrent vulvovaginal candidiasis (RVVC). RVVC is more common in women with diabetes or weak immune systems, such as with HIV, but it can also happen in otherwise healthy women.

Doctors most often treat RVVC with antifungal medicine for up to six months. Researchers also are studying the effects of a vaccine to help prevent RVVC.

Section 25.4

Molluscum Contagiosum

This section includes text excerpted from "Molluscum Contagiosum," Centers for Disease Control and Prevention (CDC), May 11, 2015.

Molluscum contagiosum is an infection caused by a poxvirus (molluscum contagiosum virus). The result of the infection is usually a benign, mild skin disease characterized by lesions (growths) that may appear anywhere on the body. Within 6–12 months, Molluscum contagiosum typically resolves without scarring but may take as long as 4 years.

The lesions, known as Mollusca, are small, raised, and usually white, pink, or flesh-colored with a dimple or pit in the center. They often have a pearly appearance. They're usually smooth and firm. In most people, the lesions range from about the size of a pinhead to as large as a pencil eraser (2 to 5 millimeters in diameter). They may become itchy, sore, red, and/or swollen.

Mollusca may occur anywhere on the body including the face, neck, arms, legs, abdomen, and genital area, alone or in groups. The lesions are rarely found on the palms of the hands or the soles of the feet.

Transmission

The virus that causes molluscum spreads from direct person-to-person physical contact and through contaminated fomites. Fomites are inanimate objects that can become contaminated with virus; in the instance of molluscum contagiosum this can include linens such as clothing and towels, bathing sponges, pool equipment, and toys. Although the virus might be spread by sharing swimming pools, baths, saunas, or other wet and warm environments, this has not been proven. Researchers who have investigated this idea think it is more likely the virus is spread by sharing towels and other items around a pool or sauna than through water.

Someone with molluscum can spread it to other parts of their body by touching or scratching a lesion and then touching their body somewhere else. This is called autoinoculation. Shaving and electrolysis can also spread mollusca to other parts of the body.

Molluscum can spread from one person to another by sexual contact. Many, but not all, cases of molluscum in adults are caused by sexual contact.

Conflicting reports make it unclear whether the disease may be spread by simple contact with seemingly intact lesions or if the breaking of a lesion and the subsequent transferring of core material is necessary to spread the virus.

The molluscum contagiosum virus remains in the top layer of skin (epidermis) and does not circulate throughout the body; therefore, it cannot spread through coughing or sneezing.

Since the virus lives only in the top layer of skin, once the lesions are gone the virus is gone and you cannot spread it to others. Molluscum contagiosum is not like herpes viruses, which can remain dormant ("sleeping") in your body for long periods and then reappear.

Risk Factors

Who Is at Risk for Infection?

Molluscum contagiosum is common enough that you should not be surprised if you see someone with it or if someone in your family becomes infected. Although not limited to children, it is most common in children 1 to 10 years of age.

People at increased risk for getting the disease include:

- People with weakened immune systems (i.e., HIV-infected persons or persons being treated for cancer) are at higher risk for getting molluscum contagiosum. Their growths may look different, be larger, and be more difficult to treat.

- Atopic dermatitis may also be a risk factor for getting molluscum contagiosum due to frequent breaks in the skin. People with this condition also may be more likely to spread molluscum contagiousm to other parts of their body for the same reason.

- People who live in warm, humid climates where living conditions are crowded.

In addition, there is evidence that molluscum infections have been on the rise in the United States since 1966, but these infections are not routinely monitored because they are seldom serious and routinely disappear without treatment.

Treatment Options

What Are the Treatment Options?

Because molluscum contagiosum is self-limited in healthy individuals, treatment may be unnecessary. Nonetheless, issues such as lesion visibility, underlying atopic disease, and the desire to prevent transmission may prompt therapy.

Treatment for molluscum is usually recommended if lesions are in the genital area (on or near the penis, vulva, vagina, or anus). If lesions are found in this area it is a good idea to visit your healthcare provider as there is a possibility that you may have another disease spread by sexual contact.

Be aware that some treatments available through the internet may not be effective and may even be harmful.

Physical removal

Physical removal of lesions may include cryotherapy (freezing the lesion with liquid nitrogen), curettage (the piercing of the core and scraping of caseous or cheesy material), and laser therapy. These options are rapid and require a trained health care provider, may require local anesthesia, and can result in post-procedural pain, irritation, and scarring.

It is not a good idea to try and remove lesions or the fluid inside of lesions yourself. By removing lesions or lesion fluid by yourself you may unintentionally autoinoculate other parts of the body or risk spreading it to others. By scratching or scraping the skin you could cause a bacterial infection.

Oral therapy

Gradual removal of lesions may be achieved by oral therapy. This technique is often desirable for pediatric patients because it is generally less painful and may be performed by parents at home in a less threatening environment. Oral cimetidine has been used as an alternative treatment for small children who are either afraid of the pain associated with cryotherapy, curettage, and laser therapy or because the possibility of scarring is to be avoided. While cimetidine is safe, painless, and well tolerated, facial mollusca do not respond as well as lesions elsewhere on the body.

Topical therapy

Podophyllotoxin cream (0.5%) is reliable as a home therapy for men but is not recommended for pregnant women because of presumed toxicity to the fetus. Each lesion must be treated individually as the therapeutic effect is localized. Other options for topical therapy include iodine and salicylic acid, potassium hydroxide, tretinoin, cantharidin (a blistering agent usually applied in an office setting), and imiquimod (T cell modifier). These treatments must be prescribed by a health care professional.

Therapy for immunocompromised persons

Most therapies are effective in immunocompetent patients; however, patients with HIV/AIDS or other immunosuppressing conditions often do not respond to traditional treatments. In addition, these treatments are largely ineffective in achieving long-term control in HIV patients.

Low CD4 cell counts have been linked to widespread facial mollusca and therefore have become a marker for severe HIV disease. Thus far, therapies targeted at boosting the immune system have proven the most effective therapy for molluscum contagiosum in immunocompromised persons. In extreme cases, intralesional interferon has been used to treat facial lesions in these patients. However, the severe and unpleasant side effects of interferon, such as influenza-like symptoms, site tenderness, depression, and lethargy, make it a less-than-desirable treatment. Furthermore, interferon therapy proved most effective in otherwise healthy persons. Radiation therapy is also of little benefit.

Prevention

How Can I Keep It from Spreading?

The best way to avoid getting molluscum is by following good hygiene habits. Remember that the virus lives only in the skin and once the lesions are gone, the virus is gone and you cannot spread the virus to others.

Wash Your Hands

There are ways to prevent the spread of molluscum contagiosum. The best way is to follow good hygiene (cleanliness) habits. Keeping your hands clean is the best way to avoid molluscum infection, as well as many other infections. Hand washing removes germs that may have been picked up from other people or from surfaces that have germs on them.

Don't Scratch or Pick at Molluscum Lesions

It is important not to touch, pick, or scratch skin that has lesions, that includes not only your own skin but anyone else's. Picking and scratching can spread the virus to other parts of the body and makes it easier to spread the disease to other people too.

Keep Molluscum Lesions Covered

It is important to keep the area with molluscum lesions clean and covered with clothing or a bandage so that others do not touch the lesions and become infected. Do remember to keep the affected skin clean and dry.

Any time there is no risk of others coming into contact with your skin, such as at night when you sleep, uncover the lesions to help keep your skin healthy.

Be Careful during Sports Activities

Do not share towels, clothing, or other personal items.

People with molluscum should not take part in contact sports like wrestling, basketball, and football unless all lesions can be covered by clothing or bandages.

Activities that use shared gear like helmets, baseball gloves and balls should also be avoided unless all lesions can be covered.

Swimming should also be avoided unless all lesions can be covered by watertight bandages. Personal items such as towels, goggles, and swim suits should not be shared. Other items and equipment such as kick boards and water toys should be used only when all lesions are covered by clothing or watertight bandages.

Other Ways to Avoid Sharing Your Infection

Do not shave or have electrolysis on areas with lesions.

Don't share personal items such as unwashed clothes, hair brushes, wrist watches, and bar soap with others.

If you have lesions on or near the penis, vulva, vagina, or anus, avoid sexual activities until you see a health care provider.

Long-Term Effects

What Are the Long-Term Effects?

Recovery from one molluscum infection does not prevent future infections. Molluscum contagiosum is not like herpes viruses which can remain dormant ("sleeping") in your body for long periods of time and then reappear. If you get new molluscum contagiosum lesions after you are cured, it means you have come in contact with an infected person or object again.

Complications

The lesions caused by molluscum are usually benign and resolve without scarring. However scratching at the lesion, or using scraping and scooping to remove the lesion, can cause scarring. For this reason, physically removing the lesion is not often recommended in otherwise healthy individuals.

The most common complication is a secondary infection caused by bacteria. Secondary infections may be a significant problem in immunocompromised patients, such as those with HIV/AIDS or those taking immunosuppressing drug therapies. In these cases, treatment to prevent further spread of the infection is recommended.

Section 25.5

Proctitis, Proctocolitis, and Enteritis: Sexually Transmitted Gastrointestinal Syndromes

This section includes text excerpted from "Proctitis, Proctocolitis, and Enteritis," Centers for Disease Control and Prevention (CDC), June 4, 2015.

Proctitis, Proctocolitis, and Enteritis

Sexually transmitted gastrointestinal syndromes include proctitis, proctocolitis, and enteritis. Evaluation for these syndromes should include appropriate diagnostic procedures (e.g., anoscopy or sigmoidoscopy, stool examination, and culture).

Proctitis is inflammation of the rectum (i.e., the distal 10–12 cm) that can be associated with anorectal pain, tenesmus, or rectal discharge. *N. gonorrhoeae, C. trachomatis* (including LGV serovars), T. pallidum, and HSV are the most common sexually transmitted pathogens involved. In persons with HIV infection, herpes proctitis can be especially severe. Proctitis occurs predominantly among persons who participate in receptive anal intercourse.

Proctocolitis is associated with symptoms of proctitis, diarrhea or abdominal cramps, and inflammation of the colonic mucosa extending to 12 cm above the anus. Fecal leukocytes might be detected on stool examination, depending on the pathogen. Pathogenic organisms include Campylobacter sp., Shigella sp., Entamoeba histolytica, and LGV serovars of *C. trachomatis*. CMV or other opportunistic agents can be involved in immunosuppressed HIV-infected patients. Proctocolitis can be acquired through receptive anal intercourse or by oral-anal contact, depending on the pathogen.

Enteritis usually results in diarrhea and abdominal cramping without signs of proctitis or proctocolitis; it occurs among persons whose sexual practices include oral-anal contact. In otherwise healthy persons, *Giardia lamblia* is most frequently implicated. When outbreaks of gastrointestinal illness occur among social or sexual networks of MSM, clinicians should consider sexual transmission as a mode of spread and provide counseling accordingly. Among persons with HIV infection, enteritis can be caused by pathogens that may not be sexually transmitted, including CMV, Mycobacterium avium–intracellulare, Salmonella sp., Campylobacter sp., Shigella sp., Cryptosporidium, Microsporidium, and Isospora. Multiple stool examinations might be necessary to detect Giardia, and special stool preparations are required to diagnose cryptosporidiosis and microsporidiosis. In addition, enteritis can be directly caused by HIV infection. Diagnostic and treatment recommendations for all enteric infections are beyond the scope of these guidelines.

Diagnostic Considerations for Acute Proctitis

Persons who present with symptoms of acute proctitis should be examined by anoscopy. A Gram-stained smear of any anorectal exudate from anoscopic or anal examination should be examined for polymorphonuclear leukocytes. All persons should be evaluated for HSV (by PCR or culture), *N. gonorrhoeae* (NAAT or culture), *C. trachomatis* (NAAT), and *T. pallidum* (Darkfield if available and serologic testing). If the *C. trachomatis* test is positive on a rectal swab, a molecular test PCR for LGV should be performed, if available, to confirm an LGV diagnosis.

Treatment for Acute Proctitis

Acute proctitis of recent onset among persons who have recently practiced receptive anal intercourse is usually sexually acquired. Presumptive therapy should be initiated while awaiting results of laboratory tests for persons with anorectal exudate detected on examination or polymorphonuclear leukocytes detected on a Gram-stained smear of anorectal exudate or secretions; such therapy also should be initiated when anoscopy or Gram stain is unavailable and the clinical presentation is consistent with acute proctitis in persons reporting receptive anal intercourse.

Bloody discharge, perianal ulcers, or mucosal ulcers among MSM with acute proctitis and either a positive rectal chlamydia NAAT or HIV infection should be offered presumptive treatment for LGV with doxycycline 100 mg twice daily orally for a total of 3 weeks. If painful perianal ulcers are present or mucosal ulcers are detected on anoscopy, presumptive therapy should also include a regimen for genital herpes.

Other Management Considerations

To minimize transmission and reinfection, men treated for acute proctitis should be instructed to abstain from sexual intercourse until they and their partner(s) have been adequately treated (i.e., until completion of a 7-day regimen and symptoms resolved). All persons with acute proctitis should be tested for HIV and syphilis.

Follow-Up

Follow-up should be based on specific etiology and severity of clinical symptoms. For proctitis associated with gonorrhea or chlamydia, retesting for the respective pathogen should be performed 3 months after treatment.

Management of Sex Partners

Partners who have had sexual contact with persons treated for GC, CT, or LGV within the 60 days before the onset of the persons symptoms should be evaluated, tested, and presumptively treated for the respective pathogen. Partners of persons with sexually transmitted enteric infections should be evaluated for any diseases diagnosed in the person with acute proctitis. Sex partners should abstain from sexual intercourse until they and their partner with acute proctitis are adequately treated.

Allergy, Intolerance, and Adverse Reactions

Allergic reactions with third-generation cephalosporins (e.g., ceftriaxone) are uncommon in persons with a history of penicillin allergy. In those persons with a history of an IgE mediated penicillin allergy (e.g., those who have had anaphylaxis, Stevens Johnson syndrome, or toxic epidermal necrolysis), the use of ceftriaxone is contraindicated.

HIV Infection

Persons with HIV infection and acute proctitis may present with bloody discharge, painful perianal ulcers, or mucosal ulcers. Presumptive treatment should include a regimen for genital herpes and LGV.

351

Section 25.6

Pubic Lice

This section includes text excerpted from "Parasites-Lice-
Pubic "Crab" Lice," Centers for Disease Control and
Prevention (CDC), September 24, 2013.

What Are Pubic Lice?

Also called crab lice or "crabs," pubic lice are parasitic insects found primarily in the pubic or genital area of humans. Pubic lice infestation is found worldwide and occurs in all races, ethnic groups, and levels of society.

What Do Pubic Lice Look Like?

Pubic lice have three forms: the egg (also called a nit), the nymph, and the adult.

Nit: Nits are lice eggs. They can be hard to see and are found firmly attached to the hair shaft. They are oval and usually yellow to white. Pubic lice nits take about 6–10 days to hatch.

Nymph: The nymph is an immature louse that hatches from the nit (egg). A nymph looks like an adult pubic louse but it is smaller. Pubic lice nymphs take about 2–3 weeks after hatching to mature into adults capable of reproducing. To live, a nymph must feed on blood.

Adult: The adult pubic louse resembles a miniature crab when viewed through a strong magnifying glass. Pubic lice have six legs; their two front legs are very large and look like the pincher claws of a crab. This is how they got the nickname "crabs." Pubic lice are tan to grayish-white in color. Females lay nits and are usually larger than males. To live, lice must feed on blood. If the louse falls off a person, it dies within 1–2 days.

What Are the Signs and Symptoms of Pubic Lice?

Signs and symptoms of pubic lice include

- Itching in the genital area
- Visible nits (lice eggs) or crawling lice

How Did I Get Pubic Lice?

Pubic lice usually are spread through sexual contact and are most common in adults. Pubic lice found on children may be a sign of sexual exposure or abuse. Occasionally, pubic lice may be spread by close personal contact or contact with articles such as clothing, bed linens, or towels that have been used by an infected person. A common misconception is that pubic lice are spread easily by sitting on a toilet seat. This would be extremely rare because lice cannot live long away from a warm human body and they do not have feet designed to hold onto or walk on smooth surfaces such as toilet seats.

Persons infested with pubic lice should be examined for the presence of other sexually transmitted diseases.

How Is a Pubic Lice Infestation Diagnosed?

A pubic lice infestation is diagnosed by finding a "crab" louse or egg (nit) on hair in the pubic region or, less commonly, elsewhere on the body (eyebrows, eyelashes, beard, mustache, armpit, perianal area, groin, trunk, scalp). Pubic lice may be difficult to find because there may be only a few. Pubic lice often attach themselves to more than one hair and generally do not crawl as quickly as head and body lice. If crawling lice are not seen, finding nits in the pubic area strongly suggests that a person is infested and should be treated. If you are unsure about infestation or if treatment is not successful, see a health care provider for a diagnosis. Persons infested with pubic lice should be investigated for the presence of other sexually transmitted diseases.

Although pubic lice and nits can be large enough to be seen with the naked eye, a magnifying lens may be necessary to find lice or eggs.

How Is a Pubic Lice Infestation Treated?

1. Wash the infested area; towel dry.

2. Carefully follow the instructions in the package or on the label. Thoroughly saturate the pubic hair and other infested

353

areas with lice medication. Leave medication on hair for the time recommended in the instructions. After waiting the recommended time, remove the medication by following carefully the instructions on the label or in the box.

3. Following treatment, most nits will still be attached to hair shafts. Nits may be removed with fingernails or by using a fine-toothed comb.

4. Put on clean underwear and clothing after treatment.

5. To kill any lice or nits remaining on clothing, towels, or bedding, machine-wash and machine-dry those items that the infested person used during the 2–3 days before treatment. Use hot water (at least 130°F) and the hot dryer cycle.

6. Items that cannot be laundered can be dry-cleaned or stored in a sealed plastic bag for 2 weeks.

7. All sex partners from within the previous month should be informed that they are at risk for infestation and should be treated.

8. Persons should avoid sexual contact with their sex partner(s) until both they and their partners have been successfully treated and reevaluated to rule out persistent infestation.

9. Repeat treatment in 9–10 days if live lice are still found.

10. Persons with pubic lice should be evaluated for other sexually transmitted diseases (STDs).

Section 25.7

Scabies

This section includes text excerpted from "Sexually
Transmitted Diseases Treatment Guidelines," Centers for
Disease Control and Prevention (CDC), June 5, 2015.

What Is Scabies?

The predominant symptom of scabies is pruritus. Sensitization to
Sarcoptes scabiei occurs before pruritus begins. The first time a person
is infested with *S. scabiei*, sensitization takes up to several weeks to
develop. However, pruritus might occur within 24 hours after a subsequent reinfestation. Scabies in adults frequently is sexually acquired,
although scabies in children usually is not.

Treatment

Permethrin is effective, safe, and less expensive than ivermectin.
One study demonstrated increased mortality among elderly, debilitated persons who received ivermectin, but this observation has not
been confirmed in subsequent reports. Ivermectin has limited ovicidal
activity and may not prevent recurrences of eggs at the time of treatment; therefore, a second dose of ivermectin should be administered 14
days after the first dose. Ivermectin should be taken with food because
bioavailability is increased, thereby increasing penetration of the drug
into the epidermis. Adjustments to ivermectin dosing are not required
in patients with renal impairment, but the safety of multiple doses in
patients with severe liver disease is not known.

Lindane is an alternative regimen because it can cause toxicity; it
should only be used if the patient cannot tolerate the recommended
therapies or if these therapies have failed. Lindane should not be
used immediately after a bath or shower, and it should not be used by
persons who have extensive dermatitis or children aged <10 years. Seizures have occurred when lindane was applied after a bath or used by
patients who had extensive dermatitis. Aplastic anemia after lindane
use also has been reported. Lindane resistance has been reported in
some areas of the world, including parts of the United States.

Other Management Considerations

Bedding and clothing should be decontaminated (i.e., either machine-washed, machine-dried using the hot cycle, or dry cleaned) or removed from body contact for at least 72 hours.

Fumigation of living areas is unnecessary. Persons with scabies should be advised to keep fingernails closely trimmed to reduce injury from excessive scratching.

Crusted Scabies

Crusted scabies (i.e., Norwegian scabies) is an aggressive infestation that usually occurs in immunodeficient, debilitated, or malnourished persons, including persons receiving systemic or potent topical glucocorticoids, organ transplant recipients, persons with HIV infection or human T-lymphotrophic virus-1-infection, and persons with hematologic malignancies.

Crusted scabies is transmitted more easily than scabies. No controlled therapeutic studies for crusted scabies have been conducted, and the appropriate treatment remains unclear. Substantial treatment failure might occur with a single-dose topical scabicide or with oral ivermectin treatment. Combination treatment is recommended with a topical scabicide, either 25% topical benzyl benzoate or 5% topical permethrin cream (full-body application to be repeated daily for 7 days then 2x weekly until discharge or cure), and treatment with oral ivermectin 200 ug/kg on days 1,2,8,9, and 15. Additional ivermectin treatment on days 22 and 29 might be required for severe cases. Lindane should be avoided because of the risks for neurotoxicity with heavy applications or denuded skin.

Follow-Up

The rash and pruritus of scabies might persist for up to 2 weeks after treatment. Symptoms or signs persisting for >2 weeks can be attributed to several factors. Treatment failure can occur as a result of resistance to medication or faulty application of topical scabicides. These medications do not easily penetrate into thick, scaly skin of persons with crusted scabies, perpetuating the harboring of mites in these difficultto-penetrate layers. In the absence of appropriate contact treatment and decontamination of bedding and clothing, persisting symptoms can be attributed to reinfection by family members or fomites. Finally, other household mites can cause symptoms to persist as a result of cross reactivity between antigens. Even when treatment is successful, reinfection is avoided, and cross reactivity does not occur, symptoms can persist or worsen as a result of allergic dermatitis. Retreatment 2 weeks after the initial treatment regimen can be considered for those persons who are still symptomatic or when live mites are observed. Use of an alternative regimen is recommended for those persons who do not respond initially to the recommended treatment.

Management of Sex Partners and Household Contacts

Persons who have had sexual, close personal, or household contact with the patient within the month preceding scabies infestation should be examined. Those found to be infested should be provided treatment.

Management of Outbreaks in Communities, Nursing Homes, and Other Institutional Settings

Scabies epidemics frequently occur in nursing homes, hospitals, residential facilities, and other communities. Control of an epidemic can only be achieved by treating the entire population at risk. Ivermectin can be considered in these settings, especially if treatment with topical scabicides fails. Epidemics should be managed in consultation with a specialist.

Special Considerations

Infants, Young Children, and Pregnant or Lactating Women

Infants and young children should be treated with permethrin; the safety of ivermectin in children who weigh <15 kg has not been determined. Infants and young children aged <10 years should not be treated with lindane. Ivermectin likely poses a low risk to pregnant women and is likely compatible with breastfeeding; however, because of limited data regarding its use in pregnant and lactating women, permethrin is the preferred treatment.

HIV Infection

Persons with HIV infection who have uncomplicated scabies should receive the same treatment regimens as those who are HIV negative. Persons with HIV infection and others who are immunosuppressed are at increased risk for crusted scabies. Such persons should be managed in consultation with a specialist.

Chapter 26

Cervicitis

What Is Cervicitis?

Cervicitis is an inflammation of the cervix characterized by purulent or mucopurulent endocervical exudate visible in the endocervical canal or on an endocervical swab specimen.

Two major diagnostic signs characterize cervicitis: 1) a purulent or mucopurulent endocervical exudate visible in the endocervical canal or on an endocervical swab specimen (commonly referred to as mucopurulent cervicitis) and 2) sustained endocervical bleeding easily induced by gentle passage of a cotton swab through the cervical os. Either or both signs might be present. Cervicitis frequently is asymptomatic, but some women complain of an abnormal vaginal discharge and intermenstrual vaginal bleeding (e.g., after sexual intercourse).

A finding of leukorrhea (>10 WBC per high-power field on microscopic examination of vaginal fluid) has been associated with chlamydial and gonococcal infection of the cervix. In the absence of the major diagnostic signs of inflammatory vaginitis, leukorrhea might be a sensitive indicator of cervical inflammation with a high negative predictive value (i.e., cervicitis is unlikely in the absence of leucorrhea). The criterion of using an increased number of WBCs on endocervical Gram stain in the diagnosis of cervicitis has not been standardized and therefore is not helpful. In addition, it has a low positive-predictive value (PPV) for infection with *C. trachomatis* and *N. gonorrhoeae* and

This chapter includes text excerpted from "Diseases Characterized by Urethritis and Cervicitis," Centers for Disease Control and Prevention (CDC), June 4, 2015.

is not available in most clinical settings. Finally, although the presence of gram negative intracellular diplococci on Gram stain of endocervical fluid may be specific for the diagnosis of gonococcal cervical infection when evaluated by an experienced laboratorian, it is not a sensitive indicator of infection.

Etiology

When an etiologic organism is isolated in the presence of cervicitis, it is typically *C. trachomatis* or *N. gonorrhoeae*. Cervicitis also can accompany trichomoniasis and genital herpes (especially primary HSV-2 infection). However, in most cases of cervicitis, no organism is isolated, especially in women at relatively low risk for recent acquisition of these STDs (e.g., women aged >30 years). Limited data indicate that infection with *M. genitalium* or BV and frequent douching might cause cervicitis. For reasons that are unclear, cervicitis can persist despite repeated courses of antimicrobial therapy. Because most persistent cases of cervicitis are not caused by recurrent or reinfection with *C. trachomatis* or *N. gonorrhoeae*, other factors (e.g., persistent abnormality of vaginal flora, douching [or exposure to other types of chemical irritants], or idiopathic inflammation in the zone of ectopy) might be involved.

Diagnostic Considerations

Because cervicitis might be a sign of upper-genital–tract infection (endometritis), women with a new episode of cervicitis should be assessed for signs of PID and should be tested for *C. trachomatis* and for *N. gonorrhoeae* with NAAT; such testing can be performed on either vaginal, cervical, or urine samples.

Women with cervicitis also should be evaluated for the presence of BV and trichomoniasis, and if these are detected, they should be treated. Because the sensitivity of microscopy to detect *T. vaginalis* is relatively low (approximately 50%), symptomatic women with cervicitis and negative microscopy for trichomonads should receive further testing (i.e., culture, NAAT or other FDA approved diagnostic test). A finding of >10 WBC per high power field in vaginal fluid, in the absence of trichomoniasis, might indicate endocervical inflammation caused specifically by *C. trachomatis* or *N. gonorrhoeae*. Although HSV-2 infection has been associated with cervicitis, the utility of specific testing (i.e., PCR, culture or serologic testing) for HSV-2 is unknown. FDA-cleared diagnostic tests for *M. genitalium* are not available.

Treatment

Several factors should affect the decision to provide presumptive therapy for cervicitis. Presumptive treatment with antimicrobials for *C. trachomatis* and *N. gonorrhoeae* should be provided for women at increased risk (e.g., those aged <25 years and those with a new sex partner, a sex partner with concurrent partners, or a sex partner who has a sexually transmitted infection), especially if follow-up cannot be ensured or if testing with NAAT is not possible. Trichomoniasis and BV should also be treated if detected. For women at lower risk of STDs, deferring treatment until results of diagnostic tests are available is an option. If treatment is deferred and NAATs for *C. trachomatis* and *N. gonorrhoeae* are negative, a follow-up visit to see if the cervicitis has resolved can be considered.

Other Considerations

To minimize transmission and reinfection, women treated for cervicitis should be instructed to abstain from sexual intercourse until they and their partner(s) have been adequately treated (i.e., for 7 days after single-dose therapy or until completion of a 7-day regimen) and symptoms have resolved. Women who receive a diagnosis of cervicitis should be tested for HIV and syphilis.

Follow-Up

Women receiving treatment should return to their provider for a follow-up visit, allowing the provider to determine whether cervicitis has resolved. For women who are not treated, a follow-up visit gives providers an opportunity to communicate results of tests obtained as part of the cervicitis evaluation. Additional follow-up should be conducted as recommended for the infections identified. Women with a specific diagnosis of chlamydia, gonorrhea, or trichomonas should be offered partner services and instructed to return in 3 months after treatment for repeat testing because of high rates of reinfection, regardless of whether their sex partners were treated. If symptoms persist or recur, women should be instructed to return for re-evaluation.

Management of Sex Partners

Management of sex partners of women treated for cervicitis should be appropriate for the specific STD identified or suspected. All sex partners in the past 60 days should be referred for evaluation, testing, and presumptive treatment if chlamydia, gonorrhea, or trichomoniasis was identified or suspected in the women with cervicitis. EPT or other effective partner referral strategies are alternative approaches to treating male partners of women who have chlamydia or gonococcal infection. To avoid reinfection, sex partners should abstain from sexual intercourse until they and their partner(s) are adequately treated.

Persistent or Recurrent Cervicitis

Women with persistent or recurrent cervicitis despite having been treated should be reevaluated for possible re-exposure or treatment failure to gonorrhea or chlamydia. If relapse and/or reinfection with a specific STD have been excluded, BV is not present, and sex partners have been evaluated and treated, management options for persistent cervicitis are undefined; in addition, the utility of repeated or prolonged administration of antibiotic therapy for persistent symptomatic cervicitis remains unknown.

The etiology of persistent cervicitis including the potential role of *M. genitalium* is unclear. *M. genitalium* might be considered for cases of clinically significant cervicitis that persist after azithromycin or doxycycline therapy in which re-exposure to an infected partner or medical nonadherence is unlikely. In settings with validated assays, women with persistent cervicitis could be tested for *M. genitalium* with the decision to treat with moxifloxacin based on results of diagnostic testing. In treated women with persistent symptoms that are clearly attributable to cervicitis, referral to a gynecologic specialist can be considered.

Special Considerations

HIV Infection

Women with cervicitis and HIV infection should receive the same treatment regimen as those who are HIV negative. Cervicitis increases cervical HIV shedding. Treatment of cervicitis in women with HIV infection reduces HIV shedding from the cervix and might reduce HIV transmission to susceptible sex partners.

Pregnancy

Diagnosis and treatment of cervicitis in pregnant women does not differ from that in women that are not pregnant.

Chapter 27

Congenital Syphilis

What Is Congenital Syphilis (CS)?

Congenital syphilis (CS) is a disease that occurs when a mother with syphilis passes the infection on to her baby during pregnancy.

How Can CS Affect My Baby?

CS can have major health impacts on your baby. How CS affects your baby's health depends on how long you had syphilis and if—or when—you got treatment for the infection.

CS can cause:

- Miscarriage (losing the baby during pregnancy),
- Stillbirth (a baby born dead), or
- Death shortly after birth.

Up to 40% of babies born to women with untreated syphilis may be stillborn, or die from the infection as a newborn.

Babies born with CS can have:

- Deformed bones,
- Severe anemia (low blood count),
- Enlarged liver and spleen,

This chapter includes text excerpted from "Congenital Syphilis—CDC Fact Sheet," Centers for Disease Control and Prevention (CDC), November 10, 2015.

- Jaundice (yellowing of the skin or eyes),
- Nerve problems, like blindness or deafness,
- Meningitis, and
- Skin rashes.

Do All Babies Born with CS Have Signs or Symptoms?

No. It is possible that a baby with CS won't have any symptoms at birth. But without treatment, the baby may develop serious problems. Usually, these health problems develop in the first few weeks after birth, but they can also happen years later.

Babies who do not get treatment for CS and develop symptoms later on can die from the infection. They may also be developmentally delayed or have seizures.

How Common Is CS?

After a steady decline from 2008–2012, data show a sharp increase in CS rates. In 2014, the number of CS cases was the highest it's been since 2001.

Public health professionals across the country are very concerned about the growing number of congenital syphilis cases in the United States. That's why it's so important to make sure you get tested for syphilis during your pregnancy.

I'm Pregnant. Do I Need to Get Tested for Syphilis?

Yes. All pregnant women should be tested for syphilis at the first prenatal visit (the first time you see your doctor for health care during pregnancy). If you don't get tested at your first visit, make sure to ask your doctor about getting tested during a future checkup.

Keep in mind that you can have syphilis and not know it. Symptoms of syphilis may be very mild, or be similar to signs of other health problems. The only way to know for sure if you have syphilis is to get tested.

Is There Treatment for Syphilis?

Yes. Doctors can treat pregnant women who have syphilis with antibiotics. If you test positive for syphilis during pregnancy, be sure to get treatment right away.

If you are diagnosed with and treated for syphilis, your doctor should do follow-up testing for at least one year to make sure that your treatment is working. Ask your doctor about the number of syphilis cases in your area to determine if you need to get tested again at the beginning of the third trimester, and again when your baby is born.

How Will My Doctor Know If My Baby Has CS?

Your doctor must consider several factors to determine if your baby has CS. These factors will include the results of your syphilis blood test and, if you were diagnosed with syphilis, whether you received treatment for syphilis during your pregnancy. Your doctor may also want to test your baby's blood, perform a physical exam of your baby, or do other tests, such as a spinal tap or an X-ray, to determine if your baby has CS.

My Baby Was Born with CS. Is There a Way to Treat the Infection?

Yes. There is treatment for CS. Babies who have CS need to be treated right away or they can develop serious health problems. Depending on the type of CS infection your baby has, it may receive antibiotics in a hospital for 10 days, or, in some cases, the infection can be cured with one injection of antibiotic.

It's also important that babies treated for CS get follow-up care to make sure that the treatment worked.

How Can I Reduce the Risk of My Baby Getting CS or Having Health Problems Associated with CS?

Your baby will not get CS if you do not have syphilis. There are two important things you can do to protect your baby from getting CS and the health problems associated with the infection:

- Get a syphilis test at your first prenatal visit.

- Reduce your risk of getting syphilis before and during your pregnancy.

Talk with your doctor about your risk for syphilis. Have an open and honest conversation about your sexual history and STD testing. Your doctor can give you the best advice on any testing and treatment that you may need.

Get a Syphilis Test at Your First Prenatal Visit

If you are pregnant, and infected with syphilis, you can still reduce your risk of CS complications in your unborn baby. Getting tested, and treated, for syphilis can prevent serious health complications that may otherwise result in infection to both mother and baby.

Prenatal care is essential to the overall health and wellness of you and your unborn child. The sooner you begin receiving medical care during pregnancy, the better the health outcomes will be for you and your unborn baby.

At your first prenatal visit, ask your doctor about getting tested for syphilis. It is important that you have an open and honest conversation with your doctor at this time. Discuss any new or unusual physical symptoms you may be experiencing, as well as any drugs you are using, and whether you have new or multiple sex partners. This information will allow your doctor to make the appropriate testing recommendations. Even if you have been tested for syphilis in the past, you should be tested again when you become pregnant.

If you test positive for syphilis, you will need to be treated right away. Do not wait for your next prenatal visit. It is also important that your sex partner(s) receive treatment. In addition, having syphilis once does not protect you from getting it again. Even after you've been successfully treated, you can still be reinfected. For this reason you must continue to take actions that will reduce your risk of getting a new infection.

Reduce Your Risk of Getting Syphilis Before and During Your Pregnancy

Preventing syphilis in women and their sex partners is the best way to prevent CS.

If you are sexually active, you can do the following things to lower your chances of getting syphilis:

- Get into a long-term mutually monogamous relationship with a partner who has been tested and has received negative syphilis test results.

- Using latex condoms the right way every time you have sex. Although condoms can prevent transmission of syphilis by preventing contact with a sore, you should know that sometimes syphilis sores occur in areas not covered by a condom, and contact with these sores can still transmit syphilis.

366

Also, talk with your doctor about your risk for syphilis. Have an open and honest conversation with your doctor about your sexual history and about STD testing. Your doctor can give you the best advice on any testing and treatment that you may need.

Remember that it's possible to be infected with syphilis and not know it, because sometimes the infection causes only very mild symptoms, or symptoms that mimic other illnesses.

Chapter 28

Epididymitis

What Is Epididymitis?

Epididymitis is swelling (inflammation) of the tube that connects the testicle with the vas deferens. The tube is called the epididymis.

Among sexually active men aged <35 years, acute epididymitis is most frequently caused by *C. trachomatis* or *N. gonorrhoeae*. Acute epididymitis caused by sexually transmitted enteric organisms (e.g., *Escherichia coli*) also occurs among men who are the insertive partner during anal intercourse. Sexually transmitted acute epididymitis usually is accompanied by urethritis, which frequently is asymptomatic. Other nonsexually transmitted infectious causes of acute epididymitis (e.g., Fournier's gangrene) are uncommon and should be managed in consultation with a urologist.

In men aged ≥35 years who do not report insertive anal intercourse, sexually transmitted acute epididymitis is less common. In this group, the epididymis usually becomes infected in the setting of bacteruria secondary to bladder outlet obstruction (e.g., benign prostatic hyperplasia). In older men, nonsexually transmitted acute epididymitis is also associated with prostate biopsy, urinary tract instrumentation or surgery, systemic disease, and/or immunosuppression.

Chronic epididymitis is characterized by a ≥6 week history of symptoms of discomfort and/or pain in the scrotum, testicle, or epididymis. Chronic infectious epididymitis is most frequently seen in conditions

---

This chapter includes text excerpted from "Epididymitis," Centers for Disease Control and Prevention (CDC), June 4, 2015.

associated with a granulomatous reaction; *Mycobacterium tuberculosis* (TB) is the most common granulomatous disease affecting the epididymis and should be suspected, especially in men with a known history of or recent exposure to TB. The differential diagnosis of chronic non-infectious epididymitis, sometimes termed "orchalgia/epididymalgia" is broad (i.e., trauma, cancer, autoimmune, and idiopathic conditions); men with this diagnosis should be referred to a urologist for clinical management.

Diagnostic Considerations

Men who have acute epididymitis typically have unilateral testicular pain and tenderness, hydrocele, and palpable swelling of the epididymis. Although inflammation and swelling usually begins in the tail of the epididymis, it can spread to involve the rest of the epididymis and testicle. The spermatic cord is usually tender and swollen. Spermatic cord (testicular) torsion, a surgical emergency, should be considered in all cases, but it occurs more frequently among adolescents and in men without evidence of inflammation or infection. In men with severe, unilateral pain with sudden onset, those whose test results do not support a diagnosis of urethritis or urinary-tract infection, or men in whom diagnosis of acute epididymitis is questionable, immediate referral to a urologist for evaluation of testicular torsion is important because testicular viability might be compromised.

Bilateral symptoms should raise suspicion of other causes of testicular pain. Radionuclide scanning of the scrotum is the most accurate method to diagnose epididymitis, but it is not routinely available. Ultrasound should be primarily used for ruling out torsion of the spermatic cord in cases of acute, unilateral, painful scrotum swelling. However, because partial spermatic cord torsion can mimic epididymitis on scrotal ultrasound, when torsion is not ruled out by ultrasound, differentiation between spermatic cord torsion and epididymitis must be made on the basis of clinical evaluation.

Although ultrasound can demonstrate epididymal hyperemia and swelling associated with epididymitis, it provides minimal utility for men with a clinical presentation consistent with epididymitis, because a negative ultrasound does not alter clinical management. Ultrasound should be reserved for men with scrotal pain who cannot receive an accurate diagnosis by history, physical examination, and objective laboratory findings or if torsion of the spermatic cord is suspected.

All suspected cases of acute epididymitis should be evaluated for objective evidence of inflammation by one of the following point-of-care tests.

- Gram or methylene blue or gentian violet (MB/GV) stain of urethral secretions demonstrating ≥2 WBC per oil immersion field (478). These stains are preferred point-of-care diagnostic tests for evaluating urethritis because they are highly sensitive and specific for documenting both urethral inflammation and the presence or absence of gonococcal infection. Gonococcal infection is established by documenting the presence of WBC-containing intracellular Gram-negative or purple diplococci on urethral Gram stain or MB/GV smear, respectively.

- Positive leukocyte esterase test on first-void urine.

- Microscopic examination of sediment from a spun first-void urine demonstrating ≥10 WBC per high power field.

All suspected cases of acute epididymitis should be tested for *C. trachomatis* and for *N. gonorrhoeae* by NAAT. Urine is the preferred specimen for NAAT testing in men. Urine cultures for chlamydia and gonococcal epididymitis are insensitive and are not recommended. Urine bacterial culture might have a higher yield in men with sexually transmitted enteric infections and in older men with acute epididymitis caused by genitourinary bacteruria.

Treatment

To prevent complications and transmission of sexually transmitted infections, presumptive therapy is indicated at the time of the visit before all laboratory test results are available. Selection of presumptive therapy is based on risk for chlamydia and gonorrhea and/or enteric organisms.

The goals of treatment of acute epididymitis are

1. microbiologic cure of infection,

2. improvement of signs and symptoms,

3. prevention of transmission of chlamydia and gonorrhea to others, and

4. a decrease in potential chlamydia/gonorrhea epididymitis complications (e.g., infertility and chronic pain).

Recommended Regimens

For acute epididymitis most likely caused by sexually transmitted chlamydia and gonorrhea

Ceftriaxone 250 mg IM in a single dose

PLUS

Doxycycline 100 mg orally twice a day for 10 days

For acute epididymitis most likely caused by sexually-transmitted chlamydia and gonorrhea and enteric organisms (men who practice insertive anal sex)

Ceftriaxone 250 mg IM in a single dose

PLUS

Levofloxacin 500 mg orally once a day for 10 days

OR

Ofloxacin 300 mg orally twice a day for 10 days

For acute epididymitis most likely caused by enteric organisms

Levofloxacin 500 mg orally once daily for 10 days

OR

Ofloxacin 300 mg orally twice a day for 10 days

Although most men with acute epididymitis can be treated on an outpatient basis, referral to a specialist and hospitalization should be considered when severe pain or fever suggests other diagnoses (e.g., torsion, testicular infarction, abscess, and necrotizing fasciitis) or when men are unable to comply with an antimicrobial regimen. Because high fever is uncommon and indicates a complicated infection, hospitalization for further evaluation is recommended.

Therapy including levofloxacin or ofloxacin should be considered if the infection is most likely caused by enteric organisms and gonorrhea has been ruled out by gram, MB, or GV stain. This includes men who have undergone prostate biopsy, vasectomy, and other urinary-tract instrumentation procedures. As an adjunct to therapy, bed rest, scrotal elevation, and nonsteroidal anti-inflammatory drugs are recommended until fever and local inflammation have subsided. Complete resolution of discomfort might not occur until a few weeks after completion of the antibiotic regimen.

Other Management Considerations

Men who have acute epididymitis confirmed or suspected to be caused by *N. gonorrhoeae* or *C. trachomatis* should be advised to abstain from sexual intercourse until they and their partners have been adequately treated and symptoms have resolved. All men with acute epididymitis should be tested for other STDs, including HIV.

Follow-Up

Men should be instructed to return to their health-care providers if their symptoms fail to improve within 72 hours of the initiation of treatment. Signs and symptoms of epididymitis that do not subside within 3 days require re-evaluation of the diagnosis and therapy. Men who experience swelling and tenderness that persist after completion of antimicrobial therapy should be evaluated for alternative diagnoses, including tumor, abscess, infarction, testicular cancer, tuberculosis, and fungal epididymitis.

Management of Sex Partners

Men who have acute sexually transmitted epididymitis confirmed or suspected to be caused by *N. gonorrhoeae* or *C. trachomatis* should be instructed to refer for evaluation, testing, and presumptive treatment all sex partners with whom they have had sexual contact within the 60 days preceding onset of symptoms If the last sexual intercourse was >60 days before onset of symptoms or diagnosis, the most recent sex partner should be treated.

Arrangements should be made to link female partners to care. EPT and enhanced referral are effective strategies for treating female sex partners of men who have chlamydia or gonorrhea for whom linkage to care is anticipated to be delayed. Partners should be instructed to abstain from sexual intercourse until they and their sex partners are adequately treated and symptoms have resolved.

Special Considerations

Allergy, Intolerance, and Adverse Reactions

The cross reactivity between penicillins and cephalosporins is <2.5% in persons with a history of penicillin allergy. The risk for penicillin cross-reactivity is highest with first-generation cephalosporins, but is negligible between most second-generation (cefoxitin) and all third-generation (ceftriaxone) cephalosporins. Alternative regimens have not been studied; therefore, clinicians should consult infectious-disease specialists if such regimens are required.

HIV Infection

Men with HIV infection who have uncomplicated acute epididymitis should receive the same treatment regimen as those who are HIV negative. Other etiologic agents have been implicated in acute epididymitis in men with HIV infection, including CMV, salmonella, toxoplasmosis, *Ureaplasma urealyticum*, *Corynebacterium* sp., *Mycoplasma* sp., and *Mima polymorpha*. Fungi and mycobacteria also are more likely to cause acute epididymitis in men with HIV infection than in those who are immunocompetent.

Chapter 29

Infertility Linked to STD Infection

Diseases and Conditions That Influence Fertility

Many different health issues can affect a woman's ability to get pregnant.

Endometriosis

Endometriosis occurs when the cells that normally line the uterine cavity, called endometrium, grow outside the uterus instead.

Research has found a link between infertility and endometriosis. Studies show that between 25% and 50% of infertile woman have endometriosis and between 30% and 40% of women with endometriosis are infertile. Scientists do not know the exact cause of infertility in women with endometriosis.

Some current theories on how endometriosis causes infertility include the following:

- Changes in the structure of the female reproductive organs may occur and affect the release of the egg after ovulation or interrupt the egg's movement through the fallopian tube.

This chapter includes text excerpted from "Diseases and Conditions That Influence Fertility," National Institute of Child Health and Human Development (NICHD), February 7, 2013.

- The lining of the abdomen, which is called the peritoneum, may go through changes that affect its function:

- In women with endometriosis, the amount of fluid inside the peritoneum often increases.

- The fluid in the peritoneum contains substances that can negatively affect the functions of the egg, sperm, and fallopian tubes.

- Chemical changes in the lining of the uterus that occur as a result of endometriosis may affect an embryo's ability to implant properly and make it difficult for a woman to stay pregnant after conception.

Polycystic Ovary Syndrome (PCOS)

PCOS is one of the most common causes of female infertility. It is a condition in which a woman's ovaries, and in some cases the adrenal glands, produce more androgens (a type of hormone) than normal. High levels of these hormones interfere with the development of ovarian follicles and release of eggs during ovulation. As a result, fluid-filled sacs, or cysts, can develop within the ovaries.

Researchers estimate that 5% to 10% of women in the United States have PCOS. The exact cause of PCOS is unknown, but current research suggests that a combination of genetic and environmental factors leads to the disease.

Primary Ovary Insufficiency (POI)

POI is a condition in which a woman's ovaries stop producing hormones and producing eggs at a young age. Women with POI do not ovulate regularly, or sometimes not at all, and may have abnormal levels of hormones due to problems with their ovaries.

Women with POI often have trouble getting pregnant. However, pregnancy is still possible. About 5% to 10% of women with POI get pregnant without medical treatment.

Uterine Fibroids

Uterine fibroids are noncancerous tumors that form inside the uterus. Uterine fibroids can cause symptoms in some cases, depending on their size and location. Scientists do not know what causes fibroids to form, but it is believed that there may be a genetic basis.

Fibroids can contribute to infertility and are found in 5% to 10% of infertile women. Fibroids located in the uterine cavity (as opposed to those that grow within the uterine wall) or those that are larger than centimeters in diameter are more likely to have a negative effect on fertility. Fibroids are more likely to affect a woman's fertility if they:

- Change the position of the cervix, which can reduce the number of sperm that enter the uterus
- Change the shape of the uterus, which can interfere with the movement of sperm or implantation
- Block the fallopian tubes, which prevents sperm from reaching the egg and keeps a fertilized egg from moving to the uterus
- Interfere with blood flow to the uterus, which can prevent the embryo from implanting.

General Causes of Infertility

General causes of infertility include:

- Failure to ovulate
- Structural problems of the reproductive system
- Infections
- Failure of an egg to mature properly
- Implantation failure
- Autoimmune disorders

Failure to Ovulate

The most common overall cause of infertility is the failure to ovulate, which occurs in 40% of women with infertility issues. Not ovulating can result from:

- POI
- PCOS
- Aging
- **Diminished ovarian reserve.** This refers to a low number of eggs remaining in a woman's ovaries due to normal aging. This situation may result in hormone levels that can affect ovulation.
- **Endocrine disorders.** These disorders affect the hormones produced by the body. Abnormal hormone levels can disrupt ovulation. Some endocrine disorders known to affect ovulation are:
- **Hypothalamic amenorrhea**, in which a structure in the brain called the hypothalamus produces abnormal levels of hormones

- **Hyperprolactinemia**, in which levels of the hormone prolactin are too high

- **Thyroid disease**, which affects the levels of hormones released by the thyroid, a gland in the neck

- **Adrenal disease**, which affects the levels of hormones released by the adrenal glands that sit on top of each kidney

- **Tobacco use.** Smoking or other use of tobacco can also affect ovulation and can cause complications with pregnancy.

Structural Problems of the Reproductive System

Structural problems usually involve the presence of abnormal tissue in the fallopian tubes or uterus.

If the fallopian tubes are blocked, eggs are not able to move from the ovaries to the uterus and sperm is not able to reach the egg for fertilization. Blockage of the fallopian tubes can be associated with:

- Endometriosis

- Uterine fibroids

- **Pelvic inflammatory disease**, an infection of the female reproductive structures that is often caused by bacteria resulting from a common sexually transmitted infection (STI), such as gonorrhea or chlamydia

- **Tubal ligation**, a surgical procedure that closes a woman's fallopian tubes permanently.

In addition, some women are born with blockages in their fallopian tubes.

Structural problems with the uterus that may lead to infertility include:

- **Uterine fibroids**, which are growths that appear within and around the wall of the uterus. Most women with fibroids do not have problems with fertility and can get pregnant. However, some women with fibroids may not be able to get pregnant naturally or may have multiple miscarriages or preterm labor.

- **Polyps**, which are noncancerous growths on the inside surface of the uterus. Polyps can interfere with the function of the uterus and make it difficult for a woman to remain pregnant after conception. Surgical removal of the polyps can increase the chances for a woman to get pregnant.

- Scarring in the uterus from previous injuries or surgery. Scarring may increase the risk of miscarriage and infertility.

- An unusually shaped uterus, which can affect a woman's ability to remain pregnant after conception.

Infections

Infections can also cause infertility. Chlamydia is one of the most common sexually transmitted infections that affect female fertility.

Chronic infections in the cervix can also reduce the amount or quality of cervical mucus, the sticky or slippery substance that collects on the cervix and in the vagina. Reduced amount or quality of cervical mucus can make it difficult for women to get pregnant.

Failure of an Egg to Mature Properly

For some women, the egg does not mature properly, resulting in fertilization failure. This can be caused by:

- Hormonal problems, ranging from PCOS to problems with the hypothalamus or the pituitary gland. The hypothalamus sends signals from the brain to the pituitary gland, which then produces the hormones necessary to start the process of egg maturation. Any problems during this process can prevent the egg from maturing properly.

- Lack of proteins called cyclin-dependent kinases. New studies suggest this protein may be involved in the process of egg maturation.

- Injury to the ovaries. Scarred ovaries from multiple surgeries or repeated ovarian cysts can prevent the egg from maturing.

- POI

Implantation Failure

Implantation failure is a common cause of infertility among couples trying to conceive with assisted reproductive techniques (ART). Causes of implantation failure include:

- Genetic defects

- Thin endometrium

- Embryonic defects, such as problems with male or female or sperm defects

- Endometriosis

Autoimmune Disorders

Autoimmune disorders cause the body's immune system to attack normal body tissues it would normally ignore. Autoimmune disorders, such as lupus or rheumatoid arthritis, may cause a woman's immune system to reject the egg and prevent it from implanting or cut off the blood supply to an implanted embryo. Autoimmune disorders may also attack sperm or the reproductive organs.

Chapter 30

Neurosyphilis

What Is Neurosyphilis?

Neurosyphilis is a disease of the coverings of the brain, the brain itself, or the spinal cord. It can occur in people with syphilis, especially if they are left untreated. Neurosyphilis is different from syphilis because it affects the nervous system, while syphilis is a sexually transmitted disease with different signs and symptoms. There are five types of neurosyphilis:

1. asymptomatic neurosyphilis

2. meningeal neurosyphilis

3. meningovascular neurosyphilis

4. general paresis

5. tabes dorsalis

Asymptomatic neurosyphilis means that neurosyphilis is present, but the individual reports no symptoms and does not feel sick. *Meningeal syphilis* can occur between the first few weeks to the first few years of getting syphilis. Individuals with meningeal syphilis can have headache, stiff neck, nausea, and vomiting. Sometimes there can also be loss of vision or hearing. *Meningovascular syphilis* causes the same symptoms as meningeal syphilis but affected individuals also have strokes. This

This chapter includes text excerpted from "NINDS Neurosyphilis Information Page," National Institute of Neurological Disorders and Stroke (NINDS), October 29, 2009. Reviewed April 2016.

form of neurosyphilis can occur within the first few months to several years after infection. General paresis can occur between 3–30 years after getting syphilis. People with general paresis can have personality or mood changes. *Tabes dorsalis* is characterized by pains in the limbs or abdomen, failure of muscle coordination, and bladder disturbances. Other signs include vision loss, loss of reflexes and loss of sense of vibration, poor gait, and impaired balance. *Tabes dorsalis* can occur anywhere from 5–50 years after initial syphilis infection. General paresis and *tabes dorsalis* are now less common than the other forms of neurosyphilis because of advances made in prevention, screening, and treatment. People with HIV/AIDS are at higher risk of having neurosyphilis.

Is There Any Treatment?

Penicillin, an antibiotic, is used to treat syphilis. Individuals with neurosyphilis can be treated with penicillin given by vein, or by daily intramuscular injections for 10–14 days. If they are treated with daily penicillin injections, individuals must also take probenecid by mouth four times a day.

Some medical professionals recommend another antibiotic called ceftriaxone for neurosyphilis treatment. This drug is usually given daily by vein, but it can also be given by intramuscular injection. Individuals who receive ceftriaxone are also treated for 10–14 days. People with HIV/AIDS who get treated for neurosyphilis may have different outcomes than individuals without HIV/AIDS.

What Is the Prognosis?

Prognosis can change based on the type of neurosyphilis and how early in the course of the disease people with neurosyphilis get diagnosed and treated. Individuals with asymptomatic neurosyphilis or meningeal neurosyphilis usually return to normal health. People with meningovascular syphilis, general paresis, or *tabes dorsalis* usually do not return to normal health, although they may get much better. Individuals who receive treatment many years after they have been infected have a worse prognosis. Treatment outcome is different for every person.

What Research Is Being Done?

The National Institute of Neurological Disorders and Stroke (NINDS) supports and conducts research on neurodegenerative disorders, such as neurosyphilis, in an effort to find ways to prevent, treat, and ultimately cure these disorders.

Chapter 31

Pelvic Inflammatory Disease

What Is Pelvic Inflammatory Disease?

Pelvic inflammatory disease (PID) is a clinical syndrome that results from the ascension of microorganisms from the cervix and vagina to the upper genital tract. PID can lead to infertility and permanent damage of a woman's reproductive organs.

How Do Women Get Pelvic Inflammatory Disease?

Women develop PID when certain bacteria, such as chlamydia or gonorrhea, move upward from a woman's vagina or cervix into her reproductive organs. PID is a serious complication of some sexually transmitted diseases (STDs), especially chlamydia and gonorrhea.

What Causes Pelvic Inflammatory Disease?

A number of different microorganisms can cause or contribute to PID. The sexually transmitted pathogens *Chlamydia trachomatis* (CT) and *Neisseria gonorrhoeae* (NG) have been implicated in a third to a half of PID cases. However, endogenous microorganisms, including gram positive and negative anaerobic organisms and aerobic/

This chapter includes text excerpted from "Pelvic Inflammatory Disease (PID)—CDC Fact Sheet," Centers for Disease Control and Prevention (CDC), January 24, 2014.

facultative gram positive and negative rods and cocci, found at high levels in women with bacterial vaginosis, also have been implicated in the pathogenesis of PID. Newer data suggest that *Mycoplasm genitalium* may also play a role in PID and may be associated with milder symptoms although one study failed to demonstrate a significant increase in PID following detection of *M. genitalium* in the lower genital tract. Because of the polymicrobial nature of PID, broad-spectrum regimens that provide adequate coverage of likely pathogens are recommended.

What Are the Signs and Symptoms of Pelvic Inflammatory Disease?

Women with PID present with a variety of clinical signs and symptoms that range from subtle and mild to severe. PID can go unrecognized by women and their health care providers when the symptoms are mild. Despite lack of symptoms, histologic evidence of endometritis has been demonstrated in women with subclinical PID. When present, signs and symptoms of PID are nonspecific, so other reproductive tract illnesses and diseases of both the urinary and the gastrointestinal tracts should be considered when evaluating a sexually active woman with lower abdominal pain. Pregnancy (including ectopic pregnancy) must also be excluded, as PID can occur concurrently with pregnancy.

When symptoms are present, the most common symptoms of PID are

- Lower abdominal pain
- Mild pelvic pain
- Increased vaginal discharge
- Irregular menstrual bleeding
- Fever (>38°C)
- Pain with intercourse
- Painful and frequent urination
- Abdominal tenderness
- Pelvic organ tenderness
- Uterine tenderness
- Adnexal tenderness

- Cervical motion tenderness
- Inflammation

What Are the Complications of Pelvic Inflammatory Disease?

Complications of PID include

- Tubo-ovarian abscess (TOA)
- Tubal factor infertility
- Ectopic pregnancy
- Chronic pelvic pain

Recurrent episodes of PID and increased severity of tubal inflammation detected by laparoscopy are associated with greater risk of infertility following PID. However, even subclinical PID has been associated with infertility. This emphasizes the importance of following screening and treatment recommendations for chlamydia and gonorrhea to prevent PID when possible, and promptly and appropriately treating cases of PID that do occur.

Tubo-ovarian abscess (TOA) is a serious short-term complication of PID that is characterized by an inflammatory mass involving the fallopian tube, ovary, and, occasionally, other adjacent pelvic organs. The microbiology of TOAs is similar to PID and the diagnosis necessitates initial hospital admission. Treatment includes broad-spectrum antibiotics with or without a drainage procedure, with surgery often reserved for patients with suspected rupture or who fail to respond to antibiotics. Women infected with HIV may be at higher risk for TOA. Mortality from PID is less than 1% and is usually secondary to rupture of a TOA or to ectopic pregnancy.

How Is Pelvic Inflammatory Disease Diagnosed?

The wide variation in symptoms and signs associated with PID can make diagnosis challenging. No single historical, physical, or laboratory finding is both sensitive and specific for the diagnosis of PID. Clinicians should therefore maintain a low threshold for the diagnosis of PID, particularly in young, sexually active women.

Criteria have been developed for the diagnosis of PID. Presumptive treatment for PID should be initiated in sexually active young women and other women at risk for STDs if they are experiencing pelvic or lower abdominal pain, if no cause for the illness other than PID can be identified, and if one or more of the following minimum clinical criteria are present on pelvic examination:

- cervical motion tenderness

  or

- uterine tenderness

  or

- adnexal tenderness

The requirement that all three minimum criteria be present before the initiation of empiric treatment could result in insufficient sensitivity for the diagnosis of PID. After deciding whether to initiate empiric treatment, clinicians should also consider the risk profile for STDs.

More elaborate diagnostic evaluation frequently is needed because incorrect diagnosis and management of PID might cause unnecessary morbidity. For example, the presence of signs of lower-genital–tract inflammation (predominance of leukocytes in vaginal secretions, cervical exudates, or cervical friability), in addition to one of the three minimum criteria, increases the specificity of the diagnosis. One or more of the following additional criteria can be used to enhance the specificity of the minimum clinical criteria and support a diagnosis of PID:

- oral temperature >101°F (>38.3°C);

- abnormal cervical mucopurulent discharge or cervical friability;

- presence of abundant numbers of WBC on saline microscopy of vaginal fluid;

- elevated erythrocyte sedimentation rate;

- elevated C-reactive protein; and

- laboratory documentation of cervical infection with *N. gonorrhoeae* or *C. trachomatis*.

Most women with PID have either mucopurulent cervical discharge or evidence of WBCs on a microscopic evaluation of a saline preparation of vaginal fluid (i.e., wet prep). If the cervical discharge appears normal and no WBCs are observed on the wet prep of vaginal fluid, the diagnosis of PID is unlikely, and alternative causes of pain should be considered. A wet prep of vaginal fluid also can detect the presence of concomitant infections (e.g., BV and trichomoniasis).

The most specific criteria for diagnosing PID include:

- endometrial biopsy with histopathologic evidence of endometritis;

- transvaginal sonography or magnetic resonance imaging techniques showing thickened, fluid-filled tubes with or without free pelvic fluid or tubo-ovarian complex, or Doppler studies suggesting pelvic infection (e.g., tubal hyperemia); or

- laparoscopic findings consistent with PID.

A diagnostic evaluation that includes some of these more extensive procedures might be warranted in some cases. Endometrial biopsy is warranted in women undergoing laparoscopy who do not have visual evidence of salpingitis, because endometritis is the only sign of PID for some women.

A serologic test for human immunodeficiency virus (HIV) is also recommended. A pregnancy test should always be performed to exclude ectopic pregnancy and because PID can occur concurrently with pregnancy. When the diagnosis of PID is questionable, or when the illness is severe or not responding to therapy, further investigation may be warranted using other invasive procedures (endometrial biopsy, transvaginal ultrasonography, magnetic resonance imaging, or laparoscopy).

How Is Pelvic Inflammatory Disease Treated?

PID is treated with broad spectrum antibiotics to cover likely pathogens. Several types of antibiotics can cure PID. Antibiotic treatment does not, however, reverse any scarring that has already been caused by the infection. For this reason, it is critical that a woman receive care immediately if she has pelvic pain or other symptoms of PID. Prompt antibiotic treatment could prevent severe damage to the reproductive organs.

Health care providers should emphasize to their patients that although their symptoms may go away before the infection is cured, they should finish taking all of the prescribed medicine. Additionally, a woman's sex partner(s) should be treated to decrease the risk of re-infection, even if the partner(s) has no symptoms. Although sex partners may have no symptoms, they may still be infected with the organisms that can cause PID.

What Should a Patient Do after Being Diagnosed with Pelvic Inflammatory Disease?

A patient should abstain from sexual intercourse until she and her partner(s) have completed treatment. Female latex condoms are also an option if a woman prefers them or if her male partner chooses not to use male condoms. Women who are told they have an STD and are treated for it should notify all of their recent sex partners so they can see a health care provider and be evaluated for STDs.

The diagnosis of PID provides an opportunity to educate adolescent and young women about prevention of STDs, including abstinence, consistent use of barrier methods of protection, immunization, and the importance of receiving periodic screening for STDs and HIV.

How Can Pelvic Inflammatory Disease Be Prevented?

Latex condoms may reduce the risk of PID by preventing STDs. Since STDs play a major role in PID, screening of women at risk for infection and treatment of infected women and their sex partners can help to minimize the risk of PID. Screening of young sexually active women for chlamydia has been shown to decrease the incidence of PID.

CDC recommends that providers screen the following populations for chlamydia and gonorrhea: all sexually active women younger than 25 years, as well as older women with risk factors such as new or multiple sex partners, or a sex partner who has a sexually transmitted infection.

What Are the Risk Factors for Developing Pelvic Inflammatory Disease?

Risk factors for PID include factors associated with STD acquisition, such as younger age, having a new or multiple sex partners, having a sex partner who has other concurrent sex partners, and inconsistent use of condoms during sex. Other factors that have been associated with PID include a history of STDs or prior PID, and vaginal douching. A small increased risk of PID associated with intrauterine device (IUD) use is primarily confined to the first three weeks after IUD insertion.

Is the Number of Women in the United States Being Diagnosed with Pelvic Inflammatory Disease Increasing?

No. Over the last decade, there have been several studies published suggesting overall declines in PID diagnosis in both hospital and ambulatory settings. While no single explanation exists for this declining trend, some have suggested that changes in sexually transmitted disease (STD) rates, increases in chlamydia screening coverage, availability of antimicrobial therapies that increase adherence to treatment, and more sensitive diagnostic technologies, could be impacting PID rates.

Despite declining trends, PID is a frequent and important infection that occurs among women of reproductive age. Based on a nationally representative sample from 2006–2010, 5% of U.S. women have reported being treated for PID in their lifetime.

The significant burden of disease attributed to PID comes predominantly from the long-term reproductive sequelae of tubal infection: tubal factor infertility, ectopic pregnancy, and pelvic adhesions, which can lead to chronic pelvic pain. Our knowledge of the longitudinal outcomes for affected women who experience PID is primarily derived from data published using a Scandinavian cohort of inpatients diagnosed with PID. Data from this study indicated that those women with PID were more likely to have ectopic pregnancy (6 times increased rate), tubal factor infertility (ranging 8% after first episode to as high as 40% after three episodes) and chronic pelvic pain (18% following first episode).

What Is the Economic Burden of Pelvic Inflammatory Disease in the United States?

A decline in incidence of PID is also reflected in the most recent cost estimates of PID and its sequelae. Direct medical expenditures for PID and its sequelae were estimated at $1.88 billion in 1998, compared to approximately $2.7 billion estimated in 1990. Based on a nationally representative sample from 2006–2010, approximately 4.2% of U.S. women have reported being treated for PID in their lifetime.

Chapter 32

Pregnancy
Complications and STDs

Chapter Contents

Section 32.1

STDs during Pregnancy

This section includes text excerpted from "Sexually
Transmitted Infections, Pregnancy, and Breastfeeding,"
Office on Women's Health (OWH), August 31, 2015;
text under heading "Should I Get Tested for HIV
If I Am Pregnant?" only is excerpted from "Pregnancy
and Childbirth," U.S. Department of Health and
Human Services (HHS), September 28, 2015.

How Do STIs Affect Pregnant Women?

STIs can cause many of the same health problems in pregnant
women as in women who are not pregnant. But having an STI also
can hurt the unborn baby's health.

Having an STI during pregnancy can cause:

- Premature labor (labor before 37 weeks of pregnancy). Early
  (preterm) birth is the number one cause of infant death and
  can lead to long-term developmental and health problems in
  children.

- Infection in the uterus (womb) after birth.

Should I Get Tested for HIV If I Am Pregnant?

Yes. Get tested for HIV when you are planning a pregnancy or as
soon as possible after you find out you are pregnant, even if you have
been tested before.

CDC also recommends that some women receive a second HIV test
in their third trimester if they meet certain criteria, such as continuing
to engage in behaviors that put you at high risk for getting HIV.

Not all health care facilities offer an automatic HIV test for pregnant women. Be sure to request one if it isn't offered.

Of course, some women go into labor before they have been tested.
If a pregnant woman goes into labor without having had an HIV test,

392

CDC recommends that she be given a rapid HIV test in the labor and delivery room. That way, if the test is positive, the doctors can work with her to help prevent passing HIV to the baby.

Can I Pass an STI to My Baby?

Yes. Some STIs can be passed from a pregnant woman to the baby before and during the baby's birth.

- Some STIs, such as syphilis, cross the placenta and infect the baby in the womb.

- Other STIs, like gonorrhea, chlamydia, hepatitis B, and genital herpes, can pass from the mother to the baby as the baby passes through the birth canal.

- HIV can cross the placenta during pregnancy and infect the baby during delivery

What Are the Harmful Effects of Passing an STI to a Baby?

The harmful effects to babies may include:

- Low birth weight (less than 5 pounds)

- Eye infection

- Pneumonia

- Infection in the baby's blood

- Brain damage

- Lack of coordination in body movements

- Blindness

- Deafness

- Acute hepatitis

- Meningitis

- Chronic liver disease, which can lead to scarring of the liver (cirrhosis)

- Stillbirth

I'm Pregnant. What Can I Do to Prevent Problems from STIs?

You can prevent some of the health problems caused by STIs and pregnancy with regular prenatal care. Your doctor will test you for STIs early in your pregnancy and again closer to childbirth, if needed.

- **STIs caused by bacteria**, such as chlamydia and gonorrhea, can be cured with antibiotics. Some antibiotics are safe to take during pregnancy. Your doctor can prescribe antibiotics for chlamydia, gonorrhea, syphilis, and trichomoniasis during pregnancy.

- **STIs caused by viruses**, such as genital herpes and HIV, have no cure.

  - If you have herpes, antiviral medicine may help reduce symptoms. If you have symptoms of herpes or active genital herpes sores at the start of labor, you may need a cesarean section (C-section). This can help lower the risk of passing the infection to your baby.

  - If you have HIV, antiviral medicines can lower the risk of giving HIV to your baby to less than 1%. You also may need to have a C-section.

You also can take steps to lower your risk of getting an STI during pregnancy.

Can I Breastfeed If I Have an STI?

Maybe. Some STIs affect breastfeeding, and some don't. The following are some general guidelines, but talk to your doctor, nurse, or a lactation consultant about the risk of passing the STI to your baby while breastfeeding:

- **If you have HIV**, do not breastfeed. You can pass the virus to your baby. In countries like the United States where clean water is available, using a breastmilk substitute like formula is recommended.

- **If you have chlamydia, gonorrhea, or HPV**, you can breastfeed your baby.

- **If you have trichomoniasis**, you can take the antibiotic metronidazole if you are breastfeeding. You may need to wait 12 to 24 hours after taking the medicine to breastfeed.

- **If you have syphilis or herpes**, you can breastfeed as long as your baby or pumping equipment does not touch a sore. It is possible to spread syphilis or herpes to any part of your breast, including your nipple and areola. If you have sores on your breast, pump or hand-express your milk until the sores heal. Pumping will help keep up your milk supply and prevent your breast from getting overly full and painful. You can store your milk to give to your baby in a bottle for another feeding. But if parts of your breast pump also touch the sore(s) while pumping, you should throw the milk away.

Are STI Treatments Safe to Use While Breastfeeding?

If you are being treated for an STI, ask your doctor about the possible effects of the medicine on your breastfeeding baby. Most treatments for STIs are safe to take while breastfeeding.

Section 32.2

Treatment for STDs during Pregnancy

This section includes text excerpted from "Special Populations," Centers for Disease Control and Prevention (CDC), June 4, 2015.

Pregnant Women

Intrauterine or perinatally transmitted STDs can have severely debilitating effects on pregnant women, their partners, and their fetuses. All pregnant women and their sex partners should be asked about STDs, counseled about the possibility of perinatal infections, and provided access to screening and treatment, if needed.

Recommendations to screen pregnant women for STDs are based on disease severity and sequelae, prevalence in the population, costs, medico-legal considerations (e.g., state laws), and other factors.

Recommended Screening Tests

- All pregnant women in the United States should be screened for HIV infection at the first prenatal visit, even if they have been previously tested. Screening should be conducted after the woman is notified of the need to be screened for HIV as part of the routine panel of prenatal tests, unless she declines (i.e., opt-out screening). For women who decline HIV testing, providers should address their objections, and when appropriate, continue to encourage testing. Women who decline testing because they have had a previous negative HIV test should be informed of the importance of retesting during each pregnancy. Testing pregnant women and treating those who are infected are vital not only to maintain the health of the woman, but to reduce perinatal transmission of HIV through available antiretroviral and obstetrical interventions. Retesting in the third trimester (preferably before 36 weeks' gestation) is recommended for women at high risk for acquiring HIV infection (e.g., women who use illicit drugs, have STDs during pregnancy, have multiple sex partners during pregnancy, live in areas with high HIV prevalence, or have partners with HIV infection). Rapid HIV screening should be performed on any woman in labor who has not been screened for HIV during pregnancy unless she declines. If a rapid HIV test result is positive in these women, antiretroviral prophylaxis should be administered without waiting for the results of the confirmatory test.

- A serologic test for syphilis should be performed for all pregnant women at the first prenatal visit. When access to prenatal care is not optimal, rapid plasma reagin (RPR) card test screening (and treatment, if that test is reactive) should be performed at the time that a pregnancy is confirmed. Women who are at high risk for syphilis or live in areas of high syphilis morbidity should be screened again early in the third trimester (at approximately 28 weeks' gestation) and at delivery. Some states require all women to be screened at delivery. Neonates should not be discharged from the hospital unless the syphilis serologic status of the mother has been determined at least one time during pregnancy and preferably again at delivery if at risk. Any woman who delivers a stillborn infant should be tested for syphilis.

- All pregnant women should be routinely tested for hepatitis B surface antigen (HBsAg) at the first prenatal visit even if they have been previously vaccinated or tested. Women who were not screened prenatally, those who engage in behaviors that put them at high risk for infection (e.g., having had more than one sex partner in the previous 6 months, evaluation or treatment for an STD, recent or current injection-drug use, and an HBsAg-positive sex partner) and those with clinical hepatitis should be retested at the time of admission to the hospital for delivery. Pregnant women at risk for HBV infection also should be vaccinated. To avoid misinterpreting a transient positive HBsAg result during the 21 days after vaccination, HBsAg testing should be performed before vaccine administration. All laboratories that conduct HBsAg tests should test initially reactive specimens with a licensed neutralizing confirmatory test. When pregnant women are tested for HBsAg at the time of admission for delivery, shortened testing protocols can be used, and initially reactive results should prompt expedited administration of immunoprophylaxis to neonates. Pregnant women who are HBsAg positive should be reported to the local or state health department to ensure that they are entered into a case-management system and that timely and appropriate prophylaxis is provided to their infants. Information concerning the pregnant woman's HBsAg status should be provided to the hospital in which delivery is planned and to the health-care provider who will care for the newborn. In addition, household and sex contacts of women who are HBsAg positive should be vaccinated. Women who are HBsAg positive should be provided with, or referred for, appropriate counseling and medical management.

- All pregnant women aged <25 years and older women at increased risk for infection (e.g., those who have a new sex partner, more than one sex partner, a sex partner with concurrent partners, or a sex partner who has a sexually transmitted infection) should be routinely screened for Chlamydia trachomatis at the first prenatal visit. Women aged <25 years and those at increased risk for chlamydia also should be retested during the third trimester to prevent maternal postnatal complications and chlamydial infection in the neonate. Pregnant women found to have chlamydial infection should have a test-of-cure to document chlamydial eradication (preferably by nucleic acid amplification testing [NAAT]) 3–4 weeks after treatment and then retested within 3 months. Screening during the first trimester might prevent the adverse effects of chlamydia during pregnancy, but evidence for such screening is lacking.

- All pregnant women aged <25 years and older women at increased risk for gonorrhea (e.g., those with a new sex partner, more than one sex partner, a sex partner with concurrent partners, or a sex partner who has a sexually transmitted infection) should be screened for *N. gonorrhoeae* at the first prenatal visit. Additional risk factors for gonorrhea include inconsistent condom use among persons not in mutually monogamous relationships, previous or coexisting sexually transmitted infection, and exchanging sex for money or drugs. Clinicians should consider the communities they serve and might choose to consult local public health authorities for guidance on identifying groups that are at increased risk. Gonococcal infection, in particular, is concentrated in specific geographic locations and communities. Women found to have gonococcal infection should be treated immediately and retested within 3 months. Pregnant women who remain at high risk for gonococcal infection also should be retested during the third trimester to prevent maternal postnatal complications and gonococcal infection in the neonate.

- All pregnant women at risk for HCV infection should be screened for hepatitis C antibodies at the first prenatal visit. The most important risk factor for HCV infection is past or current injection drug use. Additional risk factors include having had a blood transfusion before July 1992, receipt of an unregulated tattoo, having been on long-term hemodialysis, intranasal drug use, and other percutaneous exposures. No established treatment regimen exists for pregnant women infected with HCV. However, all women with HCV infection should receive appropriate counseling and supportive care as needed. No vaccine is available to prevent HCV transmission.

- Pregnant women should undergo a Papanicolau (Pap) test at the same frequency as nonpregnant women, although recommendations for management of abnormal Pap tests in pregnancy differ.

Other Tests

- Evidence does not support routine screening for BV in asymptomatic pregnant women at high risk for preterm delivery. Symptomatic women should be evaluated and treated.

- Evidence does not support routine screening for Trichomonas vaginalis in asymptomatic pregnant women. Women who report symptoms should be evaluated and treated appropriately.

- Evidence does not support routine HSV-2 serologic screening among asymptomatic pregnant women. However, type-specific serologic tests might be useful for identifying pregnant women at risk for HSV infection and guiding counseling regarding the risk for acquiring genital herpes during pregnancy. In the absence of lesions during the third trimester, routine serial cultures for HSV are not indicated for women in the third trimester who have a history of recurrent genital herpes.

Chapter 33

Vaginitis

What Is Vaginitis?

Vaginitis is an inflammation of the vagina. It is often caused by infections, some of which are associated with serious diseases. The most common vaginal infections are

- Bacterial Vaginosis

- Trichomoniasis

- Vaginal Yeast Infection

Some vaginal infections are transmitted through sexual contact, but others, such as yeast infections, probably are not.

Other Causes of Vaginitis

Although most vaginal infections in women are due to bacterial vaginosis, trichomoniasis, or yeast, there may be other causes as well. These causes include other sexually transmitted diseases, allergic reactions, and irritations.

Allergic symptoms can be caused by spermicides, vaginal hygiene products, detergents, and fabric softeners. Inflammation of the cervix (opening to the womb) also is associated with abnormal vaginal

---

This chapter includes text excerpted from "Vaginitis," National Institute of Allergy and Infectious Diseases (NIAID), National Institutes of Health (NIH), September 25, 2015.

discharge. Healthcare providers can tell them apart from true vaginal infections by doing lab tests.

Research

To control vaginitis, research is under way to determine the factors that promote the growth and disease-causing potential of vaginal microbes (germs). This information could help improve efforts to treat and prevent vaginitis. Vaginitis is the object of serious studies as scientists try to clarify its role in such conditions as pelvic inflammatory disease and pregnancy-related complications.

Vaginitis refers to disorders of the vagina caused by infection, inflammation, or changes in the normal vaginal flora. Symptoms include vaginal discharge, odor, itching, and/or discomfort. The three most common diseases diagnosed among women with these symptoms include bacterial vaginosis (40–45 percent), vulvovaginal candidiasis (20–25 percent), and trichomoniasis (15–20 percent). In some cases, there may be more than one disease present. Recurrent vaginitis is also common.

Research is under way to determine the factors that promote the growth and disease-causing potential of vaginal microbes and their role in vaginitis. These microbes include the sexually transmitted pathogen *Trichomonas vaginalis*, *Candida* species, and microbes associated with bacterial vaginosis, such as *Gardnerella vaginalis*.

NIAID-supported research has led to advances in knowledge about the normal microflora of the vagina, reproductive behavior of yeast, and the genetic code of *T. vaginalis*. For example, researchers have discovered an association between certain lactobacilli species in the normal microflora in the vagina and protection from bacterial vaginosis (BV). They are investigating a lactobacillus vaginal suppository aimed to help these beneficial bacteria grow in the vagina. Researchers also are studying the use of combination treatment with vaginal lactobacilli suppositories and oral medication to treat BV and prevent its recurrence.

Other NIAID-funded researchers have sequenced the genome of *T. vaginalis*. Understanding the genome of this pathogen will help researchers understand how it evolves, spreads, and causes disease. *T. vaginalis* is particularly interesting to medical researchers because it increases both transmission and acquisition of HIV among women. Additionally, both *T. vaginalis* and BV are associated with adverse pregnancy outcomes including preterm birth and low birth weight. Knowledge gained from ongoing research could help improve efforts to treat and prevent vaginitis and also prevent its potential complications.

Part Four

STD Testing and Treatment Concerns

Chapter 34

Frequently Asked Questions about STD and HIV Testing

What Are Sexually Transmitted Diseases and Should I Be Tested?

CDC estimates that there are approximately 19 million new sexually transmitted disease (STD) infections each year—almost half of them among young people 15 to 24 years of age. Most infections have no symptoms and often go undiagnosed and untreated, which may lead to severe health consequences, especially for women.

Knowing your STD status is a critical step to stopping STD transmission. If you know you are infected you can take steps to protect yourself and your partners. Many STDs can be easily diagnosed and treated. If either you or your partner is infected, both of you may need to receive treatment at the same time to avoid getting re-infected.

What Is HIV and Should I Be Tested?

HIV stands for human immunodeficiency virus. It is the virus that can lead to acquired immunodeficiency syndrome, or AIDS. Unlike some other viruses, the human body cannot get rid of HIV. That means that once you have HIV, you have it for life. The only way to know if

This chapter includes text excerpted from "National HIV, STD, and Hepatitis Testing," Centers for Disease Control and Prevention (CDC), August 4, 2014.

you are infected with HIV is to be tested. With proper medical care, HIV can be controlled.

One in six people with HIV are unaware of their infection. That's why CDC recommends that everyone between the ages of 13 and 64 get tested at least once and that high-risk groups get tested more often.

What Is Viral Hepatitis and Should I Be Tested?

Viral Hepatitis refers to a group of viral infections that affect the liver. The most common types are hepatitis A, hepatitis B, and hepatitis C.

Hepatitis A, hepatitis B, and hepatitis C are diseases caused by three different viruses. Although each can cause similar symptoms, they have different modes of transmission and can affect the liver differently. Hepatitis A appears only as an acute or newly occurring infection and does not become chronic. People with hepatitis A usually improve without treatment. hepatitis B and hepatitis C can also begin as acute infections, but in some people, the virus remains in the body, resulting in chronic disease and long-term liver problems. There are vaccines to prevent hepatitis A and B; however, there is not one for hepatitis C. Recommendations for testing depend on many different factors and on the type of hepatitis.

What Puts Me at Risk for HIV, Viral Hepatitis, and STDs?

Risks for HIV

The most common ways HIV is transmitted in the United States is through anal or vaginal sex or sharing drug injection equipment with a person infected with HIV. Although the risk factors for HIV are the same for everyone, some racial/ethnic, gender, and age groups are far more affected than others.

What Puts Me at Risk for Hepatitis A?

Hepatitis A is usually spread when a person ingests fecal matter—even in microscopic amounts—from contact with objects, food, or drinks contaminated by the feces or stool of an infected person. Due to routine vaccination of children, hepatitis A has decreased dramatically in the United States. Although anyone can get hepatitis A, certain groups of people are at higher risk, including men who have sex with men, people who use illegal drugs, people who travel to certain international countries, and people who have sexual contact with someone who has hepatitis A.

What Puts Me at Risk for Hepatitis B?

Hepatitis B is usually spread when blood, semen, or another body fluid from a person infected with the hepatitis B virus enters the body of someone who is not infected. This can happen through sexual contact with an infected person or sharing needles, syringes, or other drug-injection equipment. hepatitis B can also be passed from an infected mother to her baby at birth.

Among adults in the United States, hepatitis B is most commonly spread through sexual contact and accounts for nearly two-thirds of acute hepatitis B cases. Hepatitis B is 50–100 times more infectious than HIV.

What Puts Me at Risk for Hepatitis C?

Hepatitis C is usually spread when blood from a person infected with the hepatitis C virus enters the body of someone who is not infected. Today, most people become infected with the hepatitis C virus by sharing needles or other equipment to inject drugs. Hepatitis C was also commonly spread through blood transfusions and organ transplants prior to the early 1990s. At that time, widespread screening of the blood supply began in the United States, which has helped ensure a safe blood supply.

Risks for Genital Herpes

Genital herpes is a common STD, and most people with genital herpes infection do not know they have it. You can get genital herpes from an infected partner, even if your partner has no herpes symptoms. There is no cure for herpes, but medication is available to reduce symptoms and make it less likely that you will spread herpes to a sex partner.

Risks for Genital Human Papillomavirus (HPV)

HPV is so common that most sexually active people get it at some point in their lives. Anyone who is sexually active can get HPV, even if you have had sex with only one person. In most cases, HPV goes away on its own and does not cause any health problems. But when HPV does not go away, it can cause health problems like genital warts and cancer. HPV is passed on through genital contact (such as vaginal and anal sex). You can pass HPV to others without knowing it.

Risks for Chlamydia

Most people who have chlamydia don't know it since the disease often has no symptoms. Chlamydia is the most commonly reported STD in the United States. Sexually active females 25 years old and younger need testing every year. Although it is easy to cure, chlamydia can make it difficult for a woman to get pregnant if left untreated.

Risks for Gonorrhea

Anyone who is sexually active can get gonorrhea, an STD that can cause infections in the genitals, rectum, and throat. It is a very common infection, especially among young people ages 15–24 years. But it can be easily cured. You can get gonorrhea by having anal, vaginal, or oral sex with someone who has gonorrhea. A pregnant woman with gonorrhea can give the infection to her baby during childbirth.

Risks for Syphilis

Any sexually active person can get syphilis. It is more common among men who have sex with men. Syphilis is passed through direct contact with a syphilis sore. Sores occur mainly on the external genitals, anus, or in the rectum. Sores also can occur on the lips and in the mouth. A pregnant women with syphilis can give the infection to her unborn baby.

Risks for Bacterial Vaginosis

BV is common among women of childbearing age. Any woman can get BV, but women are at a higher risk for BV if they have a new sex partner, multiple sex partners, use an intrauterine device (IUD), and/or douche.

Risks for Trichomoniasis

Trichomoniasis is a common STD that affects both women and men, although symptoms are more common in women. You can get trichomoniasis by having vaginal sex with someone who has it. Women can acquire the disease from men or women, but men usually contract it only from women.

How Do I Protect Myself and My Partner(S) from HIV, Viral Hepatitis, and STDs?

HIV Prevention

Your life matters and staying healthy is important. It's important for you, the people who care about you, and your community. Knowing your HIV status gives you powerful information to help you take steps to keep you and your partners healthy. You should get tested for HIV, and encourage your partners to get tested too. For people who are sexually active, there are more tools available today to prevent HIV than ever before. The list below provides a number of ways that you can lower your chances of getting HIV. The more of these actions you take, the safer you can be.

- **Get tested and treated for other STDs and encourage your partners to do the same**. All adults and adolescents from ages 13—64 should be tested at least once for HIV and high-risk groups get tested more often. STDs can have long-term health consequences. They can also increase your chance of getting HIV or transmitting it to others. It is important to have an honest and open talk with your healthcare provider and ask whether you should be tested for STDs. Your healthcare provider can offer you the best care if you discuss your sexual history openly.

- **Choose less risky sexual behaviors**. Oral sex is much less risky than anal or vaginal sex for HIV transmission. Anal sex is the highest-risk sexual activity for HIV transmission. If you are HIV-negative, insertive anal sex (topping) is less risky for getting HIV than receptive anal sex (bottoming). Sexual activities that do not involve the potential exchange of bodily fluids carry no risk for getting HIV (e.g., touching).

- **Use condoms consistently and correctly**.

- **Reduce the number of people you have sex with**. The number of sex partners you have affects your HIV risk. The more partners you have, the more likely you are to have a partner with HIV whose viral load is not suppressed or to have a sex partner with a sexually transmitted disease. Both of these factors can increase the risk of HIV transmission.

- **Talk to your doctor about pre-exposure prophylaxis (PrEP)**. CDC recommends that PrEP be considered for people who are HIV-negative and at substancial risk for HIV. For sexual transmission, this includes HIV-negative persons who are in an ongoing relationship with an HIV-positive partner. It also includes anyone who,

1. is not in a mutually monogamous* relationship with a partner who recently tested HIV-negative, and

2. is a gay or bisexual man who has had anal sex without a condom or been diagnosed with an STD in the past 6 months; or heterosexual man or woman who does not regularly use condoms during sex with partners of unknown HIV status who are at substantial risk of HIV infection (e.g., people who inject drugs or have bisexual male partners).

For people who inject drugs, this includes those who have injected illicit drugs in the past 6 months and who have shared injection equipment or been in drug treatment for injection drug use in the past 6 months.

- **Talk to your doctor right away (within 3 days) about post-exposure prophylaxis (PEP) if you have a possible exposure to HIV**. An example of a possible exposure is if you have anal or vaginal sex without a condom with someone who is or may be HIV-positive, and you are HIV-negative and not taking PrEP. Your chance of exposure to HIV is lower if your HIV-positive partner is taking antiretroviral therapy (ART) consistently and correctly, especially if his/her viral load is undetectable. Starting medicine immediately (known as post-exposure prophylaxis, or PEP) and taking it daily for 4 weeks reduces your chance of getting HIV.

- **If your partner is HIV-positive, encourage your partner to get and stay on treatment**. ART reduces the amount of HIV virus (viral load) in blood and body fluids. ART can keep people with HIV healthy for many years, and greatly reduce the chance of transmitting HIV to sex partners if taken consistently and correctly.

* Mutually monogamous means that you and your partner only have sex with each other and do not have sex outside the relationship.

Hepatitis Prevention

The best way to prevent both hepatitis A and B is by getting vaccinated. There is no vaccine available to prevent hepatitis C. The best way to prevent hepatitis C is by avoiding behaviors that can spread the disease, such as sharing needles or other equipment to inject drugs.

STD Prevention

The only way to avoid STDs is to not have vaginal, anal, or oral sex. If you are sexually active, you can do several things to lower your chances of getting an STD, including:

- Get tested for STDs and encourage your partner(s) to do the same. It is important to have an honest and open talk with your healthcare provider and ask whether you should be tested for STDs. Your healthcare provider can offer you the best care if you discuss your sexual history openly.

- Get vaccinated. Vaccines are safe, effective, and recommended ways to prevent hepatitis A, hepatitis B, and HPV.

- Be in a sexually active relationship with only one person, who has agreed to be sexually active only with you.

- Reduce your number of sex partners. By doing so, you decrease your risk for STDs. It is still important that you and your partner get tested, and that you share your test results with one another.

- Use a condom every time you have vaginal, anal, or oral sex. Correct and consistent use of the male latex condom is highly effective in reducing STD transmission.

How Do HIV, Viral Hepatitis, and STDs Relate to Each Other?

Persons who have an STD are at least two to five times more likely than uninfected persons to acquire HIV infection if they are exposed to the virus through sexual contact. In addition, if a person who is HIV positive also has an STD, that person is more likely to transmit HIV through sexual contact than other HIV-infected persons.

Hepatitis B virus (HBV) and HIV are bloodborne viruses transmitted primarily through sexual contact and injection drug use. Because of these shared modes of transmission, a high proportion of adults at risk for HIV infection are also at risk for HBV infection. HIV-positive persons who become infected with HBV are at increased risk for developing chronic HBV infection and should be tested. In addition, persons who are co-infected with HIV and HBV can have serious medical complications, including an increased risk for liver-related morbidity and mortality.

Hepatitis C Virus (HCV) is one of the most common causes of chronic liver disease in the United States. For persons who are HIV infected, co-infection with HCV can result in a more rapid occurrence of liver damage and may also impact the course and management of HIV infection.

Chapter 35

Newly Diagnosed: What You Need to Know

What Does "HIV-Positive" Mean?

If you have just been diagnosed with HIV, you may have many questions:

- What does it mean to be HIV-positive?
- Does it mean that you have AIDS?
- Is HIV manageable?
- What are some of the first things you need to think about and do?

Being diagnosed with HIV means that you have been infected with the Human Immunodeficiency Virus (HIV) and that two HIV tests—a preliminary test and a confirmatory test—have both come back positive.

Once you have been infected with HIV, you will always carry it in your body. There is no cure for HIV. It is a serious, infectious disease that can lead to death if it isn't treated. But there is good news: by getting linked to HIV medical care early, starting antiretroviral therapy (ART), adhering to your medication, and staying in care you can keep the virus under control, and live a healthy life.

This chapter includes text excerpted from "Newly Diagnosed: What You Need to Know," U.S. Department of Health and Human Services (HHS), October 4, 2015.

Being HIV-positive also means that it is possible for you to pass the virus along to others, including your sexual partners. If you are female, you could also pass it along to your unborn child. Through treatment for HIV disease, you can suppress the virus and reduce the chances of transmitting HIV to others.

Do I Have AIDS?

Being HIV-positive does NOT necessarily mean you have AIDS. AIDS is the most advanced stage of HIV disease. If you are diagnosed early, start treatment, and adhere to your medication, you can stay healthy and prevent the virus from developing into AIDS. Ask your healthcare provider for more specifics about exactly what stage of HIV infection you have.

Is HIV Manageable?

Yes, today HIV is a manageable disease. HIV medications have significantly changed the course of HIV infection since the early days of the epidemic and with the proper care and treatment, you can live a healthy life.

The sooner you take steps to protect your health, the better. Early treatment with antiretroviral drugs and a healthy lifestyle can help you stay well. Prompt medical care prevents the onset of AIDS and some life-threatening AIDS-related conditions.

Newly Diagnosed Checklist

Here is a checklist to help you take the first steps toward managing your infection.

- **Don't panic—just breathe.** This is life-changing news but you have options to protect your health. There are HIV medicines to treat HIV infection and help you stay healthy.

- **Find an HIV care provider, even if you don't feel sick.** Your HIV care provider will be the person who partners with you to manage your HIV. He or she will monitor your health on an ongoing basis and work with you to develop a treatment plan. It's never too early to start treatment. Current guidelines recommend treatment with ART for all people with HIV, including those with early infection. If you don't have a regular doctor, your HIV testing location or your local health department can help you find an HIV care provider. Or, you can use the AIDS. gov HIV Testing and Care Services Locator to find a provider near you.

- **Prepare for your first appointment.** Your first appointment with your HIV care provider can cause anxiety. Make a list of questions before you go. Making a list is a good way to organize your thoughts. The Department of Veterans Affairs offers a list of sample questions you can bring with you. Remember: there are no stupid questions! **Do some research.** After you have listed your questions, take some time to understand what it means to have HIV.

- **Find a support system.** This is one of the most important pieces of managing a new HIV diagnosis. You can find support among friends, family, or members of your community. If you are not ready to tell other people about your HIV diagnosis, that's ok. Look to community resources and professional organizations that offer support groups for newly diagnosed people, one-on-one counseling, peer counselors, or health educators.

- **Begin thinking about whom you want to tell.** Disclosing can be one of the hardest parts about managing a new diagnosis of HIV. It's important to remember that you do not need to tell everyone all at once, and that there are systems in place to help you. At this time, it is important to disclose your HIV status to your healthcare providers and sexual partners.

Prevent HIV Transmission

You also need to take steps to avoid giving HIV to anyone else:

- **Use ART.** ART reduces the amount of virus (viral load) in your blood and body fluids. ART can keep you healthy for many years, and reduce your chance of transmitting HIV to your sex partners if taken consistently and correctly.

- **If you are taking ART, follow your health care provider's advice.** Visit your health care provider regularly and always take your medication as directed.

- **Use condoms consistently and correctly with every sexual contact.** When used consistently and correctly, condoms are highly effective at preventing HIV. **If your steady partner is HIV-negative, talk to him or her about** pre-exposure prophylaxis (PrEP), taking HIV medicines daily to prevent HIV infection. The CDC recommends PrEP be considered for people who are HIV-negative and at substantial risk for HIV infection. This includes HIV-negative individuals who are in an ongoing relationship with an HIV-positive partner, as well as others at high risk.

- **Talk to your partners about post-exposure prophylaxis (PEP) if you think they have had a possible exposure to HIV.** An example of a possible exposure is you have anal or vaginal sex without a condom or the condom breaks and your partner is HIV-negative and not on PrEP. Your partners' chance of exposure to HIV is lower if you are taking ART consistently and correctly, especially if your viral load is undetectable. Your partners should talk to their doctors right away (within 3 days) if they think they have had a possible exposure to HIV. Starting medicine immediately (known as post-exposure prophylaxis, or PEP) and taking it daily for 4 weeks reduces your partners' chance of getting HIV.

- **Don't share needles, syringes, or other drug paraphernalia with anyone.**

- **Choose less risky sexual behaviors.** Oral sex is much less risky than anal or vaginal sex. Anal sex is the highest-risk sexual activity for HIV transmission. If you are HIV-positive, receptive anal sex ("bottoming") is less risky for transmitting HIV than insertive anal sex.

- **Get tested and treated for STDs and encourage your partners to do the same.** If you are sexually active, get tested at least once a year. STDs can have long-term health consequences. They can also increase the chance of getting HIV or transmitting it to others.

If I Am Diagnosed with HIV, Can a Healthcare Provider Tell Who Gave Me the Infection?

No. HIV tests cannot determine who gave you the infection.

If I Am Diagnosed with HIV, Can I Tell When I Got It?

In general, no. A skilled healthcare provider can generally estimate how long you have been infected by looking at the levels of virus in your body, your CD4 (T-cell) count, and whether or not you have had any opportunistic infections. If you are currently suffering from symptoms of acute HIV infection, a healthcare provider can usually conclude that infection occurred within the past few weeks.

If I Am Diagnosed with HIV, Will I Have a Normal Lifespan?

Life expectancy for many people living with HIV who start treatment early, remain adherent to HIV medications and stay in care is similar to that of HIV-negative individuals.

Chapter 36

STD and HIV Screening Recommendations

STD and HIV Screening Recommendations

If you are sexually active, getting tested for STDs is one of the most important things you can do to protect your health. Make sure you have an open and honest conversation about your sexual history and STD testing with your doctor and ask whether you should be tested for STDs. If you are not comfortable talking with your regular health care provider about STDs, there are many clinics that provide confidential and free or low-cost testing.

Below is a brief overview of STD testing recommendations.

All adults and adolescents from ages 13 to 64 should be tested at least once for HIV.

Annual chlamydia screening of all sexually active women younger than 25 years, as well as older women with risk factors such as new or multiple sex partners, or a sex partner who has a sexually transmitted infection

This chapter contains text excerpted from the following sources: Text under the heading "STD & HIV Screening Recommendations" is excerpted from "STD & HIV Screening Recommendations," Centers for Disease Control and Prevention (CDC), June 30, 2014; Text under the heading "Screening Recommendations Referenced in Treatment Guidelines and Original Recommendation Sources" is excerpted from "Screening Recommendations Referenced in Treatment Guidelines and Original Recommendation Sources," Centers for Disease Control and Prevention (CDC), June 4, 2015.

Annual gonorrhea screening for all sexually active women younger than 25 years, as well as older women with risk factors such as new or multiple sex partners, or a sex partner who has a sexually transmitted infection.

Syphilis, HIV, chlamydia, and hepatitis B screening for all pregnant women, and gonorrhea screening for at-risk pregnant women starting early in pregnancy, with repeat testing as needed, to protect the health of mothers and their infants.

Screening at least once a year for syphilis, chlamydia, and gonorrhea for all sexually active gay, bisexual, and other men who have sex with men (MSM). MSM who have multiple or anonymous partners should be screened more frequently for STDs (i.e., at 3-to-6 month intervals).

Anyone who has unsafe sex or shares injection drug equipment should get tested for HIV at least once a year. Sexually active gay and bisexual men may benefit from more frequent testing (e.g., every 3 to 6 months).

Screening Recommendations Referenced in Treatment Guidelines and Original Recommendation Sources

Chlamydia

Women

- Sexually active women under 25 years of age.

- Sexually active women aged 25 years and older if at increased risk.

- Retest approximately 3 months after treatment.

Pregnant Women

- All pregnant women under 25 years of age.

- Pregnant women, aged 25 and older if at increased risk.

- Retest during the 3rd trimester for women under 25 years of age or at risk.

- Pregnant women with chlamydial infection should have a test-of-cure 3–4 weeks after treatment and be retested within 3 months.

Men

- Consider screening young men in high prevalence clinical settings or in populations with high burden of infection (e.g. MSM)

Men Who have Sex With Men (MSM)

- At least annually for sexually active MSM at sites of contact (urethra, rectum) regardless of condom use.

- Every 3 to 6 months if at increased risk.

Persons with HIV

- For sexually active individuals, screen at first HIV evaluation, and at least annually thereafter.

- More frequent screening for might be appropriate depending on individual risk behaviors and the local epidemiology.

Syphilis

Pregnant Women

- All pregnant women at the first prenatal visit.

- Retest early in the third trimester and at delivery if at high risk.

Men Who have Sex With Men (MSM)

- At least annually for sexually active MSM.

- Every 3 to 6 months if at increased risk.

Persons with HIV

- For sexually active individuals, screen at first HIV evaluation, and at least annually thereafter.

- More frequent screening might be appropriate depending on individual risk behaviors and the local epidemiology.

Trichomonas

Women

- Consider for women receiving care in high-prevalence settings (e.g., STD clinics and correctional facilities) and for women at high risk for infection (e.g., women with multiple sex partners, exchanging sex for payment, illicit drug use, and a history of STD).

Persons with HIV

- Recommended for sexually active women at entry to care and at least annually thereafter.

Herpes

Women

- Type-specific HSV serologic testing should be considered for women presenting for an STD evaluation (especially for women with multiple sex partners).

Pregnant Women

- Evidence does not support routine HSV-2 serologic screening among asymptomatic pregnant women. However, type-specific serologic tests might be useful for identifying pregnant women at risk for HSV infection and guiding counseling regarding the risk for acquiring genital herpes during pregnancy.

Men

- Type-specific HSV serologic testing should be considered for men presenting for an STD evaluation (especially for men with multiple sex partners).

Men Who have Sex with Men (MSM)

- Type-specific serologic tests can be considered if infection status is unknown in MSM with previously undiagnosed genital tract infection.

Persons with HIV

- Type-specific HSV serologic testing should be considered for persons presenting for an STD evaluation (especially for those persons with multiple sex partners), persons with HIV infection, and MSM at increased risk for HIV acquisition.

HIV

Women

- All women aged 13–64 years
- All women who seek evaluation and treatment for STDs

Pregnant Women

- All pregnant women should be screened at first prenatal visit (opt-out)
- Retest in the third trimester if at high risk

Men

- All men aged 13–64
- All men who seek evaluation and treatment for STDs

Men Who have Sex with Men (MSM)

- At least annually for sexually active MSM if HIV status is unknown or negative and the patient himself or his sex partner(s) have had more than one sex partner since most recent IIIV test.

Cervical Cancer

Women

- Women 21–29 years of age every 3 years with cytology.
- Women 30–65 years of age every 3 years with cytology, or every 5 years with a combination of cytology and HPV testing.

Pregnant Women

- Pregnant women should be screened at same intervals as non-pregnant women.
- Men at increased risk.

Persons with HIV

- Women should be screened within 1 year of sexual activity or initial HIV diagnosis using conventional or liquid-based cytology; testing should be repeated 6 months later.

Hepatitis B Screening

Women

- Women at increased risk.

Pregnant Women

- Test for HBsAg at first prenatal visit of each pregnancy regardless of prior testing; retest at delivery if at high risk.

Men

- Men at increased risk.
- Men Who have Sex With Men (MSM).
- All MSM should be tested for HbsAg.

Persons with HIV

- Test for HBsAg and anti-HBc and/or anti-HBs.

Hepatitis C Screening

Women

- Women born between 1945–1965.
- Other women If risk factors are present.

Pregnant Women

- Pregnant women born between 1945–1965.
- Other pregnant women if risk factors are present.

Men

- Men born between 1945–1965.
- Other men If risk factors are present.
- Men Who have Sex with Men (MSM).
- MSM born between 1945–1965.
- Other MSM if risk factors are present.
- Annual HCV testing in MSM with HIV infection.

Persons with HIV

- Serologic testing at initial evaluation.
- Annual HCV testing in MSM with HIV infection.

Chapter 37

Talking to Your Health Care Professional about STDs

Chapter Contents

Section 37.1

Talking about Your Health

This section includes text excerpted from "Questions to Ask
Your Doctor," Agency for Heathcare Research and Quality
(AHRQ), U.S. Department of Health and Human Services
(HHS), September 2012. Reviewed April 2016.

Questions Are the Answers

Asking questions and providing information to your doctor and
other care providers can improve your care. Talking with your
doctor builds trust and leads to better results, quality, safety, and
satisfaction.

Quality health care is a team effort. You play an important role.
One of the best ways to communicate with your doctor and health care
team is by asking questions. Because time is limited during medical
appointments, you will feel less rushed if you prepare your questions
before your appointment.

Your Doctor Wants Your Questions

Doctors know a lot about a lot of things, but they don't always know
everything about you or what is best for you. Your questions give your
doctor and health care team important information about you, such
as your most important health care concerns. That is why they need
you to speak up.

Questions You Should Know

A simple question can help you feel better, let you take better care
of yourself, or save your life. The questions below can get you started.

- What is the test for?

- How many times have you done this procedure?

- When will I get the results?

- Why do I need this treatment?

- Are there any alternatives?

- What are the possible complications?

- Which hospital is best for my needs?

- How do you spell the name of that drug?

- Are there any side effects?

- Will this medicine interact with medicines that I'm already taking?

Before Your Appointment

You can make sure you get the best possible care by being an active member of your health care team. Being involved means being prepared and asking questions.

Asking questions about your diagnoses, treatments, and medicines can improve the quality, safety, and effectiveness of your health care. Taking steps before your medical appointments will help you to make the most of your time with your doctor and health care team.

Prepare Your Questions

Time is limited during doctor visits. Prepare for your appointment by thinking about what you want to do during your next visit. Do you want to:

- Talk about a health problem?

- Get or change a medicine?

- Get medical tests?

- Talk about surgery or treatment options?

Write down your questions to bring to your appointment. The answers can help you make better decisions, get good care, and feel better about your health care.

During Your Appointment

During your appointment, make sure to ask the questions you prepared before your appointment. Start by asking the ones that are most important to you. To get the most from your visit, tell the nurse or person at the front desk that you have questions for your doctor. If your doctor does not ask you if you have questions, ask your doctor when the best time would be to ask them.

Understand the Answers and Next Steps

Asking questions is important but so is making sure you hear—and understand—the answers you get. Take notes. Or bring someone to your appointment to help you understand and remember what you heard. If you don't understand or are confused, ask your doctor to explain the answer again.

It is very important to understand the plan or next steps that your doctor recommends. Ask questions to make sure you understand what your doctor wants you to do.

The questions you may want to ask will depend on whether your doctor gives you a diagnosis; recommends a treatment, medical test, or surgery; or gives you a prescription for medicine.

Questions could include:

- What is my diagnosis?

- What are my treatment options? What are the benefits of each option? What are the side effects?

- Will I need a test? What is the test for? What will the results tell me?

- What will the medicine you are prescribing do? How do I take it? Are there any side effects?

- Why do I need surgery? Are there other ways to treat my condition? How often do you perform this surgery?

- Do I need to change my daily routine?

After Your Appointment

After you meet with your doctor, you will need to follow his or her instructions to keep your health on track.

Your doctor may have you fill a prescription or make an appointment for tests, lab work, or a follow-up visit. It is important for you to follow your doctor's instructions.

It also is important to call your doctor if you are unclear about any instructions or have more questions.

Prioritize Your Questions

Create a list of follow-up questions to ask if you:

- Have a health problem
- Need to get or change a medicine
- Need a medical test
- Need to have surgery

Other Times to Call Your Doctor

There are other times when you should follow up on your care and call your doctor. Call your doctor:

- If you experience any side effects or other problems with your medicines.
- If your symptoms get worse after seeing the doctor.
- If you receive any new prescriptions or start taking any over-the-counter medicines.
- To get results of any tests you've had. Do not assume that no news is good news.
- To ask about test results you do not understand.

Your questions help your doctor and health care team learn more about you. Your doctor's answers to your questions can help you make better decisions, receive a higher level of care, avoid medical harm, and feel better about your health care. Your questions can also lead to better results for your health.

Section 37.2

General Questions to Ask Your Health Care Professional about STDs

"Talking to Your Health Care Professional about STDs," © 2016
Omnigraphics, Inc. Reviewed April 2016.

Talking about Sexual Health

Talking to a health care professional about your sexual health may be highly intimidating and outside of your comfort zone. You may feel hesitant or scared to talk about it, but it is important to understand that talking with your healthcare professional about your sexual health is as important as talking about your physical health.

Why Should I talk to My Healthcare Provider about STDs?

The only way to be certain about whether or not you have an STD is to talk to your healthcare professional about being tested for an STD. Many STD symptoms are non-specific, meaning the symptoms could be caused by a number of STDs or a totally unrelated disease. Whether you have symptoms that lead you to believe you have an STD or if you are just unsure, the only way to be certain is to be tested specifically for an STD.

Talking to Your Healthcare Professional

When you meet with your healthcare professional, do not shy away from telling the truth. If necessary set boundaries with your professional and let them know what you are comfortable with when dealing with and discussing your body. But your provider needs to know some personal information about you like your sexual history, any symptoms you have etc...

By being honest and establishing trust with your healthcare professional you will help them diagnose the problem correctly, and provide you with the best possible treatment options. The good news is STDs are curable!

Questions to Ask Your Healthcare Professional

Preparing yourself before meeting your healthcare professional covering a wide range of topics from changes in sex drive, dealing with sex during pregnancy, pain during sex, what form of contraception would be best etc... is very important. It will help you get a complete picture of your sexual health. Some possible questions you can ask your healthcare professional include:

- What is an STD? What should I do to be absolutely sure of preventing it?
- How will I know if I have an STD?
- Some of my symptoms points towards STD. Do I have an STD?
- How will I know if my partner has an STD?
- Should my partner and I get tested for STDs before having sex?
- How often should I check for sexually transmitted infections (STIs)?
- Can contraception or vaccines protect me from getting STDs?
- There is a change in my sex drive. Do you think I may have an STD?
- What are the recommended screenings for STDs? Where can I get them done?
- What are the costs for STDs testing? Does my insurance cover them?
- Are STDs curable?
- Should I notify my partner on my STD status?
- Can I get any help from Partner Services to notify my partner on my STD status?
- Can I recover completely with proper treatment?

Remember that your healthcare professional is there to help you. Their experience will help you deal with your problem.

References

1. "Ten Questions to Ask." American Sexual Health Association, 2016.
2. "Know the Facts, Keep Yourself Healthy." Within Reach, 2015.
3. "Frequently Asked Questions about STDs." Vermont Department of Health, 2016.
4. "STD Testing." Healthline, 2014.

Section 37.3

For Teens: How Do I Discuss Embarrassing Things with My Doctor?

This section includes text excerpted from "Questions to Ask Your Doctor," Office of Women's Health (OWH), October 31, 2013.

Talking with Your Doctor

Talking freely with your doctor can make you feel better and gives your doctor the information she or he needs to give you the best care. You can even discuss personal things about your health with your doctor. Don't be afraid or embarrassed to discuss something that is bothering you.

Tips for Talking with Your Doctor

1. **Stay positive.** Go to your doctor's visits with a good attitude. Remember, your doctor and other caregivers are on your side. Think teamwork! Think positive!

2. **Keep track of how you are feeling**. Before your doctor visit, keep notes on how you are feeling. This will make it easier for you to answer questions about your symptoms and how medicines make you feel. It also makes it easier for you to bring up anything that you are worried about. Make sure to be honest about how you feel and how long you've felt that way. Also, let your doctor know if you are you scared, worried, or sad. Your care will be better if your doctor knows how you are feeling. Your doctor can also tell you about counselors and support groups to help you talk about your feelings. Find support groups.

3. **Bring your medical history, including a list of your current medicines**. If you're seeing a doctor for the first time, bring your medical history. Your medical history is a list of your illnesses, dates of operations, treatments (including medicines), names of doctors you've seen, what the doctors told you to do,

and anything else you think your doctor should know. If you take medicines that you buy at the pharmacy without a prescription (an order from the doctor), make sure to also include them in your list. That includes things like vitamins, herbal medicines, and aspirin. Also, if you are allergic to any medicines, such as penicillin, be sure to mention that to your doctor.

4. **Ask questions**. Do not be afraid to ask your doctor any questions you have. This will help you understand your own health better. Maybe you've been reading a lot about your health condition and that has caused you to think of some questions. To remember all the questions you have when you are not in the doctor's office, write them down and bring the list with you to your appointment. Be sure to talk with your parents about the things you want to ask the doctor. This will make getting answers even easier!

At your appointment, your doctor may talk about a new treatment that he or she wants you to try. It may involve medicine, surgery, changes in daily habits such as what you eat, or a few of these together. You will get the most out of your treatments if you understand what's involved and why you need them. In case your doctor talks about a new treatment at your next visit, here are some questions you can print or write down to take with you:

- How long will it take?

- What will happen? (Is it a shot, pill, or operation?)

- Will it hurt?

- How many treatments do I have to have?

- Will I be able to go to school?

- Are there things I won't be able to do, such as ride a bike?

- Is this treatment to try to cure my health problem or help take away some of my symptoms?

- Will these treatments make me tired or feel pain? How long will this last?

- What happens if I miss a treatment?

- What will we do if the treatments don't work?

- Is this the best treatment out there for me?

- What will happen to me if I don't have this treatment?

If the treatment you get makes you feel bad, ask if there are others you can try. There may not be others. But you and your doctor can talk about it.

Remember—there's no such thing as a stupid question. If you don't understand the answer to a question, ask the doctor to explain it again until you do understand

Write down what the doctor says. This will help you remember important information later on. You might even bring a tape recorder and record what the doctor says. But if you bring a tape recorder, be sure to ask the doctor first if it's okay to use it.

Talking about Personal Things

It's okay to be nervous about talking to your doctor about things that embarrass you. Who wants to talk to a strange adult about sex, feeling sad, or what you eat? But it's easier than you think. Doctors are there to talk about everything that is going on with your body. They will not think any less of you no matter what you ask or what your problem is. In fact, they are very used to personal issues (and they likely have had to seek help for their own!). Telling them everything that is going on with you is very important for your health. By not telling them about a strange smell, rash, pain, or anything else going on with your body, you could be making a health problem worse.

Talking about personal issues with your doctor can be confidential, which means that your doctor has to keep everything you say secret. Doctors might feel they have to tell your parents what you say if they think you are in danger or aren't able to make choices on your own. Ask your doctor about the privacy policy before you begin.

Chapter 38

Confidentiality Issues Associated with STD Testing

Chapter Contents

Section 38.1

Anonymous Testing for STDs Like HIV

This section includes text excerpted from "Confidential and
Anonymous Testing," U.S. Department of Health and Human
Services (HHS), May 6, 2015.

HIV Test Results and Privacy Issues

HIV test results fall under the same privacy rules as all of your medical information. Information about your HIV test cannot be released without your permission. The Health Insurance Portability and Accountability Act of 1996 (HIPAA) ensures that the privacy of individuals' health information is protected while ensuring access to care. However it is important to note that not all HIV testing sites are bound by HIPAA regulations. Before you get tested be sure to inquire about the privacy rules of the HIV test site as well those surrounding your test results.

Available Testing Services

HIV tests can be taken either confidentially or anonymously. Most states offer both anonymous and confidential testing, however some states only offer confidential testing services.

- **Confidential testing** means that your name and other identifying information will be attached to your test results. The results will go in your medical record and may be shared with your healthcare providers and your insurance company. Otherwise, the results are protected by state and Federal privacy laws.

- **Anonymous testing** means that nothing ties your test results to you. When you take an anonymous HIV test, you get a unique identifier that allows you to get your test results. Not all HIV test sites offer anonymous testing. Contact your local health department or 1-800-CDC-INFO (800-232-4636) to see if there are anonymous test sites in your area.

With confidential testing, if you test positive for HIV or another sexually transmitted infection (STI), the test result and your name will be reported to the state or local health department to help public health officials get better estimates of the rates of HIV in the state. The state health department will then remove all personal information about you (name, address, etc.) and share the remaining non-identifying information with CDC. CDC does not share this information with anyone else, including insurance companies.

If you have concerns regarding who can have access to your tests results, it is important to ask your testing center about their privacy policies and whom they are required to report a positive result to.

Frequently Asked Questions

Do the Results of My HIV Test Become Part of My Medical Records?

Yes. Unless you take an anonymous HIV test, your test results (positive or negative) are like any other medical test and are a part of your medical record.

Can My Insurance Company Find out That I Took an HIV Test, or Even Drop My Insurance Coverage for Taking One?

Usually laboratories aren't required to share test results with anyone other than the person tested and the medical professional who ordered the test. This does vary from state to state and among different insurance plans. Thanks to the Affordable Care Act (ACA), your insurance company can't turn you down, drop you, or charge you more because of a pre-existing health condition like HIV.

Section 38.2

Confidentiality for Adolescents Who Seek STD Testing and Care

This section includes text excerpted from "Special Populations,"
Centers for Disease Control and Prevention (CDC), June 4, 2015.

Adolescents

In the United States, prevalence rates of many sexually acquired
infections are highest among adolescents and young adults. For example, the reported rates of chlamydia and gonorrhea are highest among
females during their adolescent and young adult years, and many
persons acquire HPV infection at this time.

Persons who initiate sex early in adolescence are at higher risk for
STDs, along with adolescents residing in detention facilities, those
who use injection drugs, adolescents attending STD clinics, and young
men who have sex with men (YMSM). Factors contributing to this
increased risk during adolescence include having multiple sexual partners concurrently, having sequential sexual partnerships of limited
duration, failing to use barrier protection consistently and correctly,
having increased biologic susceptibility to infection, and facing multiple obstacles to accessing health care.

All 50 states and the District of Columbia explicitly allow minors
to consent for their own health services for STDs. No state requires
parental consent for STD care, although some states restrict a minor's
ability to provide consent on the basis of age or type of service (i.e., prevention, diagnosis, or treatment only). No state requires that providers
notify parents that an adolescent minor has received STD services,
except in limited or unusual circumstances. However, many states
authorize parental notification of a minor's receipt of STD services,
even where the minor can legally provide his or her own consent to the
service. Protecting confidentiality for such care, particularly for adolescents enrolled in private health insurance plans, presents multiple
problems. After a claim has been reported, many states mandate that
health plans provide a written statement to the beneficiary indicating

the service performed, the charges covered, what the insurer allows, and the amount for which the patient is responsible (i.e., explanation of benefit [EOB]). In addition, federal laws obligate notices to beneficiaries when claims are denied, including alerting beneficiaries who need to pay for care until the allowable deductible is reached. For STD detection- and treatment-related care, an EOB or medical bill that is received by a parent might disclose services provided and list STD laboratory tests performed or treatment given.

Despite the high rates of infections documented in the adolescent population, providers frequently fail to inquire about sexual behaviors, assess STD risks, provide risk-reduction counseling, and ultimately, screen for asymptomatic infections during clinical encounters. Discussions concerning sexual behavior should be appropriate for the patient's developmental level and should be aimed at identifying risk behaviors (e.g., multiple partners; unprotected oral, anal, or vaginal sex; and drug-use behaviors). Careful, nonjudgmental, and thorough counseling is particularly vital for adolescents who might not feel comfortable acknowledging their engagement in behaviors that place them at high risk for STDs.

Section 38.3

At-Home/Mail Order STD Tests Protect Patient Confidentiality

This section contains text excerpted from the following sources: Text beginning with the heading "Testing for HIV" is excerpted from "Testing for HIV," U.S. Food and Drug Administration (FDA), August 8, 2013; Text under the heading "Home Tests" is excerpted from "Home Tests," Centers for Disease Control and Prevention (CDC), October 16, 2015; Text under the heading "Home Access HIV-1 Test System" is excerpted from "Information regarding the Home Access HIV-1 Test System," U.S. Food and Drug Administration (FDA), October 2, 2012. Reviewed April 2016; Text under the heading "OraQuick In-Home HIV Test" is excerpted from "Information regarding the OraQuick In-Home HIV Test," U.S. Food and Drug Administration (FDA), June 18, 2014.

Testing for HIV

The U.S. Food and Drug Administration (FDA) regulates the tests that detect infection with Human Immunodeficiency Virus (HIV), the virus that causes AIDS. AIDS is a serious disease that can be fatal because the body has lost the ability to fight infections and cancers. There are a number of options for people to be tested for HIV, using tests approved by FDA:

1. Trained health professionals collect a sample and run the test in a professional medical setting. You receive your test results from a trained health professional.

2. You collect a sample in the home, forward the sample to a medical laboratory, and trained health professionals run the test in the medical laboratory.

3. You collect a sample, run the test, and obtain your own test results in your home.

How Do I Decide Which Test Is Best for Me?

There are many different factors to consider when deciding which test to use. These include your need for anonymity, the accuracy of the test should you be infected with HIV (the test sensitivity) or not infected with HIV (the test specificity), whether you need to have additional testing done to confirm a positive result, the type of sample needed (for example, blood vs. oral fluid), the time it takes to get a test result, and how you receive your test results (self-read and self-interpreted or from a healthcare professional). You should take the time to understand these differences and decide what factors are most important to you when choosing the way to test, whether through a healthcare professional or by using an over-the-counter HIV test.

When Should I Be Tested?

If you actively engage in behavior that puts you at risk for HIV infection, or your partner engages in such behavior, then you should consider testing on a regular basis. Most HIV tests detect antibodies to the virus. However, it can take some time for the immune system to produce enough antibodies for the test to detect, and this time period can vary from person to person. This timeframe is commonly referred to as the "window period," when a person is infected with HIV but the antibodies to the virus cannot be detected, however, the person may be able to infect others. According to the Centers for Disease Control and Prevention, although it can take up to six months to develop antibodies for HIV, most people (97%) will develop detectable antibodies in the first three months following the time of their infection.

Home Test

Currently there are only two home HIV tests: the Home Access HIV-1 Test System and the OraQuick In-home HIV test. If you buy your home test online make sure the HIV test is FDA-approved.

The Home Access HIV-1 Test System is a home collection kit, which involves pricking your finger to collect a blood sample, sending the sample to a licensed laboratory, and then calling in for results as early as the next business day. This test is anonymous. If the test is positive, a follow-up test is performed right away, and the results include the follow-up test. The manufacturer provides confidential counseling and referral to treatment. The tests conducted on the blood sample collected at home find infection later after infection than most lab-based tests using blood from a vein, but earlier than tests conducted with oral fluid.

The OraQuick In-Home HIV Test provides rapid results in the home. The testing procedure involves swabbing your mouth for an oral fluid sample and using a kit to test it. Results are available in 20 minutes. If you test positive, you will need a follow-up test. The manufacturer provides confidential counseling and referral to follow-up testing sites. Because the level of antibody in oral fluid is lower than it is in blood, oral fluid tests find infection later after exposure than do blood tests. Up to 1 in 12 infected people may test false-negative with this test.

Home Access HIV-1 Test System

What Is the Home Access HIV-1 Test System?

The Home Access HIV-1 Test System is a laboratory test sold over-the-counter (OTC) that uses fingerstick blood mailed to the testing laboratory. The test kit consists of multiple components, including materials for specimen self-collection, prepaid materials for mailing the specimen to a laboratory for testing, testing directions, an information booklet ("Things You Should Know about HIV And AIDS"), an anonymous registration system and a call center to receive your test results and follow-up counseling by telephone.

This approved system uses a finger prick process for home blood collection which results in dried blood spots on special paper. The dried blood spots are mailed to a laboratory with a confidential and anonymous unique personal identification number (PIN), and are analyzed by trained clinicians in a laboratory using the same tests that are used for samples taken in a doctor's office or clinic. Test results are obtained through a toll free telephone number using the PIN, and post-test counseling is provided by telephone when results are obtained.

When Should I Take a Test for HIV?

If you actively engage in behavior that puts you at risk for HIV infection, or your partner engages in such behavior, then you should consider testing on a regular basis. It may take some time for the immune system to produce sufficient antibodies for the test to detect, and this time period can vary from person to person. This time-frame is commonly referred to as the "window period," when a person is infected with HIV but antibodies to the virus cannot be detected, however, the person may be able to infect others. According to the Centers for Disease Control and Prevention, it can take up to 6 months to develop antibodies to HIV, although most people (97%) will develop detectable antibodies in the first 3 months following the time of their infection.

How Reliable Is the Home Access HIV-1 Test System?

Clinical studies reported to FDA showed that the sensitivity (i.e., the percentage of results that will be positive when HIV is present) was estimated to be greater than 99.9%. The specificity (i.e., the percentage of results that will be negative when HIV is not present) was also estimated to be greater than 99.9%. Results reported as positive have undergone testing using both a screening test and another test to confirm the positive result.

What about Counseling?

The Home Access HIV-1 Test System has a built-in mechanism for pre-test and post-test counseling provided by the manufacturer. This counseling is anonymous and confidential. Counseling, which uses both printed material and telephone interaction, provides the user with an interpretation of the test result. Counseling also provides information on how to keep from getting infected if you are negative, and how to prevent further transmission of disease if you are infected. Counseling provides you with information about treatment options if you are infected, and can even provide referrals to doctors who treat HIV-infected individuals in your area.

If the Test Results Are Positive, What Should I Do?

The counselors can provide you with information about treatment options and referrals to doctors who treat HIV-infected individuals in your area.

Do I Need a Confirmatory Test?

No, a positive result from the Home Access HIV-1 Test System means that antibodies to the HIV-1 virus are present in the blood sample submitted to the testing laboratory. The Home Access HIV-1 Test System includes confirmatory testing for HIV-1, and all confirmation testing is completed before the results are released and available to users of the test system.

How Quickly Will I Get the Results of the Home Access HIV-1 Test System?

You can anonymously call for the results approximately 7 business days (3 business days for the Express System) after shipping your specimen to the laboratory by using the unique PIN on the tear-off

443

label included with your test kit. This label includes both the unique PIN and the toll-free number for the counseling center.

How Are Unapproved Test Systems Different?

The manufacturers of unapproved test systems have not submitted data to FDA to review to determine whether or not their test systems can reliably detect HIV infection. Therefore, FDA cannot give the public any assurance that the results obtained using an unapproved test system are accurate.

How Can I Obtain Additional Information about the Test?

Information on the Home Access HIV-1 Test System can be found on FDA's website.

How the OraQuick In-Home HIV Test Works?

What Is the OraQuick In-Home HIV Test and How Does It Work?

The OraQuick In-Home HIV Test is a rapid self-administered over-the-counter (OTC) test. The OraQuick In-Home HIV Test kit consists of a test stick (device) to collect the specimen, a test tube (vial) to insert the test stick (device) and complete the test, testing directions, two information booklets ("HIV, Testing and Me" and "What your results mean to you"), a disposal bag and phone numbers for consumer support.

This approved test uses oral fluid to check for antibodies to HIV Type 1 and HIV Type 2, the viruses that cause AIDS. The kit is designed to allow you to take the HIV test anonymously and in private with the collection of an oral fluid sample by swabbing your upper and lower gums with the test device. After collecting the sample you insert the device into the kit's vial which contains a developer solution, wait 20–40 minutes, and read the test result. A positive result with this test does not mean that an individual is definitely infected with HIV but rather that additional testing should be done in a medical setting to confirm the test result. Additionally, a negative test result does not mean that an individual is definitely not infected with HIV, particularly when exposure may have been within the previous three months. Again an individual should obtain a confirmatory test in a medical setting.

When Should I Take a Test for HIV?

If you actively engage in behavior that puts you at risk for HIV infection, or your partner engages in such behavior, then you should consider testing on a regular basis. It can take some time for the immune system to produce enough antibodies for the test to detect, and this time period can vary from person to person. This timeframe is commonly referred to as the "window period," when a person is infected with HIV but antibodies to the virus can not be detected, however, the person may be able to infect others. According to the Centers for Disease Control and Prevention, although it can take up to 6 months to develop antibodies for HIV, most people (97%) will develop detectable antibodies in the first 3 months following the time of their infection.

How Reliable Is the OraQuick In-Home HIV Test?

As noted in the package insert, clinical studies have shown that the OraQuick In-Home HIV Test has an expected performance of approximately 92% for test sensitivity (i.e., the percentage of results that will be positive when HIV is present). This means that one false negative result would be expected out of every 12 test results in HIV infected individuals. The clinical studies also showed that the Ora-Quick In-Home HIV Test has an expected performance of 99.98% for test specificity (i.e., the percentage of results that will be negative when HIV is not present). This means that one false positive result would be expected out of every 5,000 test results in uninfected individuals.

It is extremely important for those who self-test using the OraQuick In-Home HIV Test to carefully read and follow all labeled directions. Even when used according to the labeled directions, there will be some false negative results and a small number of false positive results. The OraQuick test package contains step-by-step instructions, and there is also an OraQuick Consumer Support Center to assist users in the testing process.

Results

If the Test Says I'm HIV Positive, What Should I Do?

A positive test result does not necessarily mean that you are infected with HIV. If you test positive for HIV using the OraQuick In-Home Test, you should see your healthcare provider or call the

OraQuick Consumer Support Center, which has support center representatives available 24 hours a day/7 days a week to answer your questions and provide referrals to local healthcare providers for follow-up care. You will be advised to obtain confirmatory testing to confirm a positive result or inform you that the initial result was a false positive result. The test kit also contains an information booklet, "What your results mean to You," which is designed to instruct individuals on what to do once they have obtained their test results.

Do I Need a Confirmatory Test?

A positive test result on the OraQuick In-Home HIV Test indicates that you may be infected with HIV. Additional testing in a medical setting will either confirm a positive test result or inform you that the initial result was a false positive result.

What Is A "False Positive" Result?

A "false positive" result occurs when an individual not infected with the HIV virus receives a test result that indicates that he or she is infected with HIV.

If the Test Says I'm HIV Negative, What Should I Do?

A negative result on this test does not necessarily mean that you are not infected with HIV. The OraQuick test kit contains an information booklet, "What your results mean to You," which is designed to instruct individuals on what to do once they have obtained their test results. The test is relatively reliable if there has been sufficient time for HIV antibodies to develop in the infected person. For the OraQuick In-Home HIV Test, that period of time, called the window period, is about three months. If you have recently been engaging in behavior that puts you at high risk for HIV infection, you should take the test again at a later time. Alternatively, you should see your health care provider who can discuss other options for HIV testing.

What Is A "False Negative" Result?

A "false negative" result occurs when an HIV-infected individual receives a test result that incorrectly indicates that he or she is not infected with HIV.

How Quickly Will I Get the Results of the OraQuick Test?

You can read the results of the OraQuick In-Home HIV Test within 20 to 40 minutes.

Comparison

How Are Unapproved Test Systems Different?

The manufacturers of unapproved test systems have not submitted data to FDA in order for FDA to review and determine whether their test systems can reliably detect HIV infection. Therefore, FDA cannot give the public any assurance that the results obtained using an unapproved test system are accurate.

Chapter 39

Understanding Antibiotic Resistance and STD Treatment

Antibiotic Resistance Threats in the United States

Antibiotics are powerful tools for fighting illness and disease, but overuse of antibiotics has helped create bacteria that are outliving the drugs used to treat them.

Antibiotic resistance is a quickly growing, extremely dangerous problem. World health leaders have described antibiotic-resistant bacteria as "nightmare bacteria" that "pose a catastrophic threat" to people in every country in the world. Each year in the United States, at least 2 million people become infected with bacteria that are resistant to antibiotics, and at least 23,000 people die each year as a direct result of these infections. Many more people die from other conditions that were complicated by an antibiotic-resistant infection.

In addition, almost 250,000 people who are hospitalized or require hospitalization get Clostridium difficile each year, an infection usually related to antibiotic use. C. difficile causes deadly diarrhea and kills at least 14,000 people each year. Many C. difficile infections and drug-resistant infections can be prevented.

This chapter contains text excerpted from the following sources: Text under the heading "Antibiotic Resistance Threats in the US" is excerpted from "Antibiotic Resistance Threats in the US," Centers for Disease Control and Prevention (CDC), November 15, 2013; Text under the heading "Gonococcal Infections in Adolescents and Adults" is excerpted from "2015 Sexually Transmitted Diseases Treatment Guidelines," Centers for Disease Control and Prevention (CDC), June 4, 2015.

How Bacteria Become Resistant

When bacteria are exposed to antibiotics, they start learning how to outsmart the drugs. This process occurs in bacteria found in humans, animals, and the environment. Resistant bacteria can multiply and spread easily and quickly, causing severe infections. They can also share genetic information with other bacteria, making the other bacteria resistant as well. Each time bacteria learn to outsmart an antibiotic, treatment options are more limited, and these infections pose a greater risk to human health.

Infections Can Happen to Anyone, Anywhere

Anyone can become infected with antibiotic-resistant bacteria anywhere and anytime. Most infections occur in the community, like skin infections with MRSA and sexually transmitted diseases. However, most deaths related to antibiotic resistance occur from drug-resistant infections picked up in healthcare settings, such as hospitals and nursing homes.

What You Can Do to Protect Yourself Against Drug-Resistant Infections

There are many ways you can help prevent the creation and spread of resistance. First, when you are sick, do not demand antibiotics from your doctor or take antibiotics that were not prescribed to you directly for your specific illness. When taking antibiotics, do not skip doses, and make sure to follow the directions about dose and duration from your doctor.

- Second, like all diseases, common safety and hygiene methods can prevent disease and spread. Make sure to:
- Get updated and regular vaccinations against drug-resistant bacteria
- Wash your hands before eating and after using the restroom to avoid putting drug-resistant bacteria into your body
- Wash your hands after handling uncooked food to prevent ingesting drug-resistant bacteria that can live on food
- Cook meat and poultry thoroughly to kill bacteria, including potential drug-resistant bacteria

What Healthcare Providers Can Do to Protect Patients from Drug-Resistant Infections

There are many ways to help provide the best care to your patients while protecting them against antibiotic-resistant infections.

- Follow all necessary infection control recommendations, including hand hygiene, standard precautions, and contact precautions.

- Diagnose and treat resistant infections quickly and efficiently. Treatment options change often because resistance is complex. Make sure to follow the latest recommendations to ensure you are prescribing appropriately.

- Only prescribe antibiotics when likely to benefit the patient, and be sure to prescribe the right dose and duration.

- Be sure to clearly label dose, duration, and indication for treatment, and include appropriate laboratory diagnostic tests when placing antibiotic orders. This will help other clinicians caring for the patient to change or stop therapy when appropriate.

- Take an antibiotic time out, reassessing therapy after 48–72 hours. Once additional information is available, including microbiology, radiographic, and clinical information, a decision can be made on whether to continue the same therapy.

- When transferring patients, ensure the other facilities are notified of any infection or known colonization.

- Keep tabs on resistance patterns in your facility and in the area around your facility.

- Finally, encourage prevention methods with your patients. Make sure they understand how to protect themselves with vaccines, treatment, and infection control practices such as hand washing and safe food handling.

Chapter 40

Beware of Fake STD Treatment Products

Federal regulators say some companies are selling products that make unproven claims to treat sexually transmitted diseases—claims that could pose a threat to public health.

The Food and Drug Administration (FDA) says only prescription medicines and diagnostic tools available through a health care professional are effective for STD diagnosis and treatment.

FDA and the Federal Trade Commission (FTC) are warning manufacturers and distributors that they could face legal action if the products aren't removed from the market. The agencies say at least 15 products claim to treat, prevent, or cure STDs and are being sold online and at some retail outlets.

The products—some of which are sold as dietary supplements—claim to treat a range of sexually transmitted diseases, including herpes, chlamydia, genital warts, HIV, and AIDS. There are no non-prescription drugs or dietary supplements that can treat, cure, or prevent sexually transmitted disease. Condoms are the only non-prescription product that can prevent STDs by reducing the chance that an infected person will pass on the disease. STDs can only be diagnosed and treated under the supervision of a health care professional.

This chapter includes text excerpted from "FDA Warns: Beware of Bogus STD Products," U.S. Food and Drug Administration (FDA), July 25, 2015.

Some STDs have symptoms that include sores or a discharge, but the majority of infected people have no symptoms at all. Because of this, people who are sexually active, have had unprotected sex, or have been exposed to a sexually transmitted disease should get medical attention, especially if they have these symptoms:

- burning sensation with urination
- pelvic pain
- discharge from the penis or vagina
- blisters
- sores

There are FDA-approved medications available to treat many sexually transmitted diseases. These products have met federal standards for safety, effectiveness, and quality—and they're available only by prescription.

Part Five

STD Risks and Prevention

Chapter 41

Sexual Behaviors That Increase the Likelihood of STD Transmission

Chapter Contents

Section 41.1

Overview of Risky Sexual Behaviors

This section includes text excerpted from "Sexual Risk Behaviors: HIV, STD, and Teen Pregnancy Prevention," Centers for Disease Control and Prevention (CDC), February 16, 2016.

Sexual Risk Behaviors: HIV, STD, and Teen Pregnancy Prevention

Many young people engage in sexual risk behaviors that can result in unintended health outcomes. For example, among U.S. high school students surveyed in 2013

- 47% had ever had sexual intercourse.

- 34% had had sexual intercourse during the previous 3 months, and, of these

- 41% did not use a condom the last time they had sex.

- 15% had had sex with four or more people during their life.

- Only 22% of sexually experienced students have ever been tested for HIV.*

*CDC recommends all adolescents and adults 13–64 get tested for HIV at least once as part of routine medical care.

Sexual risk behaviors place adolescents at risk for HIV infection, other sexually transmitted diseases (STDs), and unintended pregnancy:

- Nearly 10,000 young people (aged 13–24) were diagnosed with HIV infection in the United States in 2013.

- Young gay and bisexual men (aged 13–24) accounted for an estimated 19% (8,800) of all new HIV infections in the United States, and 72% of new HIV infections among youth in 2010.

- Nearly half of the 20 million new STDs each year were among young people, between the ages of 15 to 24.

- Approximately 273,000 babies were born to teen girls aged 15–19 years in 2013.

To reduce sexual risk behaviors and related health problems among youth, schools and other youth-serving organizations can help young people adopt lifelong attitudes and behaviors that support their health and well-being—including behaviors that reduce their risk for HIV, other STDs, and unintended pregnancy. The National HIV/AIDS Strategy calls for all Americans to be educated about HIV. This includes knowing how HIV is transmitted and prevented, and knowing which behaviors place individuals at greatest risk for infection. HIV awareness and education should be universally integrated into all educational environments.

Section 41.2

HIV Risk among Sex Workers

This section includes text excerpted from "HIV Risk among Adult Sex Workers in the United States," Centers for Disease Control and Prevention (CDC), June 11, 2015.

Quick Facts

- Few population-based studies have been done on HIV risk and sex workers.

- The risk of HIV and other sexually transmitted infections is high among people who engage in sexual activity for income, employment, or non-monetary items, such as food, drugs, and shelter.

- Seeking care or reducing risk is sometimes difficult for sex workers living with HIV because of other social factors, such as poverty.

Sex work is defined as the use of sexual activity for income or employment or for non-monetary items, such as food, drugs, or shelter ("survival" sex). Sex work can increase a person's risk of becoming infected with or transmitting HIV and other sexually transmitted infections (STIs) by engaging in unsafe sexual behaviors and/or substance use.

Sex work crosses many socioeconomic groups. Adults who engage in such activities include high-end escorts; people who work in massage parlors and the adult film industry; exotic dancers; state-regulated prostitutes (in Nevada); and street-based men, women, and transgender people who participate in survival sex.

Reaching sex workers is a critical effort for public health. Not only are sex workers at risk for higher rates of HIV and other STIs, sex workers who are unaware of their HIV status can endanger their own health and increase their risk of transmitting HIV or STIs to others.

Prevention Challenges

Lack of Data

There are few population-based studies of sex workers in the United States or globally because sex work is a stigmatized occupation and is illegal throughout most of the United States and the world. Further, sex workers who work in settings where sex is encouraged and indirectly sold, such as massage parlors, the adult film industry, and exotic dance clubs, are often not included in studies. This lack of data and understanding around sex work creates a significant barrier to HIV prevention efforts and other services.

Socioeconomic Factors

Many sex workers face discrimination, poverty, and lack of access to health care and other social services—all of which pose obstacles to receiving HIV prevention efforts. Available research shows that

Sex workers may have a history of homelessness, mental health issues, incarceration, emotional/physical/ sexual abuse, and drug use. They may also be at risk for HIV infection or STIs because of multiple high-risk male partners.

Male-to-female transgender sex workers may view sex work as a viable option to earn money because of gender-based/societal discrimination and lack of employment. They may also use sex work to generate income for rent, drugs, hormones, gender-related surgeries, and to feel desired and feminine.

High-Risk Drug and Alcohol Use

There is a strong link between sex work and drug and alcohol use. Drug and alcohol use have been reported as coping mechanisms in response to stressful working conditions. Sex workers may have impaired judgment and difficulties negotiating safer sex (condom use, for example) with their customers while under the influence of drugs and alcohol.

Exchanging sex for drugs carries greater HIV risk than exchanging sex for money because sex workers often engage in riskier forms of sex work while under the influence of drugs. Specifically, sex workers who trade sex for drugs have more clients, use condoms less often, and are more likely to share needles and other drug works.

Knowledge of HIV Status

Nationally, approximately 18.1% of US adults and adolescents living with HIV infection in 2009 were unaware of their HIV infection, according to the Centers for Disease Control and Prevention (CDC). Many sex workers are not aware of available services such as HIV/STI testing and may not know if they are infected with HIV or other STIs, according to one study. They may also be uncomfortable with being tested for HIV or other STIs if questioned about their sexual and substance use histories. Some sex workers may know that they are living with HIV but may be reluctant to seek care or reduce their risk behaviors because of mistrust of the health care system, loss of income, drug dependency, and mental health issues.

Inconsistent Condom Use

Sex workers may not use condoms consistently. Several factors, including economics, partner type, and power dynamics contribute to this behavior. For example, sex workers may receive more money for unprotected than protected vaginal and anal sex. Further, sex workers report lower condom use with steady partners than with new or casual partners. Additionally, the unequal relationship between sex workers and clients, and substance use that is often associated with sex work, may make condom use challenging. Finally, in some jurisdictions in the United States, suspected sex workers who are caught with condoms in their possession can be arrested for suspicion of prostitution.

461

Section 41.3

Oral Sex and HIV Risk

This section includes text excerpted from "Oral Sex and
HIV Risk," Centers for Disease Control and
Prevention (CDC), October 27, 2015.

Quick Facts

- The risk of HIV transmission through oral sex is much less than
  that from anal or vaginal sex—but it is not zero.

- Performing oral sex on an HIV-infected man, with ejaculation in
  the mouth, is the riskiest oral sex activity.

- Factors that may increase the risk of HIV transmission through
  oral sex are oral ulcers, bleeding gums, genital sores, and the
  presence of other sexually transmitted diseases.

Oral sex involves giving or receiving oral stimulation (i.e., sucking
or licking) to the penis (fellatio), the vagina (cunnilingus), or the anus
(anilingus). HIV can be transmitted during any of these activities, but
the risk is much less than that from anal or vaginal sex. Receiving
fellatio, giving or receiving cunnilingus, and giving or receiving anilingus carry little to no risk. The highest oral sex risk is to individuals
performing fellatio on an HIV-infected man, with ejaculation in the
mouth.

Risk of HIV

Even though oral sex carries a lower risk of HIV transmission than
other sexual activities, the risk is not zero. It is difficult to measure the
exact risk because people who practice oral sex may also practice other
forms of sex during the same encounter. When transmission occurs,
it may be the result of oral sex or other, riskier sexual activities, such
as anal or vaginal sex.

If the person receiving oral sex has HIV, their blood, semen,
pre-seminal fluid, or vaginal fluid may contain the virus. If the person performing oral sex has HIV, blood from their mouth may enter

the body of the person receiving oral sex through the lining of the urethra (the opening at the tip of the penis), vagina, cervix, or anus, or through cuts and sores.

Several factors may increase the risk of HIV transmission through oral sex, including oral ulcers, bleeding gums, genital sores, and the presence of other sexually transmitted diseases (STDs).

Risk of Other Infections

In addition to HIV, other organisms can be transmitted through oral sex with an infected partner, leading to herpes, syphilis, gonorrhea, genital warts (human papillomavirus, or HPV), intestinal parasites (amebiasis), or hepatitis A or B infection.

Reducing the Risk

The following things can reduce the risk of getting HIV through oral sex:

- If giving oral sex, avoid having your partner ejaculate in your mouth.

- Use barriers, such as condoms, natural rubber latex sheets, dental dams, or cut-open nonlubricated condoms between your mouth and your partner's genitals or rectum.

The risk of getting HIV from oral sex is lower if you are already taking pre-exposure prophylaxis (PrEP) consistently and correctly or if your partner is living with HIV and is taking antiretroviral therapy (ART) consistently and correctly. PrEP is a drug (Truvada) that can be prescribed to people at substantial risk of HIV to prevent infection. ART is a combination of drugs to treat HIV in people who already have HIV.

Keep in mind that barrier methods are the only way to protect against some STDs, including gonorrhea of the throat. Although the chance of getting or transmitting HIV from rimming (mouth to rectum) is small, there is a greater chance of transmitting hepatitis A and B, parasites, and other bacteria to the partner who is doing the rimming. There are effective vaccines that protect against hepatitis A and B and the human papillomavirus infections (HPV).

Chapter 42

STDs and Substance Use

Chapter Contents

465

Section 42.1

HIV and Substance Use in the United States

This section includes text excerpted from "HIV and Substance Use in the United States," Centers for Disease Control and Prevention (CDC), October 27, 2015.

Quick Stats

- Substance use and abuse are important factors in the spread of HIV.

- Alcohol and other drugs can lower a person's inhibitions and create risk factors for HIV transmission.

- Vulnerable populations (people living in poverty, those who are mentally ill, and those with a history of abuse) are more likely to have high rates of alcohol and substance use.

Substance use, abuse, and dependence been closely associated with HIV infection since the beginning of the epidemic. Although injection drug use (IDU) is a direct route of transmission, drinking, smoking, ingesting, or inhaling drugs such as alcohol, crack cocaine, methamphetamine ("meth"), and amyl nitrite ("poppers") are also associated with increased risk for HIV infection. These substances may increase HIV risk by reducing users' inhibitions to engage in risky sexual behavior.

Substance use and addiction are public health concerns for many reasons. In addition to increasing the risk of HIV transmission, substance use can affect people's overall health and make them more susceptible to HIV infection and, in those already infected with HIV, substance use can hasten disease progression and negatively affect adherence to treatment.

Vulnerable Populations

- **People who live in poverty.** People who live in disadvantaged neighborhoods are more likely to have high rates of alcohol and illicit drug use.

466

- **Gay and bisexual men.** Alcohol and drug use among gay and bisexual men can be a reaction to homophobia, discrimination, or violence they experienced because of their sexual orientation and can contribute to other mental health problems. Compared with the general population, gay and bisexual men

  - Are more likely to use alcohol and drugs.

  - Are more likely to continue heavy drinking later in life.

  - Have higher rates of substance abuse.

- **People with a mental illness.** The coexistence of substance use and mental health disorders is common and is linked to poor impulse control and greater risk-taking and sensation-seeking behaviors.

- **People with a history of abuse.** People who have experienced sexual, physical, or emotional abuse are more likely to overuse drugs and alcohol and practice risky sexual behaviors.

Prevention Challenges

A number of factors contribute to the spread of HIV infection among substance users:

- **Sexual risk factors.** Substance use can decrease inhibitions and increase sexual risk factors for HIV transmission, including not using a condom.

- **Stigma and discrimination associated with substance use.** Often, drug use is viewed as a criminal activity rather than a medical issue that requires counseling and rehabilitation. Stigma may prevent users from seeking HIV testing, care, and treatment.

- **Differences among people who abuse drugs and alcohol.** Racial, ethnic, and gender differences, as well as differences in geographic location (urban vs. rural, region of the country), access to drug and alcohol treatment and HIV testing and counseling, and socioeconomic and cultural issues should be considered when developing and implementing prevention programs.

- **Complex health and social needs.** People who use drugs often have other complex health and social needs, including a need for treatment for substance abuse and mental disorders.

467

Comprehensive prevention strategies, including case management, are needed.

- **Effects on HIV treatment adherence.** Nonadherence can lead to medication-resistant viral strains. Because they fear dangerous side effects or dislike following a regimen that interrupts their drug-using activities, many HIV-infected substance users are less willing to start antiviral therapy than non–substance users, according to research.

Commonly Used Substances

Alcohol

Excessive alcohol consumption, notably binge drinking, is associated with multiple adverse health and social consequences and is sometimes linked to other drug use. Alcohol use can be an important risk factor for HIV infection because it is linked to less frequent use of condoms and to multiple sexual partners.

Crack Cocaine

Crack cocaine's short-lived high and addictiveness can create a compulsive cycle in which users quickly exhaust their resources and turn to other ways to get the drug, including trading sex for drugs or money, which increases HIV infection risk. African Americans account for the majority of people who use crack cocaine.

Compared to nonusers, crack cocaine users reported

- A greater number of recent and lifetime sexual partners.

- Infrequent condom use.

- Heightened sexual pleasure.

- Using more than one substance.

- Being less responsive to HIV prevention programs, according to recent studies.

Methamphetamine

"Meth" use is associated with increased HIV risk and has become a public health threat in recent years because, like alcohol and other substances, it is linked to high-risk sexual activity with nonsteady partners under the influence.

In addition,

- It is highly addictive and can be injected.

- It tends to dry out the skin on the penis and mucosal tissues in the anus and the vagina, which may lead to small tears and cuts during sex where the HIV can enter the body.

- Some gay and bisexual men combine meth with erectile dysfunction drugs that are also associated with unprotected anal sex.

The largest numbers of meth users are white males. According to one study, gay and bisexual men report using meth and other stimulants at rates approximately 9 times as high as the general population.

Inhalants

Like meth, use of amyl nitrite ("poppers") has also been associated with increased HIV risk. Nitrite inhalants have long been linked to risky sexual behaviors, illegal drug use, and sexually transmitted infections among gay and bisexual men and have recently been linked to increased use among adolescents because inhalants:

- Enhance sexual pleasure.

- Aid anal sex by increasing sensitivity and relaxing the sphincter, which may lead to more unprotected sex.

- Are commonly found, even in household products.

Section 42.2

Heroin and Risk of HIV/AIDS

This section includes text excerpted from "Why Does Heroin Use Create Special Risk for Contracting HIV/AIDS and Hepatitis B and C?" National Institute on Drug Abuse (NIDA), November 2014.

Why Does Heroin Use Create Special Risk for Contracting HIV/AIDS and Hepatitis B and C?

Heroin use increases the risk of being exposed to HIV, viral hepatitis, and other infectious agents through contact with infected blood or body fluids (e.g., semen, saliva) that results from the sharing of syringes and injection paraphernalia that have been used by infected individuals or through unprotected sexual contact with an infected person. Snorting or smoking does not eliminate the risk of infectious disease like hepatitis and HIV/AIDS because people under the influence of drugs still engage in risky sexual and other behaviors that can expose them to these diseases.

Injection drug users (IDUs) are the highest-risk group for acquiring hepatitis C (HCV) infection and continue to drive the escalating HCV epidemic: Each IDU infected with HCV is likely to infect 20 other people. Of the 17,000 new HCV infections occurring in the United States in 2010, over half (53 percent) were among IDUs. Hepatitis B (HBV) infection in IDUs was reported to be as high as 20 percent in the United States in 2010, which is particularly disheartening since an effective vaccine that protects against HBV infection is available. There is currently no vaccine available to protect against HCV infection.

Drug use, viral hepatitis and other infectious diseases, mental illnesses, social dysfunctions, and stigma are often co-occuring conditions that affect one another, creating more complex health challenges that require comprehensive treatment plans tailored to meet all of a patient's needs. For example, NIDA-funded research has found that drug abuse treatment along with HIV prevention and community-based outreach programs can help people who use drugs change the behaviors that put them at risk for contracting HIV and other infectious diseases. They can reduce drug use and drug-related risk behaviors such as needle sharing and unsafe sexual practices and, in turn, reduce the risk of exposure to HIV/AIDS and other infectious diseases. Only through coordinated utilization of effective antiviral therapies coupled with treatment for drug abuse and mental illness can the health of those suffering from these conditions be restored.

Chapter 43

Other Behaviors That Increase STD Risk

Chapter Contents

Section 43.1

Douching May Increase Risk of STDs

This section includes text excerpted from "Douching Fact Sheet,"
Office on Women's Health (OWH), November 19, 2014.

What Is Douching?

The word "douche" means to wash or soak. Douching is washing or
cleaning out the inside of the vagina with water or other mixtures of fluids. Most douches are sold in stores as prepackaged mixes of water and
vinegar, baking soda, or iodine. The mixtures usually come in a bottle or
bag. You squirt the douche upward through a tube or nozzle into your
vagina. The water mixture then comes back out through your vagina.

Douching is different from washing the outside of your vagina
during a bath or shower. Rinsing the outside of your vagina with
warm water will not harm your vagina. But, douching can lead to
many different health problems.

Most doctors recommend that women do not douche.

How Common Is Douching?

In the United States, almost one in four women 15 to 44 years old
douche.

More African-American and Hispanic women douche than white
women. Douching is also common in teens of all races and ethnicities.

Studies have not found any health benefit to douching. But, studies
have found that douching is linked to many health problems.

Why Should Women Not Douche?

Douching can change the necessary balance of vaginal flora (bacteria that live in the vagina) and natural acidity in a healthy vagina.

A healthy vagina has good and harmful bacteria. The balance of
bacteria helps maintain an acidic environment. The acidic environment protects the vagina from infections or irritation.

Douching can cause an overgrowth of harmful bacteria. This can lead to a yeast infection or bacterial vaginosis. If you already have a vaginal infection, douching can push the bacteria causing the infection up into the uterus, fallopian tubes, and ovaries. This can lead to pelvic inflammatory disease, a serious health problem.

Douching is also linked to other health problems.

What Health Problems Are Linked to Douching?

Health problems linked to douching include:

- Bacterial vaginosis (BV), which is an infection in the vagina. Women who douche often (once a week) are five times more likely to develop BV than women who do not douche.

- Pelvic inflammatory disease, an infection in the reproductive organs that is often caused by an STI

- Problems during pregnancy, including preterm birth and ectopic pregnancy

- STIs, including HIV

- Vaginal irritation or dryness

Researchers are studying whether douching causes these problems or whether women at higher risk for these health problems are more likely to douche.

Should I Douche to Get Rid of Vaginal Odor or Other Problems?

No. You should not douche to try to get rid of vaginal odor or other vaginal problems like discharge, pain, itching, or burning.

Douching will only cover up odor for a short time and will make other problems worse. Call your doctor or nurse if you have:

- Vaginal discharge that smells bad

- Vaginal itching and thick, white, or yellowish-green discharge with or without an odor

- Burning, redness, and swelling in or around the vagina

- Pain when urinating

- Pain or discomfort during sex

These may be signs of a vaginal infection, or an STI. Do not douche before seeing your doctor or nurse. This can make it hard for the doctor or nurse to find out what may be wrong.

Should I Douche to Clean Inside My Vagina?

No. You do not need to douche to clean your vagina. Your body naturally flushes out and cleans your vagina. Any strong odor or irritation usually means something is wrong.

Douching also can raise your chances of a vaginal infection or an STI.

What Is the Best Way to Clean My Vagina?

It is best to let your vagina clean itself. The vagina cleans itself naturally by making mucous. The mucous washes away blood, semen, and vaginal discharge.

If you are worried about vaginal odor, talk to your doctor or nurse. But you should know that even healthy, clean vaginas have a mild odor that changes throughout the day. Physical activity also can give your vagina a stronger, muskier scent, but this is still normal.

Keep your vagina clean and healthy by:

- Washing the outside of your vagina with warm water when you bathe. Some women also use mild soaps. But, if you have sensitive skin or any current vaginal infections, even mild soaps can cause dryness and irritation.

- Avoiding scented tampons, pads, powders, and sprays. These products may increase your chances of getting a vaginal infection.

Can Douching before or after Sex Prevent STIs?

No. Douching before or after sex does not prevent STIs. In fact, douching removes some of the normal bacteria in the vagina that protect you from infection. This can actually increase your risk of getting STIs, including HIV, the virus that causes AIDS.

Should I Douche If I Was Sexually Assaulted?

No. Douching removes some of the normal bacteria in the vagina that protect you from infection. This can increase your risk of getting STIs, including HIV. Douching also does not protect against pregnancy.

If you had sex without using protection or if the condom broke during sex, see a doctor right away. You can get medicine to help prevent HIV and unwanted pregnancy.

Can Douching after Sex Prevent Pregnancy?

No. Douching does not prevent pregnancy. It should never be used for birth control. If you had sex without using birth control or if your birth control method did not work correctly (failed), you can use emergency contraception to keep from getting pregnant.

If you need birth control, talk to your doctor or nurse about which type of birth control method is best for you.

How Does Douching Affect Pregnancy?

Douching can make it harder to get pregnant and can cause problems during pregnancy:

- **Trouble getting pregnant.** Women who douched at least once a month had a harder time getting pregnant than those women who did not douche.

- **Higher risk of ectopic pregnancy.** Douching may increase a woman's chance of damaged fallopian tubes and ectopic pregnancy. Ectopic pregnancy is when the fertilized egg attaches to the inside of the fallopian tube instead of the uterus. If left untreated, ectopic pregnancy can be life-threatening. It can also make it hard for a woman to get pregnant in the future.

- **Higher risk of early childbirth.** Douching raises your risk for premature birth. One study found that women who douched during pregnancy were more likely to deliver their babies early. This raises the risk for health problems for you and your baby.

Section 43.2

Body Art Allows Exposure to Bloodborne Pathogens Such as HIV

This section includes text excerpted from "Body Art," Centers for Disease Control and Prevention (CDC), September 25, 2013.

Body Art

Creating living art is a unique talent, but it puts tattooists and piercers at risk of coming in contact with their client's blood. This means artists may also be exposed to a bloodborne pathogen, such as hepatitis B virus, hepatitis C virus, or human immunodeficiency virus (HIV).

These viruses can be dangerous. They can make you sick and they can possibly make your family sick, if they are exposed. Some of these diseases are permanent and can be fatal.

Artists can be exposed to a bloodborne virus during the set-up, procedure, break down, and clean-up stages. These exposures can occur through needlesticks, contact with dried blood on equipment or surfaces, or blood splashes in the eyes, nose, or mouth.

Keeping a clean shop and using safe work practices, ensures a safe and professional atmosphere for artists and clients.

Get Vaccinated

There are many different bloodborne diseases, but not all of these diseases have vaccines available for protection. Currently, no vaccine exists to protect against hepatitis C or HIV. But a vaccine does exist to protect against hepatitis B.

Hepatitis B virus is one bloodborne pathogen. Hepatitis B is spread when blood or certain body fluids (e.g., semen) from an infected person get into the body of a person who is not infected. This can happen by getting stuck with a used needle, blood splashing into a person's eyes, nose or mouth, or by having sexual contact with someone who has hepatitis B.

The hepatitis B virus has been found to survive for more than a week in dried blood. This means artists can still be exposed to the virus long after an infected person has left the shop if shop counters, chairs, needles, or equipment are not properly disinfected.

Symptoms, or signs, of hepatitis B may not show up for several months after a person has been infected. Only 70% of people who are infected with hepatitis B have symptoms. This means a person could be infected, but still look and feel healthy. People who do not have symptoms can still spread the virus and may eventually develop liver cancer or liver failure. Besides liver cancer and liver failure, hepatitis B can also cause life-long infection, cirrhosis (scarring) of the liver, and death.

Here is some additional information for preventing exposures to hepatitis B and other bloodborne diseases:

- Hepatitis B vaccination can prevent infection

Hepatitis B is one virus people can be protected from. Currently, there is no vaccine to protect people from hepatitis C virus or HIV.

A doctor or nurse can provide more information about the vaccine and the vaccine dosing schedule.

- Employees can get vaccinated for free!

- Employers are required by Occupational Safety and Health Administration (OSHA) regulations to make the hepatitis B vaccine available at no cost to employees who may be exposed to blood while at work

- Employees who turn down the vaccine must sign a declination form

- Employees have the right to refuse the hepatitis B vaccine and/ or any post- exposure evaluation and follow-up. OSHA regulations require employers to keep record of a vaccine refusal by having the employee sign a hepatitis B declination form. The studio owner must keep signed hepatitis B declination forms on file.

- If later an employee changes his/her mind, OSHA regulations still require the employer to make the vaccine available at no cost

- If exposed to blood, artists should seek emergency medical treatment

If an artist is exposed to another person's blood, the artist should notify the shop owner and immediately seek medical attention. If treatment is needed, it is more likely to be effective if it begins soon after the exposure happens.

Prevent Needlestick Injuries

Exposures to bloodborne pathogens can happen by getting stuck with a used needle or getting cut by a sharp instrument that has blood on it.

Certain practices can reduce needlesticks and other sharps injuries. Here is some additional information for preventing exposures to blood in the body art industry.

- Disposable piercing needles, tattoo needles, and razors must be discarded into a sharps disposal container

- Body artists must throw away used or contaminated sharps into a sharps disposal container

- It is safer to put disposable razors into a sharps disposal container rather than the trash. This will protect the person changing or handling the trash bag from getting cut with a used razor.

- Sharps disposal containers must be kept in a safe place that is easy to reach

Sharps disposal containers must be kept in a place that is near a work area so artists can quickly and safely dispose of used sharps.

- Sharps disposal containers must be changed when they become full

- If sharps disposal containers become full, they must be replaced so the containers do not spill over. An artist could get a needlestick if he or she throws away a sharp item into a full container.

It is a good idea to replace sharps disposal containers when they are 2/3 full.

- Sharps disposal containers must be clearly marked

Sharps disposal containers must be closeable, puncture resistant, leak-proof, and labeled. These features allow for safe disposal in a container that is familiar to all workers.

- The number of times an artist's hands are in contact with a sharp should be reduced if possible

478

When handling or disposing a used sharp, tattooists and piercers should use a tool instead of their fingers to pick up or hold the sharp. This may reduce needlesticks.

- A sharps incident log should be kept for each shop

- Though OSHA regulations do not generally require a body artist to keep an injury log, a record of cuts from sharps can increase awareness of sharps-related injuries. A sharps incidence log lets artists know how often sharps-related injuries happen and under what conditions. Recording needlesticks and cuts from sharps allow artists to learn from their mistakes and others' mistakes to help reduce exposures.

- An exposure control plan must be made and kept at each shop

- As required by OSHA, an exposure control plan is written by a shop owner and describes the steps an employer will take to minimize employee exposure to blood. The details included in an exposure control plan should be specific to each shop.

Reduce Cross-Contamination

Cross-contamination is the act of spreading bacteria and viruses from one surface to another. Since bloodborne viruses can live on objects and surfaces for up to a week, germs could be spread when surfaces are not disinfected the right way or if equipment is not cleaned and sterilized between clients.

Some examples of cross-contamination are:

- A piercer places his tools on a counter that has not been disinfected and then uses the tools for a piercing procedure without sterilizing them.

- A tattooist, while working on a client, answers the phone without removing her gloves. By not removing her gloves, the artist may spread bacteria and viruses from the gloves onto the phone. Other people using the phone could then be exposed to a disease.

Here is some additional information for preventative practices that may reduce cross-contamination in the body art industry:

- Gloves should be changed when it is necessary

- Gloves must be removed and thrown away whenever a tattooist or piercer leaves his or her work area

- Gloves should be changed if they tear

- Disposable gloves must not be washed or reused

- Hands should be washed often

- Hand washing can get rid of most the disease-causing organisms on a person's hands

- When wearing gloves, heat and moisture build up. This creates the right conditions to allow bacteria to reproduce. To lessen the spread of viruses and bacteria, tattooists and piercers should wash their hands before and after wearing gloves.

- Gloves are not a substitute for hand washing

- Surfaces should be disinfected often

Body artists should disinfect surfaces, such as the client's chair and counter space, between procedures.

The Environmental Protection Agency (EPA) has a list of registered disinfectants that are made to kill certain bacteria and viruses. EPA-registered tuberculocidal disinfectants are best for cleaning surfaces contaminated with blood.

The germ that causes tuberculosis is one of the most difficult to kill. Any disinfectant that claims to be able to eliminate the tuberculosis germ can also kill HIV, hepatitis B and hepatitis C viruses.

Many disinfectants need to stay on surfaces for a specific amount of time to fully disinfect the surface before being wiped down. The instructions included with the disinfectant should note the amount of time needed to properly disinfect an area.

- Reusable tools and equipment should be cleaned before being sterilized

Cleaning is the first step in removing viruses and bacteria from equipment. Reusable tools and equipment should first be washed before being sterilized. If washing tools manually, piercers and tattooists should use a brush or similar tool whenever possible.

Ultrasonic cleaners work well to clean tools in hard-to-reach places and reduce the amount of time contaminated equipment is handled. Shop employers should check with the owner's manual to be sure the machine is cared for correctly.

- Use disposable "single-use" supplies whenever possible

Disposable supplies, such as pigment caps, razors, rinse cups, and sterilized pre-made needle bars, should be used once and disposed of.

By not reusing disposable supplies, the possibility of being exposed to blood while cleaning them is avoided.

- Sterilization machines must be regularly tested and serviced

Autoclave machines use steam, pressure, and temperature to kill bacteria, fungi, and viruses. Gauge readings and the color change of indicator strips on autoclave packaging are not reliable ways of ensuring an autoclave is sterilizing correctly.

If the machine is not well cared for, it may not reach the conditions needed to sterilize reusable equipment well.

Routine spore tests can check if an autoclave is sterilizing correctly. Employers should contact their local health department to find out how often spore tests should be done.

The employer should also ensure the autoclave is regularly serviced. The owner's manual should provide information about the maintenance schedule.

- Tattooists and piercers must attend bloodborne pathogen training at least yearly

OSHA regulations require employers to provide yearly bloodborne pathogen training at no cost to employees with the option of taking the course during work hours. If the training is done during non-working hours, employees must be compensated for their time. Record of training must be kept by employers.

Follow Regulations

Tattooing and piercing regulations and recommended practices vary from state to state.

Section 43.3

Injection Drug Use

This section includes text excerpted from "HIV and Injection Drug
Use in the United States," Centers for Disease
Control and Prevention (CDC), October 27, 2015.

HIV and Injection Drug Use in the United States

Quick Facts

- HIV infections due to injection drug use have declined, but injecting drugs remains a significant risk.

- Sharing syringes is a direct route of HIV transmission.

- In one study, two out of five people who inject drugs and were diagnosed with HIV did not know they were infected.

New HIV Infections

- In 2010, 8% (3,900) of the estimated 47,500 new HIV infections in the United States were attributed to injection drug use (IDU).

- Men accounted for 62% (2,400), and women accounted for 38% (1,500) of all IDU-associated HIV infections in 2010.

- In 2010, another 4% (1,600) of all estimated new HIV infections among men were among men who engage in both injection drug use and male-to-male sexual contact.

- Blacks/African Americans accounted for 50% (1,950) of the estimated new HIV infections among people who inject drugs (PWID) in 2010. Whites accounted for 26% (1,020) and Hispanic/Latinos represented 21% (850) of the total.

HIV Diagnoses and Deaths

- In 2013, 7% (3,096) of the estimated 47,352 diagnoses of HIV infection in the United States were attributed to IDU and another 3% (1,270) to male-to-male sexual contact/IDU.

482

- Sixty-three percent (1,942) of the 3,096 HIV diagnoses attributed to IDU in 2013 were among men. Thirty-seven percent (1,154) were among women.

- Forty-six percent (1,435) of all diagnoses of HIV infection attributed to IDU in 2013 were among African Americans, 28% (866) were among whites, and 21% (655) were among Hispanics/Latinos. American Indians/Alaska Natives, Asians, Native Hawaiians/Other Pacific Islanders, and those of multiple races made up the remaining 5% of HIV diagnoses attributed to IDU in 2013.

- Of the total 26,688 AIDS diagnoses in 2013, 10% (2,753) were attributed to IDU and another 4% (1,026) were attributed to male-to-male sexual contact/IDU.

- More than one in four (26%, 3,514) of the 13,712 deaths among people with AIDS in 2012 were attributed to IDU and another 8% (1,088) were attributed to male-to-male sexual contact/IDU.

- Through 2012, the cumulative total of deaths among people with AIDS attributed to IDU was 186,728 or 28% of the total deaths among people with AIDS (658,507) since the beginning of the epidemic. An additional 50,001 deaths among people with AIDS were attributed to male-to-male sexual contact/IDU, or 8% of the total cumulative deaths.

Prevention Challenges

- **The high-risk practice of sharing syringes and other injection equipment is common among PWID.** HIV can be transmitted by sharing needles, syringes, or other injection equipment (e.g., cookers, rinse water, cotton) that were used by a person living with HIV. According to a CDC study of cities with high levels of HIV, approximately one-third of PWID reported sharing syringes and more than half reported sharing other injection equipment in the past 12 months.

  - Some states have syringe services programs that provide new needles, syringes, and other injection equipment to reduce the risk of HIV. The North American Syringe Exchange Network has a directory of syringe services programs. If new needles and syringes are not available, cleaning used needles and syringes with bleach may reduce the risk of HIV.

- **Use of injection drugs can reduce inhibitions and increase risk behaviors.** These include not using a condom or taking preventive medicines (such as pre-exposure prophylaxis, or PrEP) as directed. In the study of cities with high levels of HIV, 72% of females who inject drugs reported having sex without a condom in the last year. People who inject drugs may also take part in risky sexual behaviors to get drugs or while under coercion.

- **Young people (aged 15–30 years) who inject drugs have many of the same risk factors for HIV found in older PWID,** including a significant risk of sexual HIV transmission among MSM who inject drugs and among PWID who exchanged sex for money or drugs. These findings suggest HIV prevention interventions for PWID should include sexual risk reduction as well as injection risk reduction.

- **Injection drug use is often viewed as a criminal activity rather than a medical issue that requires counseling and rehabilitation.** Stigma related to drug use may prevent PWID from seeking HIV testing, care, and treatment. Studies have shown that people treated for substance abuse are more likely to start and remain in HIV medical care, adopt safer behaviors, and take their HIV medications correctly than those not receiving such treatment.

- **Social and economic factors affect access to HIV treatment.** PWID are at especially high risk for getting and spreading HIV, but often have trouble getting medical treatment for HIV because of social issues. Almost two-thirds (65%) of PWID with HIV reported being homeless, 61% reported being incarcerated, and 44% reported having no health insurance in the last 12 months. Because of these issues, some providers may hesitate to prescribe HIV medications to PWID because they believe PWID will not take them correctly. Research has not supported these concerns—studies among people receiving HIV treatment have found similar rates of survival between people who don't inject drugs and people who do.

Chapter 44

Talking to Sexual Partners Can Reduce STD Risk

Chapter Contents

Section 44.1

Talking to Your Partner about Safe Sex

This section includes text excerpted from "Conversation Starters,"
Centers for Disease Control and Prevention (CDC), January 12, 2016.

Conversation Starters

It is important to have conversations with your partner about safer sex and healthy relationships, but that can be a lot easier said than done. Worried about how your new or existing guy is going to react? You're not alone, many men have those fears. Check out the advice below from other men on how to make these conversations work. These are just suggestions collected from some gay and bisexual men.

It Can Be Awkward!

Yeah, you're right it can be awkward sometimes. Try to approach the situation with confidence. Chances are if you're confident and bring it up without judgment, your partner will be open to the discussion. For all you know, he could be just as worried as you to bring it up. Just remember, nearly everyone who is having sex will have this conversation at some point, and many other guys before you have already done it.

Here are some tips that other guys have found helpful in having these conversations:

- Don't wait until the heat of the moment to start talking about HIV. It's better to talk about it earlier rather than later— certainly before you have sex.

- Some men who are living with HIV have suggested that it helps to talk about their status earlier in the relationship rather than later. Disclosing you are HIV-positive after you've become close to someone can cause your partner to feel as though you have kept something important from him.

- If you're looking for a way to start talking, show him this web page. Watch the videos together, talk about the campaign and use it as a way to start the conversation. Approaching the conversation this way doesn't make it sound like you don't trust him, but rather you've been reading about it, heard about it, were talking to a friend who brought it up, etc., and because you care, you want to make sure you're both protected.

- Don't force it. Find the right time and place to have a conversation. You can schedule a time to talk or have spontaneous conversations in a setting where you are comfortable.

- Try scheduling regular check-ins, or 'talkiversaries.' The key to a healthy relationship is having an open dialogue throughout the relationship. It can be hard to find the right time to bring these things up. If you agree to schedule them in advance, no one has to wonder about the timing of the conversations.

- A conversation does not have to be face-to-face. Whether you talk, type, or text what is important is that you start the conversation about HIV.

Testing

- I got tested for HIV and other stuff the first time about a year ago, have you ever been tested?

- I've never been tested for HIV and I'm kind of nervous to do it. Will you go with me?

- I know we haven't talked about this yet, but just so you know, I got tested for HIV last [week/month/whatever]. My test came back negative, and ever since I got the results I've committed to playing it safe. When was the last time you were tested?

- So, when was the last time you were tested for HIV? How often do you get tested for HIV and other STDs? I was tested recently, but think we should probably go together to be on the safe side. What do you think?

- I read something that said we should be getting tested for HIV at least annually, or even more often. How often do you get tested? Where do you get tested? Want to go together?

- I saw this mobile HIV testing truck last week, and it made me realize we haven't talked about HIV yet. When was the last time you were tested?

- Before we take things to the next level, I think we should get tested for HIV. No matter the results, at least we'll know how to keep each other safe and healthy.

- Have you heard about the new home HIV test? Do you want to try a home test with me?

- I was listening to the radio today and they said that you can get your HIV test results in as little as 20 minutes. I'm thinking about going. Will you go with me?

Talking about Your Status

- I was online earlier and saw a post about the importance of knowing your HIV status. Do you know yours?

- Since the last time you were tested have you had sex or shared needles with anyone?

- I don't care whether you are positive or negative, it is not going to change how I feel about you, but we need to talk about it so we can come up with ways to keep each other healthy. What's your HIV status?

- I always ask people that I am starting to date about their HIV status. What is your status?

- I am HIV negative and I want to stay that way. I really like you and want to get to know you better. Let's talk about safer sex and ways to protect each other.

- I am glad we decided to talk about HIV. I tested negative for HIV three months ago. Do you know your HIV status?

- I tested HIV negative six months ago. Let's talk about getting tested together and practicing safer sex.

Revealing Your HIV-Positive Status

- There's something I want to tell you, I've been living with HIV since [xx year]. Have you ever dated someone with HIV?

- About a year ago, I found out that I'm HIV-positive. Since then, I've been taking HIV medication consistently and correctly. The virus is controlled and at undetectable levels, and I feel good. Let's start talking about ways to keep each other healthy and safe. When was the last time you were tested for HIV?

- I really like you, and like where this is going, but before we go any further, there's something I want to tell you. I'm HIV-positive.

Learning That Your Partner Is Positive

- Thanks for telling me you are HIV-positive. I really appreciate you sharing that important information with me. I really like you and I want to make sure that we keep each other healthy. Let's talk about our options for safer sex.

- I am glad we're having this conversation. I am relieved you know that I am living with HIV and am thankful that you shared with me that you are HIV-positive, too. Let's talk about how we can help each other stay healthy.

- Thanks for feeling close enough to me that you could share your status. How long have you known? How are you doing?

Talking about Safer Sex Options

- Did you know that there are medicines that you can take that can further reduce the chance of you getting HIV? Have you heard of PrEP (pre-exposure prophylaxis)?

- Have you heard about PrEP? Maybe we should talk to our doctors to see if it's right for us.

- I can't believe the condom broke. It's a good thing there are medicines to help reduce the chance getting HIV. We should go to the doctor or emergency room right now and ask about PEP (post-exposure prophylaxis).

- If we're going to have sex, we should use condoms.

- Can we talk about sex? Safer sex is really important to me.

- You should know that for anal sex, condoms are a must. That's non-negotiable for me. Are you ok with that?

- So we haven't really talked about it, but can we agree that when the time comes, we'll use condoms to keep each other safe?

- Maybe we should consider doing things that have a lower chance of getting or transmitting HIV, like oral sex. Doing other things can be fun and are much safer than anal sex.

- I know we just met and we don't know everything about each other, but you should know that practicing safer sex is really important to me. When is the last time you were tested for HIV and other sexually transmitted diseases?

If You Are Living with HIV

- It's really important to reduce our risk and keep you negative. The fact that I'm in treatment/on meds and have an undetectable viral load helps. We can talk about how to choose things to do that are less risky.

- I'm living with HIV, and the fact that we are using condoms is great, but we need to make sure we do everything we can to keep you safe.

Section 44.2

Sharing Your HIV Status

This section includes text excerpted from "Sharing Your Status," Centers for Disease Control and Prevention (CDC), January 12, 2016.

Am I Legally Required to Share My HIV Status with Others?

Even though disclosing your HIV status may be uncomfortable, doing so allows others to protect themselves and gives you protection under the law.

Health care providers and other HIV-related service providers need to know so that they can support you and make sure you have access to the health care services that you need. Disclosing your HIV status also protects your health care provider. Even though health care providers take precautions, such as wearing gloves to avoid coming into direct contact with a patient's blood, letting them know you have HIV will remind them to be very careful about those precautions.

Sex or injection drug-use partners need to know to protect their health. Telling new partners that you have HIV before you have sex or inject drugs together allows them to make decisions that can protect their health, like going on PrEP or using PEP and using condoms consistently and correctly. In some states, there are laws that require you to share your HIV status with your sex and injection drug-use partners.

You do not have to tell your employer. But, if you have to take extended leave or alter your schedule, you may want to. By law, your disclosure is confidential.

The following resources can provide more information on sharing your HIV status with others:

- The Center for HIV Law and Policy identifies which states have HIV-specific criminal laws and provides additional resources about disclosure, confidentiality, and the law.

- Your state health department can also provide information on your state's laws and how they apply to disclosure.

How Can I Get Help Telling My Partners That They May Have Been Exposed to HIV?

If you have HIV or another sexually transmitted disease (STD) (like syphilis, gonorrhea, or chlamydia), it is very important to let your current and former sex or injection drug-use partners know that they may have been exposed. Informing partners that you have HIV lets them know that they should be tested for HIV. These conversations can be challenging because you may have become infected by one of these individuals or you may have infected one or more of them without knowing.

There are a few ways to let your partners know:

- You tell your partners:
  - You take on the responsibility of letting your current and former partners know of their exposure.
  - You give them information on local services, including counseling and testing.

- The health department tells your partners ("Partner Services"):
  - You give your current and former partners' names to the health department.

491

- Your partners are located and made aware of their exposure by health department staff. It is important to know that health department staff do not use your name when contacting your partners.

- Your partners are given or referred for counseling, testing, treatment, and other services by the health department.

- You and the health department staff work together to tell your partners ("Partner Services"):

  - You work with health department staff to let your partners know of their exposure.

  - Health department staff are there to help you during the process and provide your partners with information, access to counseling, testing, and other resources.

What Is Partner Services?

Partner Services provides many free services to people living with HIV or other STDs and their partners. Through Partner Services, health department staff notify your current and former sex and/or injection drug-use partners that they may have been exposed to HIV or another STD and provide them with testing, counseling, and referrals for other services.

Partner Services:

- Ensures that your sex or injection drug-use partners know of their possible exposure to HIV or another STD without using your name,

- Ensures that trained staff contact your partners,

- Coaches you on how to let your sex or injection drug-use partners know about their exposure, if you choose to tell your partners yourself,

- Helps your sex or injection drug-use partners get tested quickly and, if they test positive, get into care and treatment quickly, and

- Serves as another free resource for education and counseling for you to live healthier with HIV.

Partner Services programs are available through health departments and some medical offices or clinics. Your health care provider, social worker, case manager, patient navigator, or HIV testing center can help put you in touch with a Partner Services program.

492

Should I Share My HIV Status with My Friends and Family?

Sharing your HIV status with certain family members and friends has both emotional and practical benefits. Emotionally, having trusted people to talk to can help you deal with the early stages of dealing with an HIV diagnosis. They can also support you with the longer-term issues of treatment adherence and disclosing to others. Practically, trusting people with this knowledge will allow them to speak for you in case of an emergency and to help you navigate the medical system. Don't overlook the expertise of individuals you know. Many people have had these difficult conversations and they can help you work through what you will say. For example:

- Friends or family members living with HIV can share with you how they told other people in their lives.

- Your health care provider, social worker, or case manager can help you practice telling people and can share their experiences helping other patients share this information.

- Join an HIV support group in your area and hear how others told people in their lives.

What Are Some Conversation Starters to Begin Talking about Safer Sex Options with My Partners?

Some conversation starters to help you begin talking about safer sex options with your partners include:

- Talking about safer sex options with your partner(s):
  - Let's start talking about ways to keep each other healthy and safe. When was the last time you were tested for HIV?
  - It's really important to reduce our risk and keep you negative. The fact that I'm in treatment/on meds and have an undetectable viral load helps. We can talk about how to choose things to do that are less risky.
  - I'm living with HIV, and the fact that we are using condoms is great, but we need to make sure we do everything we can to keep you safe.
  - Did you know that there are medicines that you can take that can further reduce the chance of you getting HIV? Have

493

you heard of PrEP (pre-exposure prophylaxis)? Maybe we should talk to our doctors to see if it's right for us.

- I can't believe the condom broke. It's a good thing there are medicines to help reduce the chance of getting HIV. We should go to the doctor or emergency room right now and ask about PEP (post-exposure prophylaxis).

- If we're going to have sex, we should use condoms.

- Can we talk about sex? Safer sex is really important to me.

- So we haven't really talked about it, but can we agree that when the time comes, we'll use condoms to keep each other safe?

- Maybe we should consider doing things that have a lower chance of getting or transmitting HIV, like oral sex.

- I know we just met and we don't know everything about each other, but you should know that practicing safer sex is really important to me. When is the last time you were tested for HIV and other sexually transmitted diseases?

- For partners that are both living with HIV:

  - If we're going to have sex, let's get tested for other STDs together before we take that step.

  - Getting an STD could really compromise our health. Let's stay healthy and get tested for STDs regularly.

  - Let's talk about how we can practice safer sex so that we don't increase our chances of getting an STD.

Stigma

Stigma can be a complex barrier to health care for people living with HIV/AIDS. Today, with HIV treatment, many people can live a long and healthy life. However, the stigma of the disease can have a negative effect on people living with HIV.

HIV/AIDS-related stigma and discrimination refer to prejudice, negative attitudes, abuse, and maltreatment directed at people living with HIV and AIDS. Some examples of stigma and discrimination include being shunned by family, peers, and the wider community; poor treatment in health care and education settings; loss of rights; psychological damage; and a negative effect on the success of HIV testing and treatment.

HIV/AIDS stigma is not only experienced by people who are living with the disease. It also is experienced by family and friends, HIV service providers, and members of groups that have been heavily impacted by HIV/AIDS, such as gay and bisexual men, homeless individuals, street youth, and mentally ill individuals.

What Resources Are Available to Me for Support?

Know your rights. You are entitled to the same rights as any other patient in the medical system. These rights include safety, competent medical care, and confidentiality.

- The Ryan White HIV/AIDS Program helps people with HIV/AIDS who have nowhere else to turn for the care they need. If you are living with HIV, you can get medical care and some other services—even if you do not have health insurance or money to pay for health services.

- The Housing Opportunities for Persons With AIDS (HOPWA) Program is the only Federal program dedicated to the housing needs of people living with HIV/AIDS. Under the HOPWA Program, HUD makes grants to local communities, states, and non-profit organizations for projects that benefit low-income people living with HIV/AIDS and their families.

- The Americans with Disabilities Act (ADA) protects people who are discriminated against because they have HIV or have a relationship with someone who has HIV.

- If you have HIV/AIDS and cannot work, you may qualify for disability benefits from the Social Security Administration.

- The Affordable Care Act (ACA) is a law that was passed to help ensure that Americans have secure, stable, and affordable health insurance. The ACA created several changes that expand access to coverage for people living with HIV. Because coverage varies by state, talk to your health care provider or a social worker to get information about the coverage available where you live. You can find additional information about the ACA and living with HIV from the Henry J. Kaiser Family Foundation. You can also contact the ACA helpline at 1-800-318-2596 for more information.

- You may also choose to join an HIV support group of peers living with HIV. These support groups usually meet in a safe and supportive environment to provide support to other people living with HIV.

Chapter 45

Talking to Your Child or Teen about STD Prevention

The Basics

Talk with your teen about how to prevent STDs (sexually transmitted diseases), even if you don't think your teen is sexually active.

If talking about sex and STDs with your teen makes you nervous, you aren't alone. It can be hard to know where to start. But it's important to make sure your teen knows how to stay safe.

How Do I Talk with My Teen?

These tips can help you talk to your teen about preventing STDs:

- Think about what you want to say ahead of time.

- Be honest about how you feel.

- Try not to overwhelm your teen with lots of information at once.

- Use examples to start a conversation.

- Talk while you are doing something else.

- Get ideas from other parents.

This chapter includes text excerpted from "Talk with Your Teen about Preventing STDs," U.S. Department of Health and Human Services (HHS), October 21, 2015.

You can also ask your teen's doctor about STD prevention counseling.

Why Do I Need to Talk with My Teen?

All teens need accurate information about how to prevent STDs. Teens whose parents talk with them about sex are more likely to make healthy choices.

Young People Are More Likely to Get STDs.

About half of all STD cases in the United States happen in young people ages 15 to 24.

Teens, especially teen girls, are at a higher risk than adults of getting STDs for a number of reasons. For example, they may:

- Not know they need tests to check for STDs

- Be likely to have sex without a condom

- Have sexual contact with multiple partners during the same period of time

What Do I Need to Know about STDs?

STDs, or sexually transmitted diseases, are diseases that can spread from person to person during sex (vaginal, anal, or oral). Some STDs can also spread during any kind of sexual activity that involves skin-to-skin contact.

These diseases are very common. Although many STDs are curable, they can cause serious health problems if they aren't treated. Examples of STDs include herpes, chlamydia, and HIV.

STDs are sometimes called STIs, or sexually transmitted infections.

What Do I Tell My Teen about Preventing STDs?

Talk to your teen about what STDs are and how to prevent them. Use the facts and resources below to talk with your teen.

It's Important to Learn about STDs and How They Spread.

Knowing the facts helps teens protect themselves.

Complete Abstinence Is the Best Way to Prevent STDs.

Complete abstinence means not having any kind of sexual contact. This includes vaginal, anal, or oral sex and skin-to-skin contact. Complete abstinence is the only sure way to prevent STDs.

Condoms Can Help Prevent STDs.

Make sure your teen knows how to use condoms. Offer to help get condoms if your teen doesn't know where to go.

Your Teen May Need to Get Tested for STDs.

Ask your teen to talk honestly with the doctor or nurse about any sexual activity. That way, the doctor can decide which tests your teen may need. Sexually active teens may need to be tested for:

- Chlamydia and Gonorrhea
- HIV

Keep in mind that it's important to help your teen develop a trusting relationship with the doctor or nurse. Step out of the room to give your teen a chance to ask about STD testing in private.

This is an important step in teaching teens to play an active role in their health care.

It's Important for Teens to Talk with Their Partners about STDs before Having Sex.

Encourage your teen to talk with his or her partner about STD prevention before having sex. Say that you understand it may not be easy, but it's important for your teen to speak up. These tips can help:

- Talking to Your Partner About Condoms
- Talking to Your Partner About STDs
- STD Testing: Conversation starters

How Can I Talk to My Teen about Preventing Pregnancy?

It's important for teen girls and boys to know about preventing pregnancy as well as STDs.

How Can I Help My Teen Build Healthy Relationships?

Families have different rules about when it's okay for teens to start dating. Whatever your rules are, the best time to start talking about healthy relationships is before your teen starts dating.

Help your teen develop healthy expectations for relationships.

499

Does My LGBT Teen Need Information about Preventing STDs?

Yes. All teens–including LGBT (lesbian, gay, bisexual, transgender) teens–need accurate information about STDs. Remember, some STDs can spread through skin-to-skin contact.

LGBT teens may also be at higher risk for STDs than straight teens. But when LGBT teens feel valued by their parents, their risk of getting an STD goes down.

Talking to your teen is an important way to show you care.

Take Action!

Protect your teen from STDs by sharing the facts he or she needs to make healthy decisions.

Think about What You Want to Say Ahead of Time

Learn about STDs so you'll be ready to talk with your teen. You may also want to practice what you'll say to your teen with others adults, like your partner or another parent.

It's very common to be nervous when talking to your teen about something like STDs, so it can be helpful if you have an idea of what you want to say beforehand.

Be Honest about How You Feel

Talking with your teen about how to prevent STDs may not be easy for you. It's normal to feel uncomfortable–and it's okay to be honest with your teen about how you feel.

Remember, when you are honest with your teen, she's more likely to be honest with you. And keep in mind that your teen may ask a question you can't answer. Tell her you aren't sure–then look up the answer together!

Try Not to Overwhelm Your Teen with Lots of Information at Once

Remember, you have plenty of time to talk about preventing STDs. You don't need to fit everything into one conversation–it's actually better if you don't. Give your teen time to think–he may come back later and ask questions.

Make this the first conversation of many about preventing STDs.

Listen and Ask Questions

Show your teen that you are paying attention and trying to understand her thoughts and feelings. Try these tips:

- Repeat back what your teen says in your own words. For example, "So you don't think you are at risk for getting an STD?"

- Ask questions to help guide the conversation. For example, "Have you talked about preventing STDs in school?"

- Ask questions that check for your teen's understanding. For example, "Can you tell me what you learned about how STDs are spread?"

- Talk about something that happened in a movie or TV show. For example, "It looks like they had sex without protection. What do you think about that?"

Talk While You Are Doing Something Else

Sometimes it's easier to have a conversation while you are doing something else at the same time. For example, try asking your teen about sex and STDs when you are driving in the car or busy cooking dinner.

You can still show your teen that you are listening to him by nodding your head or repeating what he says.

Get Ideas from Other Parents

Remember that you aren't the only person thinking about how to talk to a teen about preventing STDs. Ask other parents what they have done. You may be able to get helpful tips and ideas.

Ask Your Teen's Doctor about STD Prevention Counseling

Counseling to prevent STDs is recommended for all teens who are sexually active. That means it's part of a doctor's job to help teens learn how to prevent STDs. The doctor may:

- Give your teen information about preventing STDs

- Refer your teen to a health educator or counselor for STD prevention counseling

STD prevention counseling includes:

- Giving your teen basic information about STDs and how they spread

- Figuring out your teen's risk of getting or spreading an STD

- Teaching your teen important skills–like how to use condoms and how to talk with a partner about STDs

What about Cost?

Thanks to the Affordable Care Act, the health care reform law passed in 2010, health insurance plans must cover prevention counseling and screening for teens at risk of getting an STD.

Depending on your insurance plan, your teen may be able to get STD counseling and screening at no cost to you.

Chapter 46

Overview of Sex Education

Key Findings

Data from the 2006–2008 National Survey of Family Growth (NSFG) says:

- Most teenagers received formal sex education before they were 18 (96% of female and 97% of male teenagers).

- Female teenagers were more likely than male teenagers to report first receiving instruction on birth control methods in high school (47% compared with 38%).

- Younger female teenagers were more likely than younger male teenagers to have talked to their parents about sex and birth control.

- Nearly two out of three female teenagers talked to their parents about "how to say no to sex" compared with about two out of five male teenagers.

Sex education in schools and other places, as well as received from parents, provides adolescents with information to make informed choices about sex at a crucial period of their development. Using data from the 2006–2008 National Survey of Family Growth (NSFG), this report examines the percentage of male and female teenagers 15–19 years who received sex education. Teenagers were asked if they received formal instruction on four topics of sex education at school,

---

This chapter includes text excerpted from "Educating Teenagers about Sex in the United States," Centers for Disease Control and Prevention (CDC), November 6, 2015.

church, a community center, or some other place before they were 18 years old and the grade they were in when this first occurred. In addition, they were asked if they talked to their parents before they were 18 about topics concerning sex, birth control, sexually transmitted diseases (STDs), and the Human Immunodeficiency Virus HIV/acquired immunodeficiency syndrome (AIDS) prevention.

What Percentage of Teenagers Received Formal Sex Education?

Most teenagers received formal sex education before they were 18 (96% of female and 97% of male teenagers).

Ninety-two percent of male and 93% of female teenagers reported being taught about STDs and 89% of male and 88% of female teenagers reported receiving instruction on how to prevent HIV/AIDS.

A larger percentage of teenagers reported receiving formal sex education on "how to say no to sex" (81% of male and 87% female teenagers) than reported receiving formal sex education on methods of birth control.

Male teenagers were less likely than female teenagers to have received instructions on methods of birth control (62% of male and 70% female teenagers).

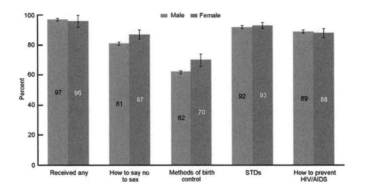

Figure 46.1. *Percentage of Teenagers Who Received Formal Sex Education*

What Grade Are Teenagers in When They First Receive Formal Sex Education?

- Among teenagers who reported receiving formal sex education from a school, church, community center, or some other place, the majority first received instruction on "how to say no to sex," STDs, or how to prevent HIV/AIDS while in middle school (grades 6–8) (Figure 46.2.).

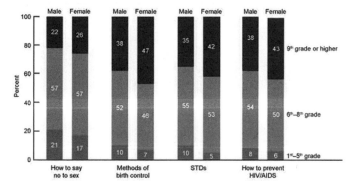

Figure 46.2. *Grade when Teenagers Their First Receive Formal Sex Education*

- Teenagers who reported first receiving sex education prior to middle school were more likely to report instruction on "how to say no to sex" than other topics. About one in five teenagers reported first receiving instruction on "how to say no to sex" while in first through fifth grade.

- Male teenagers were about as likely as female teenagers to report first receiving formal sex education on methods of birth control while in middle school (52% male teenagers compared with 46% female teenagers) and less likely than female teenagers to report first receiving instruction on methods of birth control while in high school (38% males compared with 47% females).

- Female teenagers were equally likely to report first receiving instruction on methods of birth control while in middle school or high school.

Do Teenagers Talk about Sex-Related Topics with Their Parents?

- More than two out of every three male teenagers and almost four out of every five female teenagers talked with a parent about at least one of six sex education topics ("how to say no to sex," methods of birth control, STDs, where to get birth control, how to prevent HIV/AIDS, and how to use a condom) (Figure 46.3.).

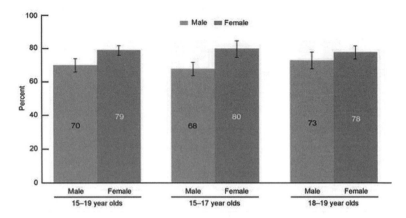

Figure 46.3. *Teenagers Who Talked about Sex-Related Education with Their Parents*

- Younger teenage (15–17 years old) females were more likely (80%) than younger male teenagers (68%) to have talked to their parents about these topics. On the other hand, there was virtually no difference for older teenage (18–19 years old) males and females in whether they talked to their parents about these topics.

Do Male and Female Teenagers Differ in Whether They Talk to Their Parents about Sex and Birth Control?

- Female teenagers were more likely than male teenagers to talk to their parents about "how to say no to sex," methods of birth control, and where to get birth control (Figure 46.4.).

- Nearly two-thirds of female teenagers have talked to their parents about "how to say no to sex" compared with about two out of five male teenagers.

- Male teenagers were more likely than female teenagers to talk to their parents about how to use a condom (38% of males compared with 29% of females).

- Female and male teenagers were equally likely to have talked with their parents about STDs and how to prevent HIV/AIDS.

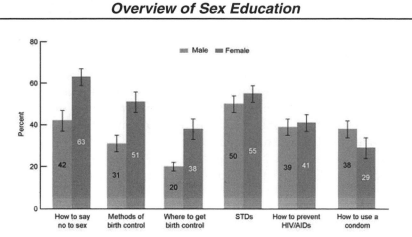

Figure 46.4. *Teenagers Who Talked with a Parent about Sex Education*

Summary

Parental communication about sex education topics with their teenagers is associated with delayed sexual initiation and increased birth control method and condom use among sexually experienced teenagers. Although the impact of formal sex education on teenagers' behavior is harder to assess and depends on its content, studies show it can be effective at reducing risk behaviors. These data show that the majority of male and female teenagers 15–19 years are receiving formal sex education on "how to say no to sex," methods of birth control, STDs, and how to prevent HIV/AIDS. About one-half of teenagers reported first receiving instruction on "how to say no to sex," STDs, and how to prevent HIV/AIDS while in middle school. Most teenagers have talked to their parents about at least one of the six sex education topics.

Female teenagers are more likely than male teenagers to talk to their parents about "how to say no to sex," methods of birth control, and where to get birth control. These findings for 2006–2008 suggest little change since 2002 in receipt of formal sex education or information from parents among teenagers. The report based on the 2006–2008 NSFG also found little change in teenagers' sexual activity and contraceptive use since the 2002 NSFG.

Definitions

Formal sex education: The analysis for this report is limited to teenagers aged 15–19 years, but males and females aged 15–24 years old were asked whether they ever had any formal sex education. There were two question variants, one for teenagers younger than 18 and one for teenagers aged 18 and older.

Now I'm interested in knowing about formal sex education you may have had. (Before you were 18, did you ever have/ have you ever had) any formal instruction at school, church, a community center, or some other place about "how to say no to sex?"

Three other sex education topics were asked about with the following wording, prefaced with the same wording as shown for "how to say no to sex," "methods of birth control," "sexually transmitted diseases," and "how to prevent HIV/AIDS." It is important to note that teenagers 15–17 who did not receive formal sex education may go on to receive sex education before they are 18.

Grade at which received instruction: For the four sex education topics, teenagers were asked what grade they were in when they first received this instruction. The grades at which first received instruction have been collapsed into grades 1–5 (elementary school), grades 6–8 (middle school), and grades 9–12 (high school) for this report. Teenagers who have not yet reached high school (9th grade and higher) will not have reported that they received sex education in these grades. Thus the "9th and higher" category only represents those teenagers already in high school.

Talking with parents about sex and birth control: The analysis for this report is limited to teenagers aged 15–19 years, but males and females aged 15–24 years old were asked whether they talked with a parent or guardian about sex and birth control with the following questions:

The next questions are about how you learned about sex and birth control. (Before you were 18 years old) which, if any, of the topics shown on Card 23 (did you ever talk/have you ever talked) with a parent or guardian about?

Teenagers could select "none of the above" or any of six sex education topics with the following wording: "how to say no to sex," methods of birth control, where to get birth control, STDs, how to prevent HIV/ AIDS, and how to use a condom. It is important to note that teenagers 15–17 years who did not talk with their parents about sex and birth control may go on to do so before they are 18.

Chapter 47

Sex Education and STD Prevention

Chapter Contents

Section 47.1

Educating Your Children about Sex

This section includes text excerpted from "Talk to Your
Kids about Sex," U.S. Department of Health and
Human Services (HHS), January 28, 2016.

The Basics

Teach your children the facts about their bodies, sex, and relationships. Talking with your kids about sex may not be easy, but it's important—and it's never too early to start. You can make a big difference in helping them stay healthy and make good choices as they grow up.

It may be hard to know where to start, especially if your parents didn't talk to you about sex when you were growing up. These tips and strategies can help.

What Do I Say?

Kids will have different questions and concerns about sex at different ages. As your child gets older, the things you talk about will change. Remember to:

- Talk early and often. You don't have to fit everything into one conversation.

- Be ready to answer questions. Children's questions can tell you a lot about what they already know.

- Listen carefully, even if you don't agree with your child's opinion.

- Try using things that come up on TV or in music to start a conversation.

- Be honest about how you are feeling. For example, if you are embarrassed or uncomfortable, it's okay to say so.

When Is the Right Time to Start Talking?

It's never too early to start talking to children about their bodies. Use the correct names for private body parts.

Be sure to keep having conversations with your child during adolescence. Adolescence is the stage between childhood and adulthood. During this time, your child will go through puberty. Puberty is when your child's body starts to change into an adult's body.

What Do I Tell My Child about Puberty?

Puberty is different for each child.

- For girls, puberty usually starts between ages 9 and 13.
- For boys, it usually begins between ages 10 and 13.

Puberty can be a confusing and overwhelming time for many kids. You can help your kids by:

- Telling them that puberty is a normal part of growing up
- Sharing facts to help them understand their changing bodies and feelings
- Talking about your own experiences when you were a kid

During puberty, kids may be less likely to ask you questions, so it's a good idea for you to start conversations with them.

What If My Child Has Questions about Being a Boy or Girl?

Some children act or feel like they are a different gender (boy or girl) than their birth sex (male or female). For example, a male child may feel like a girl, not a boy. And some kids don't feel like a boy *or* a girl.

When people act or feel like they are a different gender than their birth sex, this is called being "gender non-conforming." Children may feel this way from very early on, or they may start to feel this way during puberty.

For some kids, being gender non-conforming is temporary–for others, it's not. Either way, it's important to let your child know that you love and accept him no matter what.

How Can I Help My Child Build Healthy Relationships?

Families have different rules about when it's okay for kids to start dating. Whatever your family rules are, the best time to start talking about healthy relationships is before your child starts dating.

Start conversations about what to look for in a romantic partner. Help your kids develop realistic and healthy expectations for their relationships.

Talk about Opposite-Sex (Straight) and Same-Sex (Gay or Lesbian) Relationships.

When you talk to your child about sex and relationships, don't assume she is straight. Let your child know that it's okay to be lesbian, gay, bisexual, or straight—and that you love and accept her no matter what.

Lesbian, gay, and bisexual teens whose parents are supportive are less likely to be depressed, and more likely to make healthy choices about sex and relationships.

What Do I Tell My Child about Preventing Pregnancy and STDs?

Make sure your kids have the facts they need to make healthy decisions. This includes information about pregnancy and STDs (sexually transmitted diseases) like HIV/AIDS and chlamydia.

Both boys and girls need to know how to stay safe. Even if you think your child isn't dating or having sex, talk about ways to prevent pregnancy and STDs.

Tell your child about different birth control methods, like condoms and birth control pills. Make sure he knows which methods also help prevent STDs.

Will Talking to My Child Really Make a Difference?

Parents are the most important influence on a teen's decisions about sex and relationships. Your child may want to talk to you about sex and dating, but may not know how to start the conversation.

Teens who talk with their parents about sex are more likely to put off having sex until they are older. They are also more likely to make healthy choices, like using condoms to prevent pregnancy and STDs, if they do choose to have sex.

Take Action!

Kids need information from an adult they trust. Use these tips to start a conversation with your child today.

Talk Early and Often.

Start having conversations about your values and expectations while your child is young. Your child will get used to sharing information and opinions with you. This will make it easier for you to keep talking as your child gets older.

There's more than one way to talk to kids about sex. Try having lots of little conversations about sex instead of one big talk. And remember, if you've been putting it off, it's never too late to start a conversation about sex.

Start Small.

Try not to give your kids too much information at one time. Give them time between conversations to think. They may come back later and ask questions.

Be Ready to Answer Questions.

When your kids ask you questions, ask them what they think first. Their answers will tell you more about what they are asking and why. This will also give you time to think about your answer.

Do your best to answer questions honestly and correctly. If you don't know the answer to a question, you could say, "I'm not sure. Let's look that up together."

Keep in mind that kids get information about sex from lots of different sources–like friends, the Internet, and TV. This can be confusing for your child. That's another reason why it's important for you to answer questions clearly and accurately.

Ask Questions.

Give your kids time and space to talk about their feelings and thoughts. Ask for their opinions. Be sure to listen, even if you don't agree with your child's opinion.

Try asking questions like:

- When do you think it's okay to start dating?

- Have you talked about puberty or sex in school? Do you have any questions?

- When do you think a person is ready to have sex?

Always take your child's values and opinions seriously. This will show that you respect what your child has to say and it can help your child feel more comfortable talking to you.

Practice Active Listening.

Active listening is a way to show your kids that you are paying attention and trying to understand their thoughts and feelings. Try these tips:

- Nod your head.

- Repeat back what your child says in your own words. For example, "So you are feeling frustrated with our rules. You feel that you are old enough to make your own decisions."

Use Media to Start a Conversation.

Kids see and hear messages about sex every day in the media—like on TV, in music, and online. When something comes up in a TV show or song, use it as an opportunity to start a conversation with your child.

Talk in the Car or in the Kitchen.

It can sometimes be easier to talk about sex if you are doing something else at the same time. Try asking a question when you are driving in the car or busy cooking dinner.

You can still show your child that you are listening by nodding your head or repeating what your child says to you.

Be Honest.

It's okay to feel embarrassed or uncomfortable. Be honest with your child about how you are feeling. Remember, when you are honest with your child, your child is more likely to be honest with you.

Talk with Other Parents.

Remember that you are not the only parent thinking about how to talk to kids about sex. Ask other parents how it's going for them. You may be able to get useful tips and ideas.

Talking to parents is also a great way to learn more about the messages other kids are getting about sex and relationships.

Section 47.2

What Programs Effectively Prevent STDs in Youth?

This section includes text excerpted from "Effective HIV and STD Prevention Programs for Youth: A Summary of Scientific Evidence," Centers for Disease Control and Prevention (CDC), September 1, 2015.

Role of Schools in Preventing HIV/STD

Just as schools are critical settings for preparing students academically, they are also vital partners in helping young people take responsibility for their own health. School health programs can help youth adopt lifelong attitudes and behaviors that support overall health and well-being—including behaviors that can reduce their risk for HIV and other sexually transmitted diseases (STDs). HIV/STD prevention programs implemented by schools include prevention education programs designed specifically to reduce sexual risk behaviors and youth asset-development programs, which provide adolescents with more general skills that help them engage in healthy behaviors and solve problems.

Effective HIV/STD Prevention Education Programs

Research shows that well-designed and well-implemented HIV/STD prevention programs can decrease sexual risk behaviors among students, including—

- Delaying first sexual intercourse.

- Reducing the number of sex partners.

- Decreasing the number of times students have unprotected sex.

- Increasing condom use.

A review of 48 research studies found that about two-thirds of the HIV/STD prevention programs studied had a significant impact on reducing sexual risk behaviors, including a delay in first sexual intercourse, a decline in the number of sex partners, and an increase in condom or contraceptive use. Notably, the HIV prevention programs were not shown to hasten initiation of sexual intercourse among adolescents, even when those curricula encouraged sexually active young people to use condoms.

In addition to determining programs that are most effective in reducing sexual health risk behaviors among youth, scientists also have identified key common attributes among these programs. Effective HIV/STD prevention programs tend to be those that

- Are delivered by trained instructors.

- Are age-appropriate.

- Include components on skill-building, support of healthy behaviors in school environments, and involvement of parents, youth-serving organizations, and health organizations.

These common traits should guide curriculum development and integration of program activities for HIV/STD prevention programs in schools and communities.

Youth Asset-Development Programs

A promising approach to HIV prevention seeks to increase the skills of children and adolescents to avoid health risks, including sexual risk behaviors. Youth asset development programs, including those conducted in schools, teach youth how to solve problems, communicate with others, and plan for the future. They also help youth develop positive connections with their parents, schools, and communities. Youth asset-development programs typically address multiple health risk behaviors and are commonly provided to children and adolescents over a number of years. Evidence indicates that these programs can be associated with long-term reductions in sexual risk behaviors.

CDC's Ongoing Efforts to Identify and Implement Effective HIV/STD Prevention Programs for Youth

CDC's Division of Adolescent and School Health (DASH) supports rigorous evaluation research and other projects to identify the types of programs and practices that can reduce sexual risk behaviors among youth:

- DASH has supported the development and evaluation of

  - All About Youth, a randomized, controlled trial testing two HIV/STD education programs for middle school students: one that emphasizes sexual abstinence until marriage, and one that emphasizes abstinence in conjunction with skill-building activities for condom and contraceptive use.

- Linking Lives, a program designed to build parents' skills to help them reduce sexual health risks among their middle school children.

- DASH and CDC's Division of Reproductive Health collaborated with partners to publish a systematic review of the growing body of evidence on positive youth development approaches for reducing HIV, sexually transmitted infections, and unintended pregnancy.

- DASH scientists

  - Analyze research on program effectiveness.

  - Develop guidelines for best practices in school based HIV prevention.

  - Create tools to help schools implement the guidelines, such as the Health Education Curriculum Analysis Tool, which integrates research findings and national health education standards to help school districts select or develop health education curricula that are most likely to reduce sexual risk behaviors among the youth they serve.

Chapter 48

Preventing STDs with Safer Sex

Chapter Contents

Section 48.1

What Is "Safer" Sex?

This section includes text excerpted from "Preventing HIV infection," Office on Women's Health (OWH), July 1, 2011. Reviewed March 2016.

Practice Safer Sex

Taking simple steps to prevent getting or spreading HIV will pay off both for you and for those you love. The only 100 percent effective way to prevent the spread of HIV through sex is to abstain—to not have sex of any kind. If you do have sex, practice safer sex methods. These are the steps you can take to help prevent HIV infection from sex:

- **Abstain from sex.** Not having vaginal, anal, or oral sex is the surest way to avoid HIV. If you do decide to have sex, you can reduce your risk of HIV by practicing safer sex.

- **Get tested.** Be sure you know yours and your partner's HIV status before ever having sex.

- **Use condoms**. Use them correctly and every time you have sex. Using a male condom for all types of sex can greatly lower your risk of getting HIV during sex. If you or your partner is allergic to latex, use polyurethane condoms. If your partner won't use a male condom, you can use a female condom. It may protect against HIV, but we don't have much evidence that it does, so it is better to use a male condom, which we know has a high rate of preventing HIV infection. Do not use a male and female condom at the same time. They do not work together and can break. **"Natural" or "lambskin" condoms don't protect against HIV.** Condoms are easy to find, and some places give them out for free. Contact your local health department or a health clinic for information about places in your area that may give away free condoms. For instance, the New York State Health Department offers a cellphone app that can help youth find free condoms in their area.

- **Talk with your partner.** Learn how to talk with your sexual partner about HIV and using condoms. It's up to you to make sure you are protected. Remember, it's your body!

- **Practice monogamy (be faithful to one partner).** Being in a sexual relationship with only one partner who is also faithful to you can help protect you.

- **Limit your number of sexual partners.** Your risk of getting HIV goes up with the number of partners you have. Condoms should be used for any sexual activity with a partner who has HIV. They should also be used with any partner outside of a long-term, faithful sexual relationship.

- **Use protection for all kinds of sexual contact.** Remember that you don't only get HIV from penile-vaginal sex. Use a condom during oral sex and during anal sex. Dental dams also can be used to help lower your risk as well as your partner's risk of getting HIV during oral-vaginal or oral-anal sex.

- **Know that other types of birth control will not protect you from HIV.** Other methods of birth control, like birth control pills, shots, implants, or diaphragms, will not protect you from HIV. If you use one of these, be sure to also use a male condom or dental dam correctly every time you have sex.

- **Don't use nonoxynol-9 (N-9).** Some contraceptives, like condoms, suppositories, foams, and gels contain the spermicide N-9. You shouldn't be using gels, foams, or suppositories to prevent against HIV—these methods only lower chances of pregnancy, not of HIV and other sexually transmitted infections (STIs). N-9 actually makes your risk of HIV infection higher, because it can irritate the vagina, which might make it easier for HIV to get into your body.

- **Get screened for STIs.** Having an STI, particularly genital herpes, increases your chances of becoming infected with HIV during sex. If your partner has an STI in addition to HIV, that also increases your risk of HIV infection. If you have an STI, you should also get tested for HIV.

- **Don't douche.** Douching removes some of the normal bacteria in the vagina that protects you from infection. This can increase your risk of getting HIV.

- **Don't abuse alcohol or drugs, which are linked to sexual risk-taking.** Drinking too much alcohol or using drugs also puts you at risk of sexual assault and possible exposure to HIV.

521

Take Time to Talk before Having Sex

Talking about sex is hard for some people. So, they don't bring up safe sex or STIs with their partners. But keep in mind that it's your body, and it's up to you to protect yourself. Before having sex, talk with your partner about his or her past and present sexual behavior and HIV status, and talk about using condoms and dental dams. Ask if he or she has been tested for HIV or other STIs. Having the talk ahead of time can help you avoid misunderstandings during a moment of passion. Let your partner know that you will not have any type of sex at any time without using a condom or dental dam. If your partner gives an excuse, be ready with a response.

Section 48.2

Condoms and Sexually Transmitted Diseases

This section contains text excerpted from the following sources:
Text under the heading "A Condom Could Save Your Life" is
excerpted from" Condoms and Sexually Transmitted Diseases,"
U.S. Food and Drug Administration (FDA), January 1, 2015;
Text under the heading "How to Use Condoms" is excerpted
from "Preventing HIV Infection," Office on Women's
Health (OWH), July 1, 2011. Reviewed April 2016.

A Condom Could Save Your Life

It's important to use condoms (rubbers, prophylactics) to help reduce the spread of sexually transmitted diseases (STDs). These diseases include the Human Immunodeficiency Virus, or HIV (the virus that causes AIDS), chlamydia, genital herpes, genital warts, gonorrhea, hepatitis B, and syphilis. You can get them through having sex–vaginal, anal, or oral.

The surest way to avoid these diseases is to not have sex altogether (abstinence). Another way is to limit sex to one partner who also limits his or her sex in the same way (monogamy). Condoms are not 100% safe, but if used properly, will reduce the risk of sexually transmitted diseases, including AIDS. Protecting yourself against the AIDS virus is of special concern because this disease is fatal and has no cure.

Many people infected with HIV in the United States got the disease during sexual intercourse with an infected partner. Experts believe that many of these people could have avoided the disease by using condoms.

Condoms are used for both birth control and reducing the risk of disease. That's why some people think that other forms of birth control—such as the IUD, diaphragm, cervical cap or pill—will protect them against diseases, too. But that's not true. So if you use any other form of birth control, you still need a condom in addition to reduce the risk of getting sexually transmitted diseases.

A condom is especially important when an uninfected pregnant woman has sex, because it can also help protect her and her unborn child from a sexually transmitted disease.

Condoms are not 100% safe, but if used properly, will reduce the risk of sexually transmitted diseases, including AIDS.

Facts about Sexually Transmitted Diseases

- Sexually transmitted diseases (STDs) affect millions of men and women in the United States each year.

- Anyone can become infected through sexual intercourse with an infected person.

- Many of those infected are teenagers or young adults.

- Changing sexual partners adds to the risk of becoming infected.

- Sometimes, early in the infection, there may be no symptoms, or symptoms may be easily confused with other illnesses.

Sexually transmitted diseases can cause:

- Tubal pregnancies, sometimes fatal to the mother and always fatal to the unborn child

- Death or severe damage to a baby born to an infected woman

- Sterility (loss of ability to get pregnant)

- Cancer of the cervix in women

- Damage to other parts of the body, including the heart, kidneys, and brain

- Death of infected individuals

See a doctor if you have any of these symptoms of STDs:

- Discharge from the vagina, penis, and/or rectum

- Pain or burning during urination and/or intercourse

- Pain in the abdomen (women), testicles (men), and buttocks and legs (both)

- Blisters, open sores, warts, rash, and/or swelling in the genital area, sex organs, and/or mouth

- Flu-like symptoms, including fever, headache, aching muscles, and/or swollen glands

Who Should Use a Condom?

A person who takes part in risky sexual behavior should always use a condom.

The highest risk comes from having intercourse—vaginal, anal, or oral—with a person who has a sexually transmitted disease. If you have sex with an infected person, you're taking a big chance. If you know your partner is infected, the best rule is to avoid intercourse (including oral sex). If you do decide to have sex with an infected partner, you should always be sure a condom is used from start to finish, every time.

And it's risky to have sex with someone who has shared needles with an infected person.

It's also risky to have sex with someone who had sex with an infected person in the past. If your partner had intercourse with a person infected with HIV (the AIDS virus), he or she could pass it on to you. That can happen even if the intercourse was a long time ago and even if you partner seems perfectly healthy.

With sexually transmitted diseases, you often can't tell whether your partner has been infected. If you're not sure about yourself or your partner, you should choose to not have sex at all. But if you do have sex, be sure to use a condom that covers the entire penis to reduce your risk of being infected. This includes oral sex where the penis is in contact with the mouth.

If you think you and your partner should be using condoms but your partner refuses, then you should say NO to sex with that person.

How Can I Get the Most Protection from Condoms?

No. Consistent and correct use of the male latex condom reduces the risk of sexually transmitted disease (STD) and human immuno-deficiency virus (HIV) transmission. However, condom use cannot provide absolute protection against any STD. The most reliable ways to avoid transmission of STDs are to abstain from sexual activity, or to be in a long-term mutually monogamous relationship with an uninfected partner. However, many infected persons may be unaware of their infection because STDs often are asymptomatic and unrecognized.

In other words, sex with condoms isn't totally "safe sex," but it is "less risky" sex.

HIV infection is, by far, the most deadly STD, and considerably more scientific evidence exists regarding condom effectiveness for prevention of HIV infection than for other STDs. The body of research on the effectiveness of latex condoms in preventing sexual transmission of HIV is both comprehensive and conclusive The ability of latex condoms to prevent transmission of HIV has been scientifically established in "real-life" studies of sexually active couples as well as in laboratory studies.

How Does a Condom Protect against Sexually Transmitted Diseases?

- Choose the right kind of condoms to prevent disease.

- Store them properly.

- Remember to use a new condom every time you have sex.

- Use the condom the right way, from start to finish.

- How does a condom protect against sexually transmitted diseases?

- A condom acts as a barrier or wall to keep blood, or semen, or vaginal fluids from passing from one person to the other during intercourse.

- These fluids can harbor germs such as HIV (the virus that causes AIDS). If no condom is used, the germs can pass from the infected partner to the uninfected partner.

How Do I Choose the Right Kind of Condoms to Prevent Disease?

Always read the label. Look for two things:

1. The condoms should be made of latex (rubber), or polyurethane condoms for people sensitive or allergic to latex. Tests have shown that latex and polyurethane condoms (including the female condom) can prevent the passage of the HIV, hepatitis and herpes viruses. But natural (lambskin) condoms may not do this.

2. The package should say that the condoms are to prevent disease. If the package doesn't say anything about preventing disease, the condoms may not provide the protection you want, even though they may be the most expensive ones you can buy.

Novelty condoms will not say anything about either disease prevention or pregnancy prevention on the package. They are intended only for sexual stimulation, not protection.

Condoms which do not cover the entire penis are not labeled for disease prevention and should not be used for this purpose. For proper protection, a condom must unroll to cover the entire penis. This is another good reason to read the label carefully.

What Does the FDA Do to Ensure Condom Quality?

Always read the label. Look for two things:

1. The condoms should be made of latex (rubber), or polyurethane condoms for people sensitive or allergic to latex. Tests have shown that latex and polyurethane condoms (including the female condom) can prevent the passage of the HIV, hepatitis and herpes viruses. But natural (lambskin) condoms may not do this.

2. The package should say that the condoms are to prevent disease. If the package doesn't say anything about preventing disease, the condoms may not provide the protection you want, even though they may be the most expensive ones you can buy.

Novelty condoms will not say anything about either disease prevention or pregnancy prevention on the package. They are intended only for sexual stimulation, not protection.

Condoms which do not cover the entire penis are not labeled for disease prevention and should not be used for this purpose. For proper protection, a condom must unroll to cover the entire penis. This is another good reason to read the label carefully.

Are Condoms Strong Enough for Anal Intercourse?

Condoms may be more likely to break during anal intercourse than during other types of sex because of the greater amount of friction and other stresses involved.

Should Spermicides Be Used with Condoms?

The active ingredient in all of the over-the-counter (OTC) vaginal contraceptive drug products (spermicides) available in the U.S. is nonoxynol 9 (N-9). N-9 vaginal contraceptive drug products are used alone to prevent pregnancy, or with barrier methods such as diaphragms or cervical caps. Some condoms include a spermicidal lubricant containing N-9.

Clinical studies have shown that N-9 spermicides do not prevent or reduce the risk of getting HIV, the virus that causes AIDS, from an infected partner, or against getting other STDs. Thus, N-9 spermicides should not be used for HIV/STD prevention or protection. Clinical studies also show that use of N-9 spermicides can cause vaginal and rectal irritation which could increase the risk of getting HIV/AIDS from an infected partner.

FDA still considers N-9 safe as a contraceptive for women at low risk for HIV and other STDs. However, FDA now requires warning statements and other labeling information for all over the counter (OTC) vaginal contraceptive drug product (also known as spermicides) containing nonoxynol 9 (N9). These warning statements advise consumers that vaginal contraceptives/spermicides containing N9 do not protect against infection from the human immunodeficiency virus (HIV), the virus that causes acquired immunodeficiency syndrome (AIDS), or against getting other sexually transmitted diseases (STDs). The warnings and labeling information also advise consumers that use of vaginal contraceptives and spermicides containing N9 can irritate the vagina and rectum and may increase the risk of getting the AIDS virus (HIV) from an infected partner.

Use a Lubricant with a Condom

Some condoms are already lubricated with dry silicone, jellies, or creams. If you buy condoms not already lubricated, it's a good idea to apply some yourself. Lubricants may help prevent condoms from breaking during use and may prevent irritation, which might increase the chance of infection.

If you use a separate lubricant, be sure to use one that's water-based and made for this purpose. If you're not sure which to choose, ask your pharmacist.

Never use a lubricant that contains oils, fats, or greases such as petroleum-based jelly (like Vaseline brand), baby oil or lotion, hand or body lotions, cooking shortenings, or oily cosmetics like cold cream. They can seriously weaken latex, causing a condom to tear easily.

Does It Matter Which Styles of Condoms I Use?

It's most important to choose condoms that say "disease prevention" on the package. Other features are a matter of personal choice.

What Do the Dates Mean on the Package?

Some packages show "DATE MFG." This tells you when the condoms were made. It is not an expiration date.

Other packages may show an expiration date. The condoms should not be purchased or used after that date.

Are Condoms from Vending Machines Any Good?

It depends. Vending machine condoms may be OK:

• If you know you are getting a latex or polyurethane condom,

• If they are labeled for disease prevention,

• If the condoms do not contain nonoxynol 9 (N9) spermicide.

• If the machine is not exposed to extreme temperature and direct sunlight.

How Should Condoms Be Stored?

You should store condoms in a cool, dry place out of direct sunlight, perhaps in a drawer or closet. If you want to keep one with you, put it in a loose pocket, wallet, or purse for no more than a few hours at a time.

Extreme temperature-especially heat-can make latex brittle or gummy (like an old balloon). So don't keep these latex products in a hot place like a glove compartment

What Defects Should I Look For?

If the condom material sticks to itself or is gummy, the condom is no good. Also check the condom tip for other damage that is obvious (brittleness, tears, and holes). Don't unroll the condom to check it because this could cause damage.

How to Use Condoms

Male and female condoms can be used to protect you from HIV. But don't use them both at the same time! If used together, they won't stay in place, and they can tear or become damaged. Read the instructions and practice a few times before using condoms for the first time.

Follow these guidelines:

Male Condom

Use male condoms made of latex, or polyurethane if you or your partner is allergic to latex. Use male condoms for vaginal, anal, or oral sex.

- Keep male condoms in a cool, dry place. Don't keep them in your wallet or in your car! This can cause them to break or tear.

- Check the wrapper for tears and for the expiration date, to make sure the condom is not too old to use. Carefully open the wrapper. Don't use your teeth or fingernails. Make sure the condom looks okay to use. Don't use a condom that's gummy, brittle, discolored, or has even a tiny hole.

- Put on the condom as soon as the penis is erect, but before it touches the vagina, mouth, or anus.

- Use lubricants only made with water, such as K-Y jelly. Oil based lubricants, such as Vaseline, can weaken the condom. The lubricant is put on the outside of the condom. It helps to keep the condom from tearing. Don't use lubricants with the spermicide N-9, which might make it easier for HIV to get into your body.

529

- After sex, pull out the penis while it is still erect, holding the condom firmly at the base of the penis so it does not slip off.

Use a new condom if you want to have sex again or in a different way. Do not wash and re-use condoms—they are for one-time use!

Female Condom

The female condom, known as the FC2, is made of a rubber-like substance that is not latex. This condom is made for vaginal sex only. FC2 has a ring on each end. The inside ring holds the condom in place inside the vagina. The outer ring stays outside the vagina so it covers the labia. Some research suggests that the female condom is effective at preventing HIV. It is not yet known whether it is as effective as the male condom. The male condom is still considered best for preventing HIV. Use female condoms for vaginal sex if your partner won't use a male condom.

Remember:

Don't use a male condom and a female condom at the same time. They could break.

You can also follow these steps:

- Check the wrapper for tears and to make sure the condom is not too old to use. Open the wrapper carefully. Don't use your teeth or fingernails. Make sure the condom looks OK to use. The condom

- will be moist and may be slippery.

- Put the condom into the vagina up to eight hours before having sex, but before the penis touches the vagina. The condom cannot disappear inside your body.

- To insert the FC2, squeeze the inner ring with the thumb and middle finger and insert it into the vagina like a tampon. Then, use the index finger to push the inner ring as far up as it will go, without twisting the condom. There should be about an inch of condom outside your vagina to allow for the condom to expand during sex.

- FC2 comes pre-lubricated. But it is okay to use water or oilbased lubricants too. The lubricant is put on the inside and outside of the condom.

- During sex, make sure the outer ring of the FC2 isn't pushed into the vagina.

- After sex, hold the condom in place while your partner withdraws his penis. Remove the condom before standing up. Grasp the outside ring and twist the condom to trap in fluid and gently remove. Or, you can hold the condom tight around your partner's penis and he can pull out his penis and the condom at the same time, being careful not to spill any fluid out of the condom.

- Use a new condom if you want to have sex again.

Section 48.3

Spermicides Alone Do Not Protect against STDs

This section includes text excerpted from "Clinical Prevention Guidance," Centers for Disease Control and Prevention (CDC), January 28, 2011. Reviewed April 2016.

Topical Microbicides and Spermicides

Studies examining nonspecific topical microbicides for the prevention of HIV and STD have demonstrated that these products are ineffective. Studies of spermicides containing N-9 have demonstrated that they should not be recommended for STDs/HIV prevention, and more recent randomized controlled trials have failed to show a protective effect against HIV acquisition for BufferGel (a vaginal buffering agent), Carraguard (a carrageenan derivative), cellulose sulfate (an HIV entry inhibitor), and SAVVY (1.0% C31G, a surfactant).

Initial results from a study in which participants used 0.5% PRO2000 vaginal gel (a synthetic polyanion polymer that blocks cellular entry of HIV) on a daily basis appeared promising, reducing the rate of HIV acquisition by 30% relative to no gel. However, a recent randomized trial of approximately 9,000 women failed to show any protective effect.

Topical antiretroviral agents for the prevention of HIV appear more promising. Use of tenofovir gel during sexual intercourse significantly reduced the rate of HIV acquisition (i.e., by 39%) in a study of South

African women. Additional studies are being undertaken to elucidate the optimal dosing regimens for this drug.

Other products remain under study, including VivaGel, a topical vaginal microbicide.

Condoms and N-9 Vaginal Spermicides

Condoms lubricated with spermicides are no more effective than other lubricated condoms in protecting against the transmission of HIV and other STDs.

Furthermore, frequent use of spermicides containing N-9 has been associated with disruption of the genital epithelium, which might be associated with an increased risk for HIV transmission. Therefore, use of condoms lubricated with N-9 is not recommended for STD/HIV prevention; in addition, spermicide-coated condoms cost more, have a shorter shelf-life than other lubricated condoms, and have been associated with urinary-tract infection in young women.

Rectal Use of N-9 Spermicides

N-9 can damage the cells lining the rectum, which might provide a portal of entry for HIV and other sexually transmissible agents. Therefore, it should not used as a microbicide or lubricant during anal intercourse by MSM or by women.

Chapter 49

Preventing STDs after Possible or Certain Exposure

Chapter Contents

Section 49.1

Expedited Partner Therapy

This section includes excerpts from "Expedited Partner Therapy," Centers for Disease Control and Prevention (CDC), January 1, 2015; and text from "Guidance on the Use of Expedited Partner Therapy in the Treatment of Gonorrhea," Centers for Disease Control and Prevention (CDC), August 20, 2015; and text from "Legal Status of Expedited Partner Therapy (EPT)," Centers for Disease Control and Prevention (CDC), June 4, 2015.

What Is Expedited Partner Therapy?

Expedited Partner Therapy (EPT) is the clinical practice of treating the sex partners of patients diagnosed with chlamydia or gonorrhea by providing prescriptions or medications to the patient to take to his/her partner without the health care provider first examining the partner.

Effective clinical management of patients with treatable sexually transmitted diseases (STDs) requires treatment of the patients' current sex partners to prevent reinfection and curtail further transmission. The standard approach to partner treatment has included clinical evaluation in a health care setting, with partner notification accomplished by the index patient, by the provider or an agent of the provider, or a combination of these methods. Provider-assisted referral is considered the optimal strategy for partner treatment, but is not available to most patients with gonorrhea or chlamydial infection because of resource limitations. The usual alternative is to advise patients to refer their partners for treatment.

CDC has concluded that EPT is a useful option to facilitate partner management, particularly for treatment of male partners of women with chlamydial infection or gonorrhea. Although ongoing evaluation will be needed to define when and how EPT can be best utilized, the evidence indicates that EPT should be available to clinicians as an option for partner treatment. EPT represents an additional strategy for partner management that does not replace other strategies such as provider-assisted referral, when available.

Expedited Partner Therapy in the Treatment of Gonorrhea

Expedited Partner Therapy (EPT) is a partner treatment approach where sex partners of patients who test positive for certain sexually transmitted diseases are provided medication without previous medical evaluation. Because of EPT's effectiveness in reducing gonorrhea reinfection rates, CDC has recommended its use since 2006 for the heterosexual partners of patients diagnosed with gonorrhea if it was unlikely the partners would seek timely evaluation and treatment.

However, as of 2012, CDC no longer recommends the routine use of orally-administered cefixime for the treatment of gonorrhea in the United States. At present, the only CDC-recommended treatment of uncomplicated urogenital, anorectal, and pharyngeal gonorrhea is combination therapy with a single intramuscular dose of ceftriaxone 250 mg plus a single dose of azithromycin 1 g orally.

Since EPT is not possible where treatment involves an injection, the current CDC gonorrhea treatment recommendations have implications for the use of EPT in the treatment of gonorrhea. CDC continues to recommend EPT for heterosexual men and women with gonorrhea for whom health department partner-management strategies are impractical or unavailable and whose providers are concerned about partners' access to prompt clinical evaluation and treatment. This section is intended to provide guidance to providers who choose to use EPT for gonorrhea, and to answer frequently asked questions.

In Light of CDC's Recent Changes to Its Gonorrhea Treatment Recommendations, Can EPT Be Used for Gonorrhea?

- Under current guidelines every effort should be made to ensure that a patient's sex partners from the past 60 days are evaluated and treated with the recommended regimen (ceftriaxone 250 mg IM plus a single dose of azithromycin 1 g orally). However, because that is not always possible, providers should still consider EPT for heterosexual partners of patients diagnosed with gonorrhea who are unlikely to access timely evaluation and treatment. EPT is not routinely recommended for MSM because of a high risk for coexisting infections, especially undiagnosed HIV infection, in their partners.

Since CDC No Longer Recommends Exclusively Oral Treatment for Gonorrhea, How Does CDC Recommend EPT Be Practiced for Gonorrhea?

- If a heterosexual partner of a gonorrhea patient cannot be linked to evaluation and treatment in a timely fashion, EPT with cefixime and azithromycin should still be considered, as not treating partners is significantly more harmful than is the use of EPT for gonorrhea. As has always been the case, medication or prescriptions provided as part of EPT should be accompanied by treatment instructions, appropriate warnings about taking medications (if the partner is pregnant or has an allergy to the medication), general gonorrhea health education and counseling, and a statement advising that partners seek personal medical evaluation, particularly women with symptoms of PID.

Section 49.2

Preventing STDs after a Sexual Assault

Text in this section is excerpted from "Sexual Assault and Abuse and STDs," Centers for Disease Control and Prevention (CDC), June 4, 2015.

Sexual Assault and Abuse and STDs

These guidelines are primarily limited to the identification, prophylaxis, and treatment of STDs and conditions among adolescent and adult female sexual assault survivors. However, some of the following guidelines might still apply to male sexual assault survivors. The documentation of findings, collection of nonmicrobiologic specimens for forensic purposes, and the management of potential pregnancy or physical and psychological trauma are beyond the scope of these guidelines.

Examinations of survivors of sexual assault should be conducted by an experienced clinician in a way that minimizes further trauma to the survivor. The decision to obtain genital or other specimens for STD diagnosis should be made on an individual basis. Care systems for survivors should be designed to ensure continuity (including timely review of test results), support adherence, and monitor adverse reactions to any prescribed therapeutic or prophylactic regimens. Laws in all 50 states strictly limit the evidentiary use of a survivor's previous sexual history, including evidence of previously acquired STDs, as part of an effort to undermine the credibility of the survivor's testimony. Evidentiary privilege against revealing any aspect of the examination or treatment also is enforced in most states. Although it rarely occurs, STD diagnoses might later be accessed, and the survivor and clinician might opt to defer testing for this reason. While collection of specimens at initial examination for laboratory STD diagnosis gives the survivor and clinician the option to defer empiric prophylactic antimicrobial treatment, compliance with follow-up visits is typically poor. Among sexually active adults, the identification of an STD might represent an infection acquired before the assault, and therefore might be more important for the medical management of the patient than for legal purposes.

Trichomoniasis, BV, gonorrhea, and chlamydial infection are the most frequently diagnosed infections among women who have been sexually assaulted. Such conditions are prevalent in the population, and detection of these infections after an assault does not necessarily imply acquisition during the assault. However, a post-assault examination presents an important opportunity to identify or prevent STDs. Chlamydial and gonococcal infections in women are of particular concern because of the possibility of ascending infection. In addition, HBV infection can be prevented through postexposure vaccination. Because female survivors also are at risk for acquiring HPV infection and the efficacy of the HPV vaccine is high, HPV vaccination is also recommended for females through age 26 years. Reproductive-aged female survivors should be evaluated for pregnancy.

Evaluating Adolescents and Adults for STDs

Initial Examination

Decisions to perform these tests should be made on an individual basis. An initial examination might include the following procedures:

- NAATs for *C. trachomatis* and *N. gonorrhoeae* at the sites of penetration or attempted penetration. These tests are preferred for the diagnostic evaluation of adolescent or adult sexual assault survivors.

- NAATs from a urine or vaginal specimen or point-of-care testing (i.e., DNA probes) from a vaginal specimen for *T. vaginalis*. Point-of-care testing and/or wet mount with measurement of vaginal pH and KOH application for the whiff test from vaginal secretions should be done for evidence of BV and candidiasis, especially if vaginal discharge, malodor, or itching is present.

- A serum sample for evaluation of HIV, hepatitis B, and syphilis infections.

Treatment

Compliance with follow-up visits is poor among survivors of sexual assault. As a result, the following routine presumptive treatment after a sexual assault is recommended:

- An empiric antimicrobial regimen for chlamydia, gonorrhea, and trichomonas.

- Emergency contraception. This measure should be considered when the assault could result in pregnancy in the survivor.

- Postexposure hepatitis B vaccination (without HBIG) if the hepatitis status of the assailant is unknown and the survivor has not been previously vaccinated. If the assailant is known to be HBsAg-positive, unvaccinated survivors should receive both hepatitis B vaccine and HBIG. The vaccine and HBIG, if indicated, should be administered to sexual assault survivors at the time of the initial examination, and follow-up doses of vaccine should be administered 1–2 and 4–6 months after the first dose. Survivors who were previously vaccinated but did not receive postvaccination testing should receive a single vaccine booster dose.

- HPV vaccination is recommended for female survivors aged 9–26 years and male survivors aged 9–21 years. For MSM with who have not received HPV vaccine or who have been incompletely vaccinated, vaccine can be administered through age 26 years. The vaccine should be administered to sexual assault survivors at the time of the initial examination, and follow-up dose administered at 1–2 months and 6 months after the first dose.

- Recommendations for HIV PEP are individualized according to risk.

If alcohol has been recently ingested or emergency contraception is provided, metronidazole or tinidazole can be taken by the sexual assault survivor at home rather than as directly observed therapy to minimize potential side effects and drug interactions. Clinicians should counsel persons regarding the possible benefits and toxicities associated with these treatment regimens; gastrointestinal side effects can occur with this combination. The efficacy of these regimens in preventing infections after sexual assault has not been evaluated. For those requiring alternative treatments, refer to the specific sections in this report relevant to the specific organism.

Other Management Considerations

At the initial examination and, if indicated, at follow-up examinations, patients should be counseled regarding symptoms of STDs and the need for immediate examination if symptoms occur. Further, they should be instructed to abstain from sexual intercourse until STD prophylactic treatment is completed.

Follow-Up

After the initial post-assault examination, follow-up examinations provide an opportunity to

1. detect new infections acquired during or after the assault;

2. complete hepatitis B and HPV vaccinations, if indicated;

3. complete counseling and treatment for other STDs; and

4. monitor side effects and adherence to postexposure prophylactic medication, if prescribed.

If initial testing was done, follow-up evaluation should be conducted within 1 week to ensure that results of positive tests can be discussed promptly with the survivor, treatment is provided if not given at the initial visit, and any follow-up for the infection(s) can be arranged. If initial tests are negative and treatment was not provided, examination for STDs can be repeated within 1–2 weeks of the assault; repeat testing detects infectious organisms that might not have reached sufficient concentrations to produce positive test results at the time of initial examination. For survivors who are treated during the initial visit, regardless of whether testing was performed, post-treatment testing should be conducted only if the survivor reports having symptoms. A follow-up examination at 1–2 months should also be considered to reevaluate for development of anogenital warts, especially among sexual assault survivors who received a diagnosis of other

STDs. If initial test results were negative and infection in the assailant cannot be ruled out, serologic tests for syphilis can be repeated at 4–6 weeks and 3 months; HIV testing can be repeated at 6 weeks and at 3 and 6 months using methods to identify acute HIV infection.

Section 49.3

Post-Exposure Prophylaxis: Taking HIV Drugs If You've Been Exposed to the Virus through Blood or Sexual Contact

This section contains text excerpted from the following sources: Text under the heading "What Is PEP?" is excerpted from "PEP," Centers for Disease Control and Prevention (CDC), January 21, 2016; Text under the heading "Who Needs PEP?" is excerpted from "Post-Exposure Prophylaxis (PEP)," U.S. Department of Health and Human Services (HHS), September 21, 2015.

What Is PEP?

PEP stands for post-exposure prophylaxis. It means taking antiretroviral medicines (ART) after being potentially exposed to HIV to prevent becoming infected.

PEP must be started within 72 hours after a recent possible exposure to HIV, but the sooner you start PEP, the better. Every hour counts. If you're prescribed PEP, you'll need to take it once or twice daily for 28 days. PEP is effective in preventing HIV when administered correctly, but not 100%.

Is PEP Right for Me?

If you're HIV-negative or don't know your HIV status, and in the last 72 hours you

1. think you may have been exposed to HIV during sex (for example, if the condom broke),

2. shared needles and works to prepare drugs (for example, cotton, cookers, water), or

3.   were sexually assaulted, talk to your health care provider or an emergency room doctor about PEP right away.

PEP should be used only in emergency situations and must be started within 72 hours after a recent possible exposure to HIV. It is not a substitute for regular use of other proven HIV prevention methods, such as pre-exposure prophylaxis (PrEP), which means taking HIV medicines daily to lower your chance of getting infected; using condoms the right way every time you have sex; and using only your own new, sterile needles and works every time you inject.

PEP is effective, but not 100%, so you should continue to use condoms with sex partners and safe injection practices while taking PEP. These strategies can protect you from being exposed to HIV again and reduce the chances of transmitting HIV to others if you do become infected while you're on PEP.

I'm a Health Care Worker, and I Think I've Been Exposed to HIV at Work. Should I Take PEP?

PEP should be considered if you've had a recent possible exposure to HIV at work. Report your exposure to your supervisor, and seek medical attention immediately.

Occupational transmission of HIV to health care workers is extremely rare, and the proper use of safety devices and barriers can help minimize the risk of exposure while caring for patients with HIV.

A health care worker who has a possible exposure should see a doctor or visit an emergency room immediately. PEP must be started within 72 hours after a recent possible exposure to HIV. The sooner, the better; every hour counts.

CDC issued updated guidelines in 2013 for the management of health care worker exposures to HIV and recommendations for PEP.

Clinicians caring for health care workers who've had a possible exposure can call the PEPline (1-888-448-4911), which offers around-the-clock advice on managing occupational exposures to HIV, as well as hepatitis B and C. Exposed health care workers may also call the PEPline, but they should seek local medical attention first.

When Should I Take PEP?

PEP must be started within 72 hours after a possible exposure. The sooner you start PEP, the better; every hour counts.

541

Starting PEP as soon as possible after a potential HIV exposure is important. Research has shown that PEP has little or no effect in preventing HIV infection if it is started later than 72 hours after HIV exposure.

If you're prescribed PEP, you'll need to take it once or twice daily for 28 days.

Does PEP Have Any Side Effects?

PEP is safe but may cause side effects like nausea in some people. These side effects can be treated and aren't life-threatening.

Where Can I Get PEP?

Your health care provider or an emergency room doctor can prescribe PEP. Talk to them right away if you think you've recently been exposed to HIV.

How Can I Pay for PEP?

If you're prescribed PEP after a sexual assault, you may qualify for partial or total reimbursement for medicines and clinical care costs through the Office for Victims of Crime, funded by the United States Department of Justice.

If you're prescribed PEP for another reason and you cannot get insurance coverage (Medicaid, Medicare, private, or employer-based), your health care provider can apply for free PEP medicines through the medication assistance programs run by the manufacturers. Online applications can be faxed to the company, or some companies have special phone lines. These can be handled urgently in many cases to avoid a delay in getting medicine.

If you're a health care worker who was exposed to HIV on the job, your workplace health insurance or workers' compensation will usually pay for PEP.

Can I Take a Round of PEP Every Time I Have Unprotected Sex?

PEP is not the right choice for people who may be exposed to HIV frequently—for example, if you often have sex without a condom with a partner who is HIV-positive. Because PEP is given after a potential exposure to HIV, more drugs and higher doses are needed to block infection than with PrEP, or pre-exposure prophylaxis. PrEP is when people at high risk for HIV take HIV medicines (sold under the brand name Truvada) daily to lower their chances of getting HIV. If you are at ongoing risk for HIV, speak to your doctor about PrEP.

Who Needs PEP?

PEP is used for anyone who may have been exposed to HIV during a single high-risk event.

Healthcare workers are evaluated for PEP if they are exposed after:

• Getting cut or stuck with a needle that was used to draw blood from a person who may have HIV infection

• Getting blood or other body fluids that may have lots of HIV in their eyes or mouth

• Getting blood or other body fluids that may have lots of HIV on their skin when it is chapped, scraped, or affected by certain rashes

The risk of getting HIV infection in these ways is extremely low— fewer than 1 in 100 for all exposures.

PEP can also be used to treat people who may have been exposed to HIV during a single high-risk event unrelated to work (e.g., during episodes of unprotected sex, needle-sharing injection drug use, or sexual assault).

Keep in mind that PEP should only be used in uncommon situations right after a potential HIV exposure. PEP is not intended for long-term use. It is not a substitute for regular use of other proven HIV prevention methods, such as pre-exposure prophylaxis (PrEP), correct and consistent condom use or use of sterile injection equipment.

Because PEP is not 100% effective, you should continue to use condoms with sex partners while taking PEP and should not share injection equipment with others. This will help avoid spreading the virus to others if you become infected. If you have repeated exposures to HIV, you should consider PrEP.

Can I Prevent HIV after I've Been Exposed?

Yes. Post-exposure prophylaxis (PEP) involves taking anti-HIV medications as soon as possible (within 3 days) after you may have been exposed to HIV to try to reduce the chance of becoming HIV positive. PEP is a month-long course of emergency medication taken to try to keep HIV from making copies of itself and spreading through your body. PEP is used by health care workers who have been exposed to HIV-infected fluids on the job or anyone who may have been exposed through unprotected sex, needle-sharing injection drug use, or sexual assault. If you think you were exposed to HIV, go immediately to a clinic or emergency room and ask for PEP.

PEP must begin within 72 hours of exposure, before the virus has time to make too many copies of itself in your body. PEP consists of 2–3 antiretroviral medications and must be taken for 28 days. Your doctor will determine what treatment is right for you based on how you were exposed to HIV. You will be asked to return for follow-up appointments and additional HIV testing.

PEP is safe but may cause side effects like nausea in some people. These side effects can be treated and are not life threatening. PEP is not 100% effective; it does not guarantee that someone exposed to HIV will not become infected with HIV.

Chapter 50

Preventing Mother-to-Child HIV Transmission

Chapter Contents

545

Section 50.1

How to Prevent HIV Transmission from Mother-to-Child

This section includes text excerpted from "Preventing Mother-to-Child Transmission of HIV," U.S. Department of Health and Human Services (HHS), August 25, 2015.

Key Points

- Mother-to-child transmission of HIV is the spread of HIV from an HIV-infected woman to her child during pregnancy, childbirth (also called labor and delivery), or breastfeeding (through breast milk). Mother-to-child transmission is the most common way that children become infected with HIV.

- Pregnant women with HIV receive HIV medicines during pregnancy and childbirth to reduce the risk of mother-to-child transmission of HIV. In some situations, a woman with HIV may have a scheduled cesarean delivery (sometimes called a C-section) to prevent mother-to-child transmission of HIV during delivery.

- Babies born to women with HIV receive HIV medicine for 6 weeks after birth. The HIV medicine reduces the risk of infection from any HIV that may have entered a baby's body during childbirth.

- Because HIV can be transmitted in breast milk, women with HIV living in the United States should not breastfeed their babies. In the United States, baby formula is a safe and healthy alternative to breast milk.

What Is Mother-to-Child Transmission of HIV?

Mother-to-child transmission of HIV is the spread of HIV from an HIV-infected woman to her child during pregnancy, childbirth (also called labor and delivery), or breastfeeding (through breast milk). Mother-to-child transmission of HIV is also called perinatal transmission of HIV.

Mother-to-child transmission is the most common way that children become infected with HIV.

Can Mother-to-Child Transmission of HIV Be Prevented?

Yes. The risk of mother-to-child transmission of HIV is low when:

- Women with HIV receive HIV medicine during pregnancy and childbirth and, in certain situations, have a scheduled cesarean delivery (sometimes called a C-section).

- Babies born to women with HIV receive HIV medicines for 6 weeks after birth and are not breastfed.

Is HIV Testing Recommended for Pregnant Women?

The Centers for Disease Control and Prevention (CDC) recommends that all pregnant women get tested for HIV as early as possible during each pregnancy.

Pregnant women who test HIV positive receive HIV medicines to reduce the risk of mother-to-child transmission of HIV and to protect their own health. (HIV medicines are recommended for everyone infected with HIV. HIV medicines help people with HIV live longer, healthier lives and reduce the risk of sexual transmission of HIV.)

How Do HIV Medicines Prevent Mother-to-Child Transmission of HIV?

HIV medicines reduce the amount of HIV in the body. Having less HIV in the body reduces a woman's risk of passing HIV to her child during pregnancy and childbirth. Having less HIV in the body also protects the woman's health.

Some of the HIV medicine passes from the pregnant woman to her unborn baby across the placenta (also called the afterbirth). This transfer of HIV medicine protects the baby from HIV infection, especially during a vaginal delivery when the baby passes through the birth canal and is exposed to any HIV in the mother's blood or other fluids. In some situations, a woman with HIV may have a cesarean delivery (sometimes called a C-section) to reduce the risk of mother-to-child transmission of HIV during delivery.

Babies born to women with HIV receive HIV medicine for 6 weeks after birth. The HIV medicine reduces the risk of infection from any HIV that may have entered a baby's body during childbirth.

Are HIV Medicines Safe to Use during Pregnancy?

Pregnant women with HIV can safely use many HIV medicines during pregnancy to prevent mother-to-child transmission of HIV and to protect their own health. Health care providers carefully consider the benefits and the risks of HIV medicines when recommending HIV medicines to use during pregnancy.

The following factors are considered when choosing HIV medicines to use during pregnancy:

- Pregnancy-related changes in the body that can affect how the body processes HIV medicines. Because of these changes, the dose of an HIV medicine may change during pregnancy.

- The risk of certain side effects from some HIV medicines during pregnancy.

- The potential short-and long-term effects of HIV medicines on babies born to women with HIV. Thus far, no HIV medicines have been clearly linked to birth defects.

Are There Other Ways to Prevent Mother-to-Child Transmission of HIV?

Because HIV can be transmitted in breast milk, HIV-infected women in the United States should not breastfeed their babies. In the United States, baby formula is a safe and healthy alternative to breast milk.

There are reports of children becoming infected with HIV by eating food that was previously chewed by a person infected with HIV. To be safe, babies should not be fed pre-chewed food.

Section 50.2

Preventing Mother-to-Child Transmission of HIV during Childbirth

This section includes text excerpted from "Preventing Mother-to-Child Transmission of HIV during Childbirth," U.S. Department of Health and Human Services (HHS), August 17, 2015.

Key Points

- Pregnant women with HIV receive HIV medicines during childbirth (also called labor and delivery) to reduce the risk of mother-to-child transmission of HIV.

- Recommendations on the use of HIV medicines during childbirth consider whether a woman is already taking HIV medicines when she goes into labor and the level of HIV in her blood (HIV viral load).

- Women who are already taking HIV medicines should continue taking their HIV medicines as much as possible during childbirth. Women who have a high or unknown HIV viral load near the time of delivery should receive zidovudine (brand name: Retrovir) by intravenous (IV) injection.

- A scheduled cesarean delivery (sometimes called a C-section) at 38 weeks of pregnancy (2 weeks before a woman's expected due date) to reduce the risk of mother-to-child transmission of HIV is recommended for women with a high or unknown HIV viral load near the time of delivery.

Childbirth (also called labor and delivery) is the process of giving birth. A pregnant woman with HIV can pass HIV to her baby at any time during pregnancy, including during childbirth. The risk of mother-to-child transmission of HIV is greatest during delivery when a baby passes through the birth canal and is exposed to any HIV in an HIV-infected mother's blood or other fluids.

How Is the Risk of Mother-to-Child Transmission of HIV Reduced during Childbirth?

During childbirth, women with HIV receive HIV medicines to prevent mother-to-child transmission of HIV.

In some situations, a pregnant woman with HIV may have a scheduled cesarean delivery (sometimes called a C-section) at 38 weeks of pregnancy (2 weeks before a woman's expected due date) to reduce the risk of mother-to-child transmission of HIV. A scheduled cesarean delivery is planned ahead of time.

All decisions regarding the use of HIV medicines during childbirth and the choice of a cesarean delivery to prevent mother-to-child transmission of HIV are made jointly by a woman and her health care providers

Which HIV Medicines Do Women with HIV Receive during Childbirth?

The choice of HIV medicines to use during childbirth depends on a woman's individual situation. Recommendations on medicines to use consider whether a woman is already taking HIV medicines and the level of HIV in her blood (HIV viral load).

Women who are already taking HIV medicines when they go into labor should continue taking their HIV medicines as much as possible during childbirth. Women who have a high or unknown viral load near the time of delivery should also receive zidovudine (brand name: Retrovir) by intravenous (IV) injection.

Women who did not take HIV medicines during their pregnancies should also receive IV zidovudine during childbirth.

How Does Zidovudine Prevent Mother-To-Child Transmission of HIV during Childbirth?

Zidovudine is an HIV medicine that passes easily from a pregnant woman to her unborn baby across the placenta (also called the afterbirth). Once in a baby's system, the HIV medicine protects the baby from infection with any HIV that passed from mother to child during childbirth. For this reason, the use of zidovudine during childbirth prevents mother-to-child transmission of HIV even in women with high viral loads near the time of delivery.

When Is a Scheduled Cesarean Delivery Recommended to Prevent Mother-to-Child Transmission of HIV?

A scheduled cesarean delivery at 38 weeks to prevent mother-to-child transmission of HIV is recommended in the following situations:

- When a woman has a viral load greater than 1,000 copies/mL near the time of delivery

- When a woman's viral load is unknown

In these situations, a woman with HIV should have a scheduled cesarean delivery even if she took HIV medicine during pregnancy. The cesarean delivery should be performed before a woman goes into labor and before her water breaks (also called rupture of membranes).

The risk of mother-to-child transmission of HIV is low for women who take HIV medicines during pregnancy and have a viral load of less than 1,000 copies/mL near the time of delivery. In this situation, a woman with HIV should have a vaginal delivery unless there are other medical reasons for a cesarean delivery.

What Happens If an HIV-Infected Woman Goes into Labor or Her Water Breaks before Her Scheduled Cesarean Delivery?

Once a woman goes into labor or her water breaks, a cesarean delivery may not reduce the risk of mother-to-child transmission of HIV. In this situation, the decision whether to deliver the baby by cesarean section depends on a woman's individual circumstances.

Section 50.3

Preventing Mother-to-Child Transmission of HIV after Birth

This section includes text excerpted from "Preventing Mother-to-Child Transmission of HIV after Birth," U.S. Department of Health and Human Services (HHS), August 17, 2015.

Key Points

- The use of HIV medicines and other strategies have greatly reduced the rate of mother-to-child transmission of HIV. Fewer than 200 babies with HIV are born each year in the United States.

- For 6 weeks after birth, babies born to women with HIV receive an HIV medicine called zidovudine (brand name: Retrovir). The HIV medicine protects the babies from infection with any HIV that passed from mother to child during childbirth.

- HIV testing for babies born to women with HIV is recommended at 14 to 21 days after birth, at 1 to 2 months, and again at 4 to 6 months. The test used (called a virologic HIV test) looks directly for HIV in the blood.

- Results on two virologic tests must be negative to be certain that a baby is not infected with HIV. The first negative result must be from a test done when a baby is 1 month or older and the second result from a test done when a baby is 4 months or older. Results on two HIV virologic tests must be positive to know for certain that a baby is infected with HIV.

- If testing shows that a baby has HIV, the baby is switched from zidovudine to a combination of HIV medicines. HIV medicines help children infected with HIV live healthier lives.

- Because HIV can spread in breast milk, HIV-infected women in the United States should not breastfeed their babies. In the United States, infant formula is a safe and healthy alternative to breast milk.

How Many Babies in the United States Are Born with HIV?

HIV can be passed from an HIV-infected mother to her child during pregnancy, childbirth, or breastfeeding (through breast milk). Fortunately, the use of HIV medicines and other strategies have greatly reduced the rate of mother-to-child transmission of HIV. Fewer than 200 babies with HIV are born each year in the United States.

The risk of mother-to-child transmission of HIV is low when:

- Women with HIV receive HIV medicine during pregnancy and childbirth and, in certain situations, have a scheduled cesarean delivery (sometimes called a C-section).

- Babies born to women with HIV receive HIV medicines for 6 weeks after birth and are not breastfed.

How Soon after Birth to Babies Born to Women with HIV Receive HIV Medicines to Prevent Mother-to-Child Transmission of HIV?

Within 6 to 12 hours after birth, babies born to women with HIV receive an HIV medicine called zidovudine (brand name: Retrovir). In general, the babies receive zidovudine for 6 weeks. In certain situations, a baby may receive other HIV medicines in addition to zidovudine. The HIV medicine protects the babies from infection with any HIV that passed from mother to child during childbirth.

Once the 6-week course of zidovudine is finished, babies born to women with HIV receive a medicine called sulfamethoxazole/trimethoprim (brand name: Bactrim). Bactrim helps prevent Pneumocystis jiroveci pneumonia (PCP), which is a type of pneumonia that can develop in people with HIV. If HIV testing shows that a baby is not infected with HIV, the Bactrim is stopped.

How Soon after Birth Are Babies Born to Women with HIV Tested for HIV?

HIV testing is recommended at 14 to 21 days after birth, at 1 to 2 months, and again at 4 to 6 months. The test used (called a virologic HIV test) looks directly for HIV in the blood.

Results from at least two HIV virologic tests are needed to know whether a baby is HIV negative or HIV positive.

- **HIV-negative (not infected with HIV):**

To know for certain that a baby is not infected with HIV, results on two virologic tests must be negative. The first negative result must be from a test done when a baby is 1 month or older, and the second result from a test done when a baby is 4 months or older.

- **HIV-positive (infected with HIV):**

To know for certain that a baby is infected with HIV, results on two HIV virologic tests must be positive.

Fortunately, few babies in the United States are born with HIV because most pregnant women with HIV and their newborn babies receive HIV medicines. If testing shows that a baby is HIV positive, the baby is switched from zidovudine to a combination of HIV medicines (called antiretroviral therapy or ART). ART helps people with HIV live longer, healthier lives.

What Other Steps Are Used to Protect Babies from HIV?

Because HIV can spread in breast milk, women with HIV who live in the United States should not breastfeed their babies. In the United States, infant formula is a safe and healthy alternative to breast milk.

There are reports of children becoming infected with HIV by eating food that was previously chewed by a person with HIV. To be safe, babies should not be fed pre-chewed food.

Do Women with HIV Continue to Take HIV Medicines after Childbirth?

Women work closely with their health care providers to decide whether to continue taking HIV medicines after childbirth. Treatment with HIV medicines is recommended for everyone infected with HIV. HIV medicines prevent HIV from advancing to AIDS and reduce the risk of sexual transmission of HIV.

A woman's decision whether to continue taking HIV medicines after childbirth depends on the following factors:

- Current recommendations for HIV treatment in adults
- The level of HIV in her body (HIV viral load)
- Any issues that may make it hard for her to take HIV medicines exactly as directed
- Whether her partner is infected with HIV
- Her personal preferences and those of her health care provider

Chapter 51

Needle Exchange Programs

Access to Sterile Syringes

Persons who inject drugs can substantially reduce their risk of getting and transmitting HIV, viral hepatitis and other blood borne infections by using a sterile needle and syringe for every injection. In many jurisdictions, persons who inject drugs can access sterile needles and syringes through syringe services programs (SSPs) and through pharmacies without a prescription. Though less common, access to sterile needles and syringes may also be possible through a prescription written by a doctor and through other health care services.

SSPs, which have also been referred to as syringe exchange programs (SEPs), needle exchange programs (NEPs) and needle-syringe programs (NSPs) are community-based programs that provide access to sterile needles and syringes free of cost and facilitate safe disposal of used needles and syringes. As described in the CDC and U.S. Department of Health and Human Services (HHS) guidance, SSPs are an effective component of a comprehensive, integrated approach to HIV prevention among PWID. These programs have also been associated with reduced risk for infection with hepatitis C virus. Most SSPs offer other prevention materials (e.g., alcohol swabs, vials of sterile water, condoms) and services, such as education on safer injection practices and wound care; overdose prevention; referral to substance use disorder treatment programs including medication-assisted treatment; and

---

This chapter includes text excerpted from "Access to Sterile Syringes," Centers for Disease Control and Prevention (CDC), April 26, 2016.

counseling and testing for HIV and hepatitis C. Many SSPs also provide linkage to critical services and programs, such as HIV care, treatment, pre-exposure prophylaxis (PrEP), and post-exposure prophylaxis (PEP) services; hepatitis C treatment, hepatitis A and B vaccinations; screening for other sexually transmitted diseases and tuberculosis; partner services; prevention of mother-to-child HIV transmission; and other medical, social, and mental health services.

Federal Funding for SSPs

The Consolidated Appropriations Act of 2016 includes language in Division H, Sec. 520 that gives states and local communities, under limited circumstances, the opportunity to use federal funds to support certain components of SSPs.

To support implementation of this change in law, HHS has released new guidance for state, local, tribal, and territorial health departments that will allow them to request permission to use federal funds to support SSPs. Federal funds can now be used to support a comprehensive set of services, but they cannot be used to purchase sterile needles or syringes for illegal drug injection.

The guidance states that eligible state, local, tribal, and territorial health departments must consult with CDC and provide evidence that their jurisdiction is experiencing, or at risk for significant increases in hepatitis infections or an HIV outbreak due to injection drug use.

After receiving a request for determination of need, CDC will have 30 business days to notify the requestor whether the evidence is sufficient to demonstrate a need for SSPs. When CDC finds there is sufficient evidence, state, local, tribal, and territorial health departments and other eligible HHS grant recipients may then apply to their respective federal agencies to direct funds to support approved SSP activities. Each federal agency (e.g., CDC, HRSA, SAMHSA) is currently developing its own guidance for its funding recipients regarding which specific programs may apply and its application process.

Chapter 52

STD Vaccines and Microbicides

Chapter Contents

Section 52.1

Vaccines for HIV

This section includes text excerpted from "Vaccines," U.S.
Department of Health and Human Services (HHS), May 12, 2014.

What Are Vaccines and What Do They Do?

A vaccine—also called a "shot" or "immunization"—is a substance
that teaches your body's immune system to recognize and defend
against harmful viruses or bacteria before you get infected. These are
called "preventive vaccines" or "prophylactic vaccines," and you get
them while you are healthy. This allows your body to set up defenses
against those dangers ahead of time. That way, you won't get sick if
you're exposed to them later. Preventive vaccines are widely used to
prevent diseases like polio, chicken pox, measles, mumps, rubella,
influenza (flu), and hepatitis A and B.

In addition to preventive vaccines, there are also therapeutic vaccines. These are vaccines that are designed to treat people who already
have a disease. Some scientists prefer to refer to therapeutic vaccines
as "therapeutic immunogens." Currently, there is only one FDA-approved therapeutic vaccine for advanced prostate cancer in men.

Is There a Vaccine for HIV?

No. There is currently no vaccine that will prevent HIV infection
or treat those who have it.

Why Do We Need an HIV Vaccine?

Recently, more people living with HIV have access to life-saving
antiretroviral therapy (ART) than ever before, which is good for their
health and reduces the likelihood that they will transmit the virus to
others if they adhere to their HIV medication. In addition, others who
are at high risk for HIV infection have access to Pre-exposure Prophylaxis (PrEP), or ART being used to prevent HIV. Yet, unfortunately,
approximately 50,000 Americans and 2.3 million people worldwide still

become newly HIV-infected each year. To control and ultimately end HIV globally, we need a powerful array of HIV prevention tools that are widely accessible to all who would benefit from them.

Vaccines historically have been the most effective means to prevent and even eradicate infectious diseases. They safely and cost-effectively prevent illness, disability and death. Like smallpox and polio vaccines, a preventive HIV vaccine could help save millions of lives.

Developing safe, effective and affordable vaccines that can prevent HIV infection in uninfected people is the best hope for controlling and/or ending the HIV epidemic.

The long-term goal is to develop a safe and effective vaccine that protects people worldwide from getting infected with HIV. However, even if a vaccine only protects some people, it could still have a major impact on the rates of transmission and help control the epidemic, particularly for populations where there is a high rate of HIV transmission. A partially effective vaccine could decrease the number of people who get infected with HIV, further reducing the number of people who can pass the virus on to others.

A therapeutic immunogen could also be beneficial for people living with HIV by helping slow the progression of the disease and prevent or delay the onset of AIDS.

Why Don't We Have an HIV Vaccine Yet?

HIV is a very complex, highly changeable virus, which makes speedy development of a successful preventive HIV vaccine very difficult, but not impossible. It also takes many years to conduct the research, including the careful clinical testing that will lead to a safe and effective vaccine.

Researchers from around the world have been working for more than two decades to create a vaccine that will protect people against HIV infection. NIAID supports the HIV Vaccine Trials Network (HVTN), an international collaboration of scientists and educators searching for an effective and safe HIV vaccine. The U.S. Military HIV Research Program (MHRP) is also engaged in HIV vaccine research and led a large collaboration of clinical scientists also funded by NIAID in implementing a vaccine trial that showed for the first time that an HIV vaccine is possible.

How Is HIV Different from Other Viruses?

In part, HIV is different from other viruses because your immune system never fully gets rid of it. Most people who are infected with a virus recover from the infection, and their immune systems "clear" the virus from their bodies. This is true even for viruses that can be deadly, like influenza.

Once your body has cleared a particular virus, you often develop immunity to it—meaning it won't make you sick the next time you are exposed to it. We've known since the late 1700s that you can create immunity by exposing people to dead or weakened viruses that will protect them from deadly diseases later.

But the human body can't seem to fully clear HIV and develop immunity to it. The antibodies your immune system makes to fight HIV are not effective—and HIV actually targets, invades, and then destroys some of the most important cells in your immune system itself. This means that, over time, HIV does serious damage to your body's ability to fight disease.

So far, no person with an established HIV infection has managed to clear the virus naturally. This has made it more difficult to develop a preventive HIV vaccine.

What's the Latest on HIV Vaccine Research?

Scientists are continuing to create and test HIV vaccines—in the lab, in animals, and even in human subjects. These vaccine trials help researchers to learn whether a vaccine will work and if it can be safely given to people.

Section 52.2

Vaccines for HPV

This section includes text excerpted from "Human Papillomavirus (HPV) Vaccines," National Cancer Institute (NCI), National Institutes of Health (NIH), February 19, 2015.

What Are Human Papillomaviruses?

Human papillomaviruses (HPVs) are a group of more than 200 related viruses. More than 40 HPV types can be easily spread through direct sexual contact, from the skin and mucous membranes of infected people to the skin and mucous membranes of their partners. They can be spread by vaginal, anal, and oral sex. Other HPV types are responsible for non-genital warts, which are not sexually transmitted.

Sexually transmitted HPV types fall into two categories:

1. Low-risk HPVs, which do not cause cancer but can cause skin warts (technically known as condylomata acuminata) on or around the genitals, anus, mouth, or throat. For example, HPV types 6 and 11 cause 90 percent of all genital warts. HPV types 6 and 11 also cause recurrent respiratory papillomatosis, a disease in which benign tumors grow in the air passages leading from the nose and mouth into the lungs.

2. High-risk HPVs, which can cause cancer. About a dozen high-risk HPV types have been identified. Two of these, HPV types 16 and 18, are responsible for most HPV-caused cancers.

HPV infections are the most common sexually transmitted infections in the United States. About 14 million new genital HPV infections occur each year. In fact, the Centers for Disease Control (CDC) estimates that more than 90 percent and 80 percent, respectively, of sexually active men and women will be infected with at least one type of HPV at some point in their lives. Around one-half of these infections are with a high-risk HPV type.

Most high-risk HPV infections occur without any symptoms, go away within 1 to 2 years, and do not cause cancer. Some HPV infections, however, can persist for many years. Persistent infections with high-risk HPV types can lead to cell changes that, if untreated, may progress to cancer.

What HPV Vaccines Are Available?

Three vaccines are approved by the FDA to prevent HPV infection: Gardasil, Gardasil 9, and Cervarix. All three vaccines prevent infections with HPV types 16 and 18, two high-risk HPVs that cause about 70 percent of cervical cancers and an even higher percentage of some of the other HPV-associated cancers. Gardasil also prevents infection with HPV types 6 and 11, which cause 90 percent of genital warts. Because Gardasil protects against infection with four HPV types, it is called a quadrivalent vaccine. Gardasil 9 prevents infection with the same four HPV types plus five additional high-risk HPV types (31, 33, 45, 52, and 58) and is therefore called a nonavalent, or 9-valent, vaccine. All three vaccines are given through a series of three injections into muscle tissue over a 6-month period.

The FDA has approved Gardasil and Gardasil 9 for use in females ages 9 through 26 for the prevention of HPV-caused cervical, vulvar, vaginal, and anal cancers; precancerous cervical, vulvar, vaginal, and anal lesions; and genital warts. Gardasil and Gardasil 9 are also approved for use in males for the prevention of HPV-cause anal cancer, precancerous anal lesions, and genital warts. Gardasil is approved for use in males ages 9 through 26, and Gardasil 9 is approved for use in males ages 9 through 15.

Females and males who have previously received Gardasil may be able to also receive Gardasil 9.

The Cervarix vaccine is produced by GlaxoSmithKline (GSK). It targets two HPV types; 16 and 18, and is called a bivalent vaccine. The FDA has approved Cervarix for use in females ages 9 through 25 for the prevention of cervical cancer caused by HPV.

In addition to providing protection against the HPV types included in these vaccines, the vaccines have been found to provide partial protection against a few additional HPV types that can cause cancer, a phenomenon called cross-protection. The vaccines do not prevent other sexually transmitted diseases, nor do they treat existing HPV infections or HPV-caused disease.

Because currently available HPV vaccines do not protect against all HPV infections that cause cancer, it is important for vaccinated women to continue to undergo cervical cancer screening. There could be some future changes in recommendations for vaccinated women.

How Do HPV Vaccines Work?

Like other immunizations that guard against viral infections, HPV vaccines stimulate the body to produce antibodies that, in future encounters with HPV, bind to the virus and prevent it from infecting cells. The current HPV vaccines are based on virus-like particles (VLPs) that are formed by HPV surface components. VLPs are not infectious, because they lack the virus's DNA. However, they closely resemble the natural virus, and antibodies against the VLPs also have activity against the natural virus. The VLPs have been found to be strongly immunogenic, which means that they induce high levels of antibody production by the body. This makes the vaccines highly effective.

The VLP technology that is used in the HPV vaccines was developed by NCI and other scientists. NCI licensed the technology to Merck and GSK to develop HPV vaccines for widespread distribution.

How Effective Are HPV Vaccines?

HPV vaccines are highly effective in preventing infection with the types of HPV they target when given before initial exposure to the virus—which means before individuals begin to engage in sexual activity. In the trials that led to approval of Gardasil and Cervarix, these vaccines were found to provide nearly 100 percent protection against persistent cervical infections with HPV types 16 and 18 and the cervical cell changes that these persistent infections can cause. Gardasil 9 is as effective as Gardasil for the prevention of diseases caused by the four shared HPV types (6, 11, 16, and 18), based on similar antibody responses in participants in clinical studies. The trials that led to approval of Gardasil 9 found it to be 97 percent effective in preventing cervical, vulvar, and vaginal disease caused by the five additional HPV types (31, 33, 45, 52, and 58) that it targets.

To date, protection against the targeted HPV types has been found to last for at least 8 years with Gardasil and at least 9 years with Cervarix. The duration of protection with Gardasil 9 is not yet known. Long-term studies of vaccine efficacy that are still in progress will help scientists better understand the total duration of protection.

A clinical trial of Gardasil in men indicated that it can prevent anal cell changes caused by persistent infection and genital warts. Analyses of data from women participating in a clinical trial of Cervarix found that this vaccine can protect women against persistent HPV 16 and 18 infections in the anus and the oral cavity.

The HPV vaccines are all designed to be given to people in three doses over a 6-month period. However, one study showed that women who received only two doses of Cervarix had as much protection from persistent HPV 16/18 infections as women who received three doses, and the protection was observed through 4 years of follow up. Even one dose provided protection. In other studies, young adolescents given two doses of Cervarix or Gardasil were found to have as strong an immune response as 15-to-25-year-olds who received three doses. Based on the evidence to date, the World Health Organization has recommended two doses as the standard delivery for these vaccines, although in the United States three doses are still recommended.

Why Are These Vaccines Important?

Widespread vaccination with Cervarix or Gardasil has the potential to reduce cervical cancer incidence around the world by as much as two-thirds, while Gardasil 9 could prevent an even higher proportion.

In addition, the vaccines can reduce the need for medical care, biopsies, and invasive procedures associated with follow-up from abnormal cervical screening, thus helping to reduce health care costs and anxieties related to follow-up procedures.

Until recently, the other cancers caused by HPV were less common than cervical cancer. However, the incidence of HPV-positive oropharyngeal cancer and anal cancer has been increasing, while the incidence of cervical cancer has declined, due mainly to highly effective cervical cancer screening programs. Therefore, the number of HPV-positive cancers located outside the cervix (non-cervical cancers) in the United States is now similar to that of cervical cancer. In addition, most of the HPV-positive non-cervical cancers arise in men. There are no formal screening programs for the non-cervical cancers, so universal vaccination could have an important public health benefit.

How Safe Are the HPV Vaccines?

Before any vaccine is licensed, the FDA must determine that it is both safe and effective. All three HPV vaccines have been tested in tens of thousands of people in the United States and many other countries. Thus far, no serious side effects have been shown to be caused by the vaccines. The most common problems have been brief soreness and other local symptoms at the injection site. These problems are similar to those commonly experienced with other vaccines. The vaccines have not been sufficiently tested during pregnancy and, therefore, should not be used by pregnant women.

A recent safety review by the FDA and the Centers for Disease Control and Prevention (CDC) considered adverse side effects related to Gardasil immunization that have been reported to the Vaccine Adverse Events Reporting System since the vaccine was licensed. The rates of adverse side effects in the safety review were consistent with what was seen in safety studies carried out before the vaccine was approved and were similar to those seen with other vaccines. However, a higher proportion of syncope (fainting) and venous thrombolic events (blood clots) were seen with Gardasil than are usually seen with other vaccines. The patients who developed blood clots had known risk factors for developing them, such as taking oral contraceptives. A safety review of Gardasil in Denmark and Sweden did not identify an increased risk of blood clots.

Falls after fainting may sometimes cause serious injuries, such as head injuries. These can largely be prevented by keeping the person seated for up to 15 minutes after vaccination. The FDA and CDC have reminded health care providers that, to prevent falls and injuries, all vaccine recipients should remain seated or lying down and be closely observed for 15 minutes after vaccination.

Who Should Get the HPV Vaccines?

All three vaccines are proven to be effective only if given before infection with HPV, so it is recommended that they be given before an individual is sexually active.

After a vaccine is licensed by the FDA, the Advisory Committee on Immunization Practices (ACIP) makes additional recommendations to the Secretary of the U.S. Department of Health and Human Services and the Director of the CDC on who should receive the vaccine, at what age, how often, the appropriate dose, and situations in which it should not be administered.

The Advisory Committee on Immunization Practices (ACIP), a group of 15 medical and public health experts that develops recommendations on how to use vaccines to control diseases in the United States, has developed the following recommendations regarding HPV vaccination:

- initiation of routine HPV vaccination at age 11 or 12 years (the vaccination series can be started beginning at age 9 years)

- vaccination of females aged 13 through 26 years and of males aged 13 through 21 years who have not been vaccinated previously or who have not completed the three-dose vaccination series. Males aged 22 through 26 years may be vaccinated.

- vaccination through age 26 years of men who have sex with men and for immunocompromised persons if not vaccinated previously

- when the HPV vaccine product previously administered is not known or unavailable or the provider is switching to use of Gardasil 9, any available HPV vaccine product can be used to continue or complete the series for females; Gardasil 9 or Gardasil may be used to continue or complete the series for males

Should the Vaccines Be Given to People Who Are Already Infected with HPV?

Although HPV vaccines have been found to be safe when given to people who are already infected with HPV, the vaccines do not treat infection. They provide maximum benefit if a person receives them before he or she is sexually active.

It is likely that someone exposed to HPV will still get some residual benefit from vaccination, even if he or she has already been infected with one or more of the HPV types included in the vaccines.

At present, there is no generally available test to show whether an individual has been exposed to HPV. The currently approved HPV tests show only whether a person has a current infection with a high-risk HPV type at the cervix and do not provide information on past infections.

Should Women Who Already Have Cervical Cell Changes Get the Vaccines?

ACIP recommends that women who have abnormal Pap test results, which may indicate HPV infection, should still receive HPV vaccination if they are in the appropriate age group because the vaccine may protect them against high-risk HPV types that they have not yet acquired. However, these women should be told that the vaccination will not cure them of current HPV infections or treat the abnormal results of their Pap test.

How Much Do These Vaccines Cost, and Will Insurance Pay for It?

The retail price of the vaccines is approximately $130 to $160 per dose. However, the actual cost for vaccination may be determined by the clinic that provides the service. Clinics may charge for staff time and the vaccination equipment, for example, or they may have sliding-scale fees that set the cost according to a person's level of income or insurance coverage.

The best way to know how much vaccination will cost is to contact the insurance plan or the clinic.

Most private insurance plans cover HPV vaccination. The federal Affordable Care Act (ACA) requires all new private insurance plans to cover recommended preventive services (including HPV vaccination) with no copay or deductible.

Medicaid covers HPV vaccination in accordance with the ACIP recommendations, and immunizations are a mandatory service under Medicaid for eligible individuals under age 21. In addition, the federal Vaccines for Children Program provides immunization services for children 18 and under who are Medicaid eligible, uninsured, underinsured, receiving immunizations through a Federally Qualified Health Center or Rural Health Clinic, or are Native American or Alaska Native.

The vaccine manufacturers also offer help for people who cannot afford HPV vaccination. GSK has the Vaccines Access Program, which provides Cervarix free of charge to women who do not have insurance and who have a low income, and who are ages 19 to 25 and therefore too old for the Medicaid Vaccines for Children Program.

Merck offers the Merck Vaccine Patient Assistance Program, which provides Gardasil for free to people over the age of 19 who do not have health insurance or cannot afford to pay for the vaccine.

Section 52.3

HPV Vaccine Information for Preteens and Teens

This section contains text excerpted from the following sources: Text beginning with the heading "HPV and Cancer" is excerpted from "HPV," Centers for Disease Control and Prevention (CDC), July 2015; Text under the heading "Why Does My Child Need HPV Vaccine?" is excerpted from "HPV Vaccines: Vaccinating Your Preteen or Teen," Centers for Disease Control and Prevention (CDC), January 26, 2015.

As parents, you do everything you can to protect your children's health for now and for the future. At present,, there is a strong weapon to prevent several types of cancer in our kids: the HPV vaccine.

HPV and Cancer

HPV is short for Human Papillomavirus, a common virus. In the United States each year, there are about 17,500 women and 9,300 men affected by HPV-related cancers. Many of these cancers **could be prevented with vaccination.** In both women and men, HPV can cause anal cancer and mouth/throat (oropharyngeal) cancer. It can also cause cancers of the cervix, vulva and vagina in women; and cancer of the penis in men. For women, screening is available to detect most cases of cervical cancer with a Pap smear. Unfortunately, there is no routine screening for other HPV-related cancers for women or men, and these cancers can cause pain, suffering, or even death. **That is why a vaccine that prevents most of these types of cancers is so important.**

More about HPV

HPV is a virus passed from one person to another during skin-to-skin sexual contact, including vaginal, oral, and anal sex. HPV is most common in people in their late teens and early 20s. Almost all sexually active people will get HPV at some time in their lives, though most will never even know it. Most of the time, the body naturally fights off HPV, before HPV causes any health problems. But in some cases, the body does not fight off HPV, and HPV can cause health problems, like cancer and genital warts. Genital warts are not a life-threatening disease, but they can cause emotional stress, and their treatment can be very uncomfortable. About 1 in 100 sexually active adults in the United States have genital warts at any given time.

HPV Vaccination Is Recommended for Preteen Girls and Boys at Age 11 or 12 Years

All preteens need HPV vaccination so they can be protected from HPV infections that cause cancer. Teens and young adults who didn't start or finish the HPV vaccine series also need HPV vaccination. Young women can get HPV vaccine until they are 27 years old and young men can get HPV vaccine until they are 22 years old. Young men who have sex with other men or who have weakened immune systems can also get HPV vaccine until they are 27. HPV vaccination is a series of shots given over several months. The best way to remember to get your child all of the shots they need is to make an appointment for the remaining shots before you leave the doctor's office or clinic.

Is the HPV Vaccine Safe?

Yes. HPV vaccination has been studied very carefully and continues to be monitored by CDC and the Food and Drug Administration (FDA). No serious safety concerns have been linked to HPV vaccination. **These studies continue to show that HPV vaccines are safe.** The most common side effects reported after HPV vaccination are mild. They include pain and redness in the area of the arm where the shot was given, fever, dizziness, and nausea. Some preteens and teens may faint after getting a shot or any other medical procedure. Sitting or lying down for about 15 minutes after getting shots can help prevent injuries that could happen if your child were to fall while fainting.

Serious side effects from HPV vaccination are rare. Children with severe allergies to yeast or latex shouldn't get certain HPV vaccines. Be sure to tell the doctor or nurse if your child has any severe allergies.

Why Does My Child Need HPV Vaccine?

HPV vaccine is important because it protects against cancers caused by human papillomavirus (HPV) infection. HPV is a very common virus; nearly 80 million people—about one in four—are currently infected in the United States. About 14 million people, including teens, become infected with HPV each year. HPV infection can cause cervical, vaginal, and vulvar cancers in women; penile cancer in men; and anal cancer, cancer of the back of the throat (oropharynx), and genital warts in both men and women.

When Should My Child Be Vaccinated?

The HPV vaccine is recommended for preteen boys and girls at age 11 or 12 so they are protected before ever being exposed to the virus. HPV vaccine also produces a more robust immune response during the preteen years. Finally, older teens are less likely to get health check-ups than preteens. If your teen hasn't gotten the vaccine yet, talk to their doctor or nurse about getting it for them as soon as possible.

The HPV vaccine is given in 3 shots. The second shot is given 1 or 2 months after the first shot. Then a third shot is given 6 months after the first shot.

Who Else Should Get the HPV Vaccine?

All kids who are 11 or 12 years old should get the three-dose series of HPV vaccine to protect against HPV. Teen boys and girls who did not start or finish the HPV vaccine series when they were younger should get it now. Young women can get HPV vaccine through age 26, and young men can get vaccinated through age 21. The vaccine is also recommended for any man who has sex with men through age 26, and for men with compromised immune systems (including HIV) through age 26, if they did not get HPV vaccine when they were younger.

Section 52.4

HPV Vaccine Information for Young Women

This section contains text excerpted from the following sources:
Text under the heading "Why Is the HPV Vaccine Important?"
is excerpted from "HPV Vaccine Information for Young Women,"
Centers for Disease Control and Prevention (CDC), March 26, 2015;
Text under the heading "Investigational Genital Herpes Vaccine"
is excerpted from "NIH Launches Trial of Investigational Genital
Herpes Vaccine," National Institutes of Health (NIH), November 8,
2013; Text under the heading "The Herpevac Trial for Women" is
excerpted from "The Herpevac Trial for Women," National
Institute of Allergy and Infectious Diseases (NIAID),
September 29, 2010. Reviewed April 2016.

Three vaccines are available to prevent the human papillomavirus (HPV) types that cause most cervical cancers as well as some cancers of the anus, vulva (area around the opening of the vagina), vagina, and oropharynx (back of throat including base of tongue and tonsils). Two of these vaccines also prevent HPV types that cause most genital warts. HPV vaccines are given in 3 shots over 6 months.

Why Is the HPV Vaccine Important?

Genital HPV is a common virus that is passed from one person to another through direct skin-to-skin contact during sexual activity. Most sexually active people will get HPV at some time in their lives, though most will never even know it. HPV infection is most common in people in their late teens and early 20s. There are about 40 types of HPV that can infect the genital areas of men and women. Most HPV types cause no symptoms and go away on their own. But some types can cause cervical cancer in women and other less common cancers— like cancers of the anus, penis, vagina, and vulva and oropharynx. Other types of HPV can cause warts in the genital areas of men and women, called genital warts. Genital warts are not life-threatening. But they can cause emotional stress and their treatment can be very uncomfortable. Every year, about 12,000 women are diagnosed with cervical cancer and 4,000 women die from this disease in the U.S.

About 1% of sexually active adults in the U.S. have visible genital warts at any point in time.

Which Girls/Women Should Receive HPV Vaccination?

HPV vaccination is recommended for 11 and 12 year-old girls. It is also recommended for girls and women age 13 through 26 years of age who have not yet been vaccinated or completed the vaccine series; HPV vaccine can also be given to girls beginning at age 9 years.

Will Sexually Active Females Benefit from the Vaccine?

Ideally females should get the vaccine before they become sexually active and exposed to HPV. Females who are sexually active may also benefit from vaccination, but they may get less benefit. This is because they may have already been exposed to one or more of the HPV types targeted by the vaccines. However, few sexually active young women are infected with all HPV types prevented by the vaccines, so most young women could still get protection by getting vaccinated.

Can Pregnant Women Get the Vaccine?

The vaccines are not recommended for pregnant women. Studies show that HPV vaccines do not cause problems for babies born to women who were vaccinated while pregnant, but more research is still needed. A pregnant woman should not get any doses of either HPV vaccine until her pregnancy is completed.

Getting the HPV vaccine when pregnant is not a reason to consider ending a pregnancy. If a woman realizes that she got one or more shots of an HPV vaccine while pregnant, she should do two things:

- Wait until after her pregnancy to finish the remaining HPV vaccine doses.

- Call the pregnancy registry [877-888-4231 for Gardasil, 800-986-8999 for Gardasil 9, or 888-825-5249 for Cervarix].

Should Girls and Women Be Screened for Cervical Cancer before Getting Vaccinated?

Girls and women do not need to get an HPV test or Pap test to find out if they should get the vaccine. However it is important that women continue to be screened for cervical cancer, even after getting all 3

571

shots of either HPV vaccine. This is because neither vaccine protects against ALL types of cervical cancer.

How Effective Are the HPV Vaccines?

All HPV vaccines target the HPV types that most commonly cause cervical cancer and can cause some cancers of the vulva, vagina, anus, and oropharynx. Two of the vaccines also protect against the HPV types that cause most genital warts. HPV vaccines are highly effective in preventing the targeted HPV types, as well as the most common health problems caused by them.

The vaccines are less effective in preventing HPV-related disease in young women who have already been exposed to one or more HPV types. That is because the vaccines prevent HPV before a person is exposed to it. HPV vaccines do not treat existing HPV infections or HPV-associated diseases.

How Long Does Vaccine Protection Last?

Research suggests that vaccine protection is long-lasting. Current studies have followed vaccinated individuals for ten years, and show that there is no evidence of weakened protection over time.

What Does the Vaccine Not Protect Against?

The vaccines do not protect against all HPV types—so they will not prevent all cases of cervical cancer. Since some cervical cancers will not be prevented by the vaccines, it will be important for women to continue getting screened for cervical cancer. Also, the vaccines do not prevent other sexually transmitted infections (STIs). So it will still be important for sexually active persons to lower their risk for other STIs.

Will Girls and Women Be Protected against HPV and Related Diseases, Even If They Don't Get All 3 Doses?

It is not yet known how much protection girls and women get from receiving only one or two doses of an HPV vaccine. So it is important that girls and women get all 3 doses.

How Safe Are the HPV Vaccines?

All three HPV vaccines have been licensed by the Food and Drug Administration (FDA). The CDC has approved these vaccines as safe and effective. The vaccines were studied in thousands of people around the world, and these studies showed no serious safety concerns. Side effects reported in these studies were mild, including pain where the shot was given, fever, dizziness, and nausea. Vaccine safety continues to be monitored by CDC and the FDA. More than 60 million doses of HPV vaccine have been distributed in the United States as of March 2014.

Fainting, which can occur after any medical procedure, has also been noted after HPV vaccination. Fainting after any vaccination is more common in adolescents. Because fainting can cause falls and injuries, adolescents and adults should be seated or lying down during HPV vaccination. Sitting or lying down for about 15 minutes after a vaccination can help prevent fainting and injuries.

Why Is HPV Vaccination Only Recommended for Women Through Age 26?

HPV vaccination is not currently recommended for women over age 26 years. Clinical trials showed that, overall, HPV vaccination offered women limited or no protection against HPV-related diseases. For women over age 26 years, the best way to prevent cervical cancer is to get routine cervical cancer screening, as recommended.

Investigational Genital Herpes Vaccine

Researchers have launched an early-stage clinical trial of an investigational vaccine designed to prevent genital herpes disease. The National Institute of Allergy and Infectious Diseases (NIAID), part of the National Institutes of Health, is sponsoring the Phase I trial, which is being conducted at the NIH Clinical Center in Bethesda, Md.

Genital herpes is one of the most common sexually transmitted infections in the United States. Most genital herpes cases are caused by infection with herpes simplex virus type 2 (HSV-2); however, herpes simplex virus type 1 (HSV-1) can also cause genital herpes. An estimated 776,000 people in the United States are infected with HSV-2 or HSV-1 each year. There is no vaccine to prevent genital herpes.

Led by principal investigator Lesia K. Dropulic, M.D., of NIAID's Laboratory of Infectious Diseases, the trial will test an investigational HSV-2 vaccine candidate, called HSV529, for safety and the ability to generate an immune system response. The investigational vaccine manufactured by Sanofi Pasteur was developed by David Knipe,

Ph.D., professor of microbiology and immunobiology at Harvard Medical School, Boston.

Preclinical testing of the candidate vaccine involved a 10-year collaborative effort between Dr. Knipe and Jeffrey Cohen, M.D., chief of NIAID's Laboratory of Infectious Diseases. The experimental product is a replication-defective vaccine, meaning that scientists have removed two key proteins from the vaccine virus so that it cannot multiply to cause genital herpes.

The clinical trial is expected to enroll 60 adults ages 18 to 40, who will be divided into three groups of 20 participants each. The first group will be of people who have been previously infected with HSV-2 and HSV-1 or solely with HSV-2; the second will have individuals who had been infected with HSV-1 only; and the third will consist of those who have not been infected with HSV-1 or HSV-2. The investigational vaccine is being tested among study participants who have previously been infected with HSV to determine if it may pose any safety issues.

Within each of the three groups, researchers will randomly assign participants to receive three doses (0.5 milliliters each) of the investigational HSV529 vaccine (15 participants) or a saline-based placebo vaccine (five participants). The three vaccinations will occur at study enrollment and again one month and six months later. Participant safety will be monitored throughout the course of the trial, and researchers will follow participants for six months after they have received their last dose of vaccine. Blood samples will be used to evaluate the candidate vaccine's ability to stimulate immune system responses to HSV-2, including production of virus-specific antibodies and T-cell responses. The study is expected to be completed by October 2016.

HSV-2 is generally transmitted through sexual contact and can spread even when the infected individual shows no symptoms. Although HSV-1 commonly infects the mouth and lips, it can also cause genital herpes. Once in the body, HSV migrates to nerve cells and remains there permanently, where it can reactivate to cause painful sores and blisters.

The Herpevac Trial for Women

What Is the Herpevac Trial for Women?

The Herpevac trial for women is a clinical study investigating a vaccine to protect women against genital herpes disease. The trial, which began in 2002 and concluded in 2010, was conducted at 50 sites in the United States and Canada and was sponsored by GlaxoSmithKline

(GSK) Biologicals in cooperation with the National Institute of Allergy and Infectious Diseases (NIAID), part of the NIH. The study chair is Robert Belshe, M.D., director of the Center for Vaccine Development at the Saint Louis University School of Medicine in Missouri.

How Many Participants Were Involved in the Study?

The Herpevac Trial for Women involved 8,323 women ages 18–30. At the time of their enrollment, the study participants were free of the two common types of herpes simplex viruses (HSV): HSV-1, the primary cause of cold sores and an increasing cause of genital herpes, and HSV-2, the common cause of genital herpes. Approximately 31,000 women were screened in order to identify eligible participants.

What Was the Study's Design?

The study was a randomized, double-blind, controlled Phase III clinical trial. Participants were randomly assigned to receive either the investigational herpes vaccine or a version of Havrix, an FDA-approved, licensed vaccine to protect against hepatitis A. This was done to give all participants an opportunity to be protected against either genital herpes or hepatitis A. GSK developed the candidate herpes vaccine and is also the manufacturer of Havrix.

The investigational herpes vaccine is a subunit vaccine containing a glycoprotein from HSV along with an adjuvant to boost immune response. The Havrix vaccine administered to study participants was provided at a lower dose and smaller volume than it is routinely provided in medical practice. This was done to ensure that the vaccine could be administered in the same number of doses as the candidate herpes vaccine. Each volunteer was vaccinated at the beginning of the study and again after one month and six months following the first injection. The participants were followed for 20 months after the initial injection and evaluated for HSV infection and genital herpes disease. Throughout the study, participants were regularly counseled on how to reduce their risk of acquiring HSV.

What Were the Results of the Trial?

The trial was successfully conducted according to protocol and met statistical targets in terms of enrollment and participant follow up. The vaccine proved to be well-tolerated and its safety profile was similar to that observed in previous trials. According to the initial data analysis publicly announced in September 2010, the trial produced a point estimate of overall vaccine effectiveness of 20 percent with a confidence interval that included zero. In other words, the vaccine was not effective at preventing genital herpes disease among the study population of women. At that time, study collaborators stated that evaluation of the trial data would continue and that a more detailed analysis would be provided at a later time.

A subsequent, more detailed analysis published in the New England Journal of Medicine on Jan. 5, 2012, found that the investigational vaccine provided some protection against HSV-1, although it did not protect against HSV-2. Specifically, there were 58 percent fewer cases of genital herpes caused by HSV-1 and 35 percent fewer HSV-1 infections among women who received the investigational vaccine, compared to those who received the control vaccine. The recent analysis also found that among women enrolled in the control group, HSV-1 caused more cases of genital herpes than HSV-2.

Why Was the Trial Important?

The Herpevac Trial for Women produced important scientific information to guide future research toward a vaccine to prevent genital herpes. It also provided emerging data about genital herpes and the changing role of HSV-1 in infection.

An estimated one in four women in the United States has genital herpes, making it one of the most common infectious diseases. HSV, the cause of genital herpes disease, may be transmitted through sexual or other skin-to-skin contact, and can be spread even when the infected individual shows no symptoms. Once in the body, HSV migrates to nerve cells and remains there permanently where it can reactivate to cause painful outbreaks in the infected individual. HSV can cause severe illness in infants born to HSV-infected women, and the virus has been identified as a risk factor for HIV transmission in adults. There is no cure for herpes infection, and there is no vaccine to prevent it.

When the investigational vaccine was tested in two earlier studies involving fewer men and women who did not have genital herpes but whose sexual partners were known to be infected, the candidate vaccine prevented genital herpes disease in more than 70 percent of the female volunteers but had no clear effect in men. Further, the candidate vaccine reduced by roughly 40 percent the risk of developing antibodies to herpes, which are used as an indicator that a person has been infected with HSV. These studies formed the basis for conducting the larger Herpevac study. Results of these two earlier studies were published in November 2002 in the New England Journal of Medicine.

Though it failed to reach its primary goal, the Herpevac Trial for Women produced important scientific information to guide future research toward a vaccine to prevent genital herpes. The researchers suspect that the differences between the 2002 studies and the Herpevac Trial were due to immunologic and behavioral differences in the populations studied, which may have affected participants' protection from HSV-1 and HSV-2.

The trial results also provided emerging data about genital herpes and the changing role of HSV-1 in infection. Although HSV-1 is typically associated with cold sores and HSV-2 with genital lesions, HSV-1 has become a growing cause of genital disease, an observation echoed in this analysis. Among women enrolled in the control group of the Herpevac trial, HSV-1 was found to cause more cases of genital herpes than HSV-2.

How Was Participant Safety Monitored during the Trial?

Participant safety was closely monitored throughout the trial, both by the study investigators and by a data and safety monitoring board (DSMB). The DSMB is an independent committee composed of clinical research experts, herpes virus experts, and statisticians that provides additional oversight of a clinical study. The DSMB regularly reviews data while a clinical trial is in progress to ensure the safety of participants and that any benefits shown in the study are quickly made available to all participants.

The investigational herpes vaccine used in the trial had been previously tested in more than 7,000 volunteers; results from these studies suggested that it was well-tolerated and safe.

Was There Any Risk to Participants That the Vaccine Could Cause Herpes Infection?

No. The herpes vaccine formulation used in the study did not contain live virus and was incapable of infecting participants with herpes virus. The candidate vaccine contained only a specific fragment of a herpes virus protein to stimulate immune responses.

Analyze the Data from the Herpevac Trial to Better Understand the Results?

Yes. Researchers will continue to examine serum samples from the Herpevac study to better understand why the vaccine protected women from genital disease caused by HSV-1, but not HSV-2.

Section 52.5

Microbicides

This section contains text excerpted from the following sources:
Text beginning with the heading "Introduction" is excerpted from
"NIAID Research on Microbicides," National Institute of Allergy and
Infectious Diseases (NIAID), National Institutes of Health (NIH),
December 1, 2015; Text under the heading "FAQs on Microbicide"
is excerpted from "Microbicides," U.S. Department of Health and
Human Services (HHS), February 27, 2012. Reviewed April 2016.

What Are Microbicides?

Microbicides are products (such as gels, films, intravaginal rings
(IVR), enemas, or suppositories) that can be formulated for use in
reproductive and gastrointestinal tracts (GI) to prevent sexual transmission of HIV and other sexually transmitted infections (STIs). An
optimal microbicide would be desirable for use by a wide variety of
individuals at risk for HIV or STIs regardless of sex, gender or age,
and would be, safe, inexpensive, long-acting and easy to use and store.
Microbicides should be available in both contraceptive and non-contraceptive formulations so that women can remain protected whether
or not they are trying to conceive a child.

Optimal Characteristics of a Microbicide

Safety

- Safe when used daily, episodically or intermittently for extended
  periods of time

- No mucosal irritation or disruption of normal vaginal or rectal/
  gut mucosal environment

Effect

- Fast onset with minimal time to achieve desired drug levels in
  tissue and/or systemically (if applicable)

- Duration of action appropriate to use

- **Non-coital:** a single dose provides a window of at least seven days of prevention of HIV infection
- **Sustained protection:** a minimum of 30 days protection from a continuous release device or a single dose
- **Coital:** for individuals with infrequent sexual activity who want on-demand protection
- May possess additional activities against STIs associated with HIV infection and disease progression
- May be contraceptive
- No reproductive toxicity or carcinogenesis

Availability

- Contraceptive and non-contraceptive formulations
- Low cost
- Easy access
- Room temperature storage in discrete, easily transportable packaging

Acceptability and Desirability

- Acceptable to the user and user's sex partner
- Unobtrusive/pleasurable
- Valued by individuals and social networks creating a desire for use
- Minimal social harms associated with use

Uses

- Vaginal
- Rectal
- Dual use; product compatibility for both vaginal and rectal use
- Compatible with
  - Condoms

- Contraception methods: hormonal, non-hormonal and barrier methods

- Other STI prevention drugs and strategies

Other Advantageous Properties

- Easily scaled-up for GMP production and distribution

- Stable for up to three years in harsh environments (high humidity and temperature)

- Small storage footprint and minimal packaging waste

- Minimal residual drug remaining in delivery device or applicator

- No effect on normal vaginal or rectal microbial ecology (normal bacteria present in vagina and rectum that are necessary for a healthy environment)

Questions on Microbicide

What Are Microbicides?

Microbicides are gels, films, or suppositories that can kill or neutralize viruses and bacteria. Researchers are studying both vaginal and rectal microbicides to see if they can prevent sexual transmission of HIV. A safe, effective, and affordable microbicide against HIV could help to prevent many new infections.

Can Microbicides Prevent HIV Infection?

The answer to this question now appears to be "Yes"—though more studies are needed to be sure.

In July 2010, researchers attending the 2010 International AIDS Conference in Vienna, Austria announced exciting news about the CAPRISA 004 Microbicide Study. In that study, researchers put an antiretroviral drug into a vaginal microbicide gel and told the women participating in the trial to use the gel before and after sex to protect against HIV transmission.

The study results found that, overall, the gel was 39% effective in reducing the women's risk of becoming infected with HIV during sex. The more frequently the women used the gel as intended, the more effective it was in protecting them from HIV infection.

The gel was also 51% effective in preventing genital herpes infections. Since having a sexually transmitted infection like herpes increases your risk of contracting HIV, this is another important result.

If other studies of microbicide gels confirm these results and the microbicides are approved for licensure by the appropriate regulatory agency and made available, microbicides could prevent millions of new HIV infections over the next decade.

Why Are Microbicides so Important?

HIV is spread predominantly through sexual transmission. Right now, the best HIV prevention options for sexually active people are being mutually monogamous with an HIV-negative partner and using condoms consistently and correctly. For many people, however, these options are not possible.

It is believed that topical microbicides might be more effective than condoms in preventing HIV infection because they would be easier to use and women would not have to negotiate their use, as they often must do with condoms. Worldwide half of the people living with HIV are women. So, public health professionals are particularly interested in developing microbicides for women who aren't able to get their male sex partners to use condoms. Microbicides would make it possible for a woman to protect herself and her partner from HIV without his cooperation or knowledge—a particularly important factor for commercial sex workers (prostitutes) or women in abusive relationships.

Microbicides might also make it possible someday for women to protect themselves from HIV while still allowing them to get pregnant if they wish.

Can I Use a Microbicide to Protect Myself from HIV Infection?

Not yet. The CAPRISA study results are exciting—but even if those results are duplicated in other clinical trials, it will probably be several years before microbicides are available to the public. Researchers will have to be sure that the product is both effective in preventing HIV infection and safe for people to use.

For now, the best forms of protection against sexual transmission of HIV continue to be:

- Being mutually monogamous with an HIV-negative partner

- HIV testing—so that you know your own HIV status and your partner's too

- Using condoms consistently and correctly

Part Six

Healthy Living with HIV

Chapter 53

HIV: Life after Diagnosis

Alternative Therapies

Many people use complementary (sometimes known as alternative) health treatments to go along with the medical care they get from their doctor.

These therapies are called "complementary" therapies because usually they are used alongside the more standard medical care you receive (such as your VA doctor visits and the anti-HIV drugs you might be taking).

They are sometimes called "alternative" because they don't fit into the more mainstream, Western ways of looking at medicine and health care. These therapies may not fit in with what you usually think of as "health care."

Some common complementary therapies include:

- Physical (body) therapies, such as yoga, massage, and acupuncture

- Relaxation techniques, such as meditation and visualization

- Herbal medicine (from plants)

With most complementary therapies, your health is looked at from a holistic (or "whole picture") point of view. Think of your body as working as one big system. From a holistic viewpoint, everything you

This chapter includes text excerpted from "Living with HIV/AIDS," U.S. Department of Veterans Affairs (VA), July 30, 2015.

do—from what you eat to what you drink to how stressed you are—affects your health and well-being.

Diet and Nutrition for People with HIV

Nutrition is important for everyone because food gives our bodies the nutrients they need to stay healthy, grow, and work properly. Foods are made up of six classes of nutrients, each with its own special role in the body:

- Protein builds muscles and a strong immune system.

- Carbohydrates (including vegetables, fruits, grains) give you energy.

- Fat gives you extra energy.

- Vitamins regulate body processes.

- Minerals regulate body processes and also make up body tissues.

- Water gives cells shape and acts as a medium where body processes can occur.

Having good nutrition means eating the right types of foods in the right amounts so you get these important nutrients.

Do I need a special diet?

There are no special diets, or particular foods, that will boost your immune system. But there are things you can do to keep your immunity up.

When you are infected with HIV, your immune system has to work very hard to fight off infections--and this takes energy (measured in calories). This means you may need to eat more food than you used to.

If you are underweight--or you have advanced HIV disease, high viral loads, or opportunistic infections--you should include more protein as well as extra calories (in the form of carbohydrates and fats). You'll find tips for doing this in the next section.

Drugs, Alcohol And HIV

If you've just found out that you are HIV positive, you might be wondering what alcohol and other "recreational" drugs will do to your body. (Recreational drugs are drugs that aren't being used for medical purposes, such as beer, cocaine, amphetamines, and pot; this also includes prescription medicines that are being used for pleasure.)

You may be wondering whether these drugs are bad for your immune system. And what about your HIV medications--can recreational drugs affect those?

Is using alcohol or other drugs is bad for you? Each person is different, and a lot depends on which drugs you use and how often you use them.

However, most experts would agree that, in large amounts, drugs and alcohol are bad for your immune system and your overall health. Remember, if you have HIV, your immune system is already weakened.

Here, you can read about what alcohol and drugs can do to your overall health.

Sex and Sexuality

If you just tested positive for HIV, you may not want to think about having sex. Some people who get HIV feel guilty or embarrassed. These are common reactions, especially if you got HIV through sex. Chances are, however, that you will want to have sex again. The good news is that there is no reason why you can't. People with HIV enjoy sex and fall in love, just like other people.

You can have a good sex life, even if you have HIV.

If you are having a hard time dealing with negative feelings like anger or fear, you can get help. Talk to your doctor about support groups or counseling. Sex is a very tough topic for many people with HIV--you are not alone.

Chapter 54

Opportunistic Infections

What Are Opportunistic Infections?

Opportunistic infections (OIs) are infections that occur more frequently and are more severe in individuals with weakened immune systems, including people with HIV. OIs are less common now than they were in the early days of HIV and AIDS because better treatments reduce the amount of HIV in a person's body and keep a person's immune system stronger. However, many people with HIV still develop OIs because they may not know of their HIV infection, they may not be on treatment, or their treatment may not be keeping their HIV levels low enough for their immune system to fight off infections.

For those reasons, it is important for individuals with HIV to be familiar with the most common OIs so that they can work with their healthcare provider to prevent them or to obtain treatment for them as early as possible.

Most Common Opportunistic Infections

When a person living with HIV gets certain infections (called opportunistic infections, or OIs), he or she will get a diagnosis of AIDS, the most serious stage of HIV infection. AIDS is also diagnosed if a type of blood cell that fights infection (known as CD4 cells) falls below a

This chapter includes text excerpted from "Opportunistic Infections," Centers for Disease Control and Prevention (CDC), January 16, 2015.

certain level in persons with HIV. These blood cells are a critical part of a person's immune system.

CDC has developed a list of OIs that indicate a person has AIDS. It does not matter how many CD4 cells a person has, receiving a diagnosis with any of these OIs means HIV infection has progressed to AIDS. HIV treatment can help restore the person's immune system.

Following is a list of the most common OIs for individuals living in the United States. For more details, including signs and symptoms of specific OIs, please refer to the Opportunistic Infection pages at AIDS.gov. Additionally, CDC, the National Institutes of Health, the HIV Medicine Association of the Infectious Disease Society of America (HIVMA/IDSA), and other experts in infectious disease have published Guidelines for the Prevention and Treatment of Opportunistic Infections in HIV-Infected Adults and Adolescents. While the guidelines are intended for healthcare professionals, some consumers may find them useful.

Candidiasis of Bronchi, Trachea, Esophagus, or Lungs

This illness is caused by infection with a common (and usually harmless) type of fungus called Candida. Candidiasis, or infection with Candida, can affect the skin, nails, and mucous membranes throughout the body. Persons with HIV infection often have trouble with Candida, especially in the mouth and vagina. However, candidiasis is only considered an OI when it infects the esophagus (swallowing tube) or lower respiratory tract, such as the trachea and bronchi (breathing tube), or deeper lung tissue.

Invasive Cervical Cancer

This is a cancer that starts within the cervix, which is the lower part of the uterus at the top of the vagina, and then spreads (becomes invasive) to other parts of the body. This cancer can be prevented by having your care provider perform regular examinations of the cervix.

Coccidioidomycosis

This illness is caused by the fungus Coccidioides immitis. It most commonly acquired by inhaling fungal spores, which can lead to a pneumonia that is sometimes called desert fever, San Joaquin Valley fever, or valley fever. The disease is especially common in hot, dry regions of the southwestern United States, Central America, and South America.

Cryptococcosis

This illness is caused by infection with the fungus Cryptococcus neoformans. The fungus typically enters the body through the lungs and can cause pneumonia. It can also spread to the brain, causing swelling of the brain. It can infect any part of the body, but (after the brain and lungs) infections of skin, bones, or urinary tract are most common.

Cryptosporidiosis, Chronic Intestinal (Greater than One Month's Duration)

This diarrheal disease is caused by the protozoan parasite Cryptosporidium. Symptoms include abdominal cramps and severe, chronic, watery diarrhea.

Cytomegalovirus Diseases (Particularly Retinitis) (CMV)

This virus can infect multiple parts of the body and cause pneumonia, gastroenteritis (especially abdominal pain caused by infection of the colon), encephalitis (infection) of the brain, and sight-threatening retinitis (infection of the retina at the back of eye). People with CMV retinitis have difficulty with vision that worsens ever time. CMV retinitis is a medical emergency because it can cause blindness if not treated promptly.

Encephalopathy, HIV-Related

This brain disorder is a result of HIV infection. It can occur as part of acute HIV infection or can result from chronic HIV infection. Its exact cause is unknown but it is thought to be related to infection of the brain with HIV and the resulting inflammation.

Herpes Simplex (HSV): Chronic Ulcer(s) (Greater than One Month's Duration); Or Bronchitis, Pneumonitis, or Esophagitis

Herpes simplex virus (HSV) is a very common virus that for most people never causes any major problems. HSV is usually acquired sexually or from an infected mother during birth. In most people with healthy immune systems, HSV is usually latent (inactive). However, stress, trauma, other infections, or suppression of the immune system, (such as by HIV), can reactivate the latent virus and symptoms

591

can return. HSV can cause painful cold sores (sometime called fever blisters) in or around the mouth, or painful ulcers on or around the genitals or anus. In people with severely damaged immune systems, HSV can also cause infection of the bronchus (breathing tube), pneumonia (infection of the lungs) and esophagitis (infection of the esophagus, or swallowing tube).

Histoplasmosis

This illness is caused by the fungus Histoplasma capsulatum. Histoplasma most often infects the lungs and produces symptoms that are similar to those of influenza or pneumonia. People with severely damaged immune systems can get a very serious form of the disease called progressive disseminated histoplasmosis. This form of histoplasmosis can last a long time and involves organs other than the lungs.

Isosporiasis, Chronic Intestinal (Greater than One Month's Duration)

This infection is caused by the parasite Isospora belli, which can enter the body through contaminated food or water. Symptoms include diarrhea, fever, headache, abdominal pain, vomiting, and weight loss.

Kaposi's Sarcoma (KS)

This cancer, also known as KS, is caused by a virus called Kaposi's sarcoma herpesvirus (KSHV) or human herpesvirus 8 (HHV-8). KS causes small blood vessels, called capillaries, to grow abnormally. Because capillaries are located throughout the body, KS can occur anywhere. KS appears as firm pink or purple spots on the skin that can be raised or flat. KS can be life-threatening when it affects organs inside the body, such the lung, lymph nodes or intestines.

Lymphoma, Multiple Forms

Lymphoma refers to cancer of the lymph nodes and other lymphoid tissues in the body. There are many different kinds of lymphomas. Some types, such as non-Hodgkin lymphoma and Hodgkin lymphoma, are associated with HIV infection.

Tuberculosis (TB)

Tuberculosis (TB) infection is caused by the bacteria Mycobacterium tuberculosis. TB can be spread through the air when a person with active TB coughs, sneezes, or speaks. Breathing in the bacteria can lead to infection in the lungs. Symptoms of TB in the lungs include cough, tiredness, weight loss, fever, and night sweats. Although the disease usually occurs in the lungs, it may also affect other parts of the body, most often the larynx, lymph nodes, brain, kidneys, or bones.

Mycobacterium Avium Complex (MAC) or Mycobacterium Kansasii, Disseminated or Extrapulmonary. Other Mycobacterium, Disseminated or Extrapulmonary.

MAC is caused by infection with different types of mycobacterium: Mycobacterium avium, Mycobacterium intracellulare, or Mycobacterium kansasii. These mycobacteria live in our environment, including in soil and dust particles. They rarely cause problems for persons with healthy immune systems. In people with severely damaged immune systems, infections with these bacteria spread throughout the body and can be life-threatening.

Pneumocystis Carinii Pneumonia (PCP)

This lung infection, also called PCP, is caused by a fungus, which used to be called Pneumocystis carinii, but now is named Pneumocystis jirovecii. PCP occurs in people with weakened immune systems, including people with HIV. The first signs of infection are difficulty breathing, high fever, and dry cough.

Pneumonia, Recurrent

Pneumonia is an infection in one or both of the lungs. Many germs, including bacteria, viruses, and fungi can cause pneumonia, with symptoms such as a cough (with mucous), fever, chills, and trouble breathing. In people with immune systems severely damaged by HIV, one of the most common and life-threatening causes of pneumonia is infection with the bacteria Streptococcus pneumoniae, also called Pneumococcus. There are now effective vaccines that can prevent infection with Streptococcus pneumoniae and all persons with HIV infection should be vaccinated.

Progressive Multifocal Leukoencephalopathy

This rare brain and spinal cord disease is caused by the JC virus. It is seen almost exclusively in persons whose immune systems have been severely damaged by HIV. Symptoms may include loss of muscle control, paralysis, blindness, speech problems, and an altered mental state. This disease often progresses rapidly and may be fatal.

Salmonella septicemia, recurrent

Salmonella are a kind of bacteria that typically enter the body through ingestion of contaminated food or water. Infection with salmonella (called salmonellosis) can affect anyone and usually causes a self-limited illness with nausea, vomiting, and diarrhea. Salmonella septicemia is a severe form of infection in which the bacteria circulate through the whole body and exceeds the immune system's ability to control it.

Toxoplasmosis of Brain

This infection, often called toxo, is caused by the parasite Toxo-plasma gondii. The parasite is carried by warm-blooded animals including cats, rodents, and birds and is excreted by these animals in their feces. Humans can become infected with it by inhaling dust or eating food contaminated with the parasite. Toxoplasma can also occur in commercial meats, especially red meats and pork, but rarely poultry. Infection with toxo can occur in the lungs, retina of the eye, heart, pancreas, liver, colon, testes, and brain. Although cats can transmit toxoplasmosis, litter boxes can be changed safely by wearing gloves and washing hands thoroughly with soap and water afterwards. All raw red meats that have not been frozen for at least 24 hours should be cooked through to an internal temperature of at least 150oF.

Wasting Syndrome due to HIV

Wasting is defined as the involuntary loss of more than 10% of one's body weight while having experienced diarrhea or weakness and fever for more than 30 days. Wasting refers to the loss of muscle mass, although part of the weight loss may also be due to loss of fat.

Preventing Opportunistic Infections

The best ways to prevent getting an OI are to get into and stay on medical care and to take HIV medications as prescribed. Sometimes, your health care provider will also prescribe medications specifically to prevent certain OIs. By staying on HIV medications, you can keep the amount of HIV in your body as low as possible and keep your immune system healthy. It is especially important that you get regular check-ups and take all of your medications as prescribed by your care giver. Taking HIV medications is a life-long commitment.

In addition to taking HIV medications to keep your immune system strong, there are other steps you can take to prevent getting an OI.

- Use condoms consistently and correctly to prevent exposure to sexually transmitted infections.

- Don't share drug injection equipment. Blood with hepatitis C in it can remain in syringes and needles after use and the infection can be transmitted to the next user.

- Get vaccinated – your doctor can tell you what vaccines you need. If he or she doesn't, you should ask.

- Understand what germs you are exposed to (such as tuberculosis or germs found in the stools, saliva, or on the skin of animals) and limit your exposure to them.

- Don't consume certain foods, including undercooked eggs, unpasteurized (raw) milk and cheeses, unpasteurized fruit juices, or raw seed sprouts.

- Don't drink untreated water such as water directly from lakes or rivers. Tap water in foreign countries is also often not safe. Use bottled water or water filters.

- Ask your doctor to review with you the other things you do at work, at home, and on vacation to make sure you aren't exposed to an OI.

Treating Opportunistic Infections

If you do develop an OI, there are treatments available, such as antibiotics or antifungal drugs. Having an OI may be a very serious medical situation and its treatment can be challenging. The development of an OI likely means that your immune system is weakened and that your HIV is not under control. That is why it is so important to be on medication, take it as prescribed, see your care provider regularly, and undergo the routine monitoring he or she recommends to ensure your viral load is reduced and your immune system is healthy.

Chapter 55

Partnering with Your Health Care Provider

What Can I Expect at My Regular Medical Visits?

Living with HIV can be challenging at times. Partnering with your health care provider will help you manage your health and HIV care. During your medical appointments, your health care provider may:

- Conduct medical exams to see how HIV is affecting your body.

- Ask you questions about your health history.

- Take a blood sample to check your CD4 count and viral load.

- Look for other kinds of infections or health problems that may weaken your body, make your HIV worse, or prevent your treatment from working as well as possible.

- Give you immunizations, if you need them.

- Discuss, prescribe, and monitor your HIV medicines, including when and how to take them, possible side effects, and continued effectiveness.

- Discuss strategies that will help you follow your HIV treatment plan and maintain your treatment.

- Help identify additional support you may need, such as finding a social worker, case manager or patient navigator; finding an

This chapter includes text excerpted from "Understanding Care," Centers for Disease Control and Prevention (CDC), January 12, 2016.

HIV support group; finding support services for mental health or substance use issues; or finding support services for transportation or housing.

- Ask you about your sex partners and discuss ways to protect them from getting HIV.

- Ask you about your plans for getting pregnant or getting your partner pregnant.

Talk regularly with your health care provider about how you are feeling and communicate openly and honestly. Tell your health care provider about any health problems you are having so that you can get proper treatment. Discuss how often you should expect to attend medical visits. Staying informed about HIV care and treatment advances and partnering with your health care provider are important steps in managing your health and HIV care.

What Tests Can Help Monitor My HIV Infection?

Your health care provider will use blood tests to monitor your HIV infection. The results of these blood tests, which measure the amount of HIV virus and the number of CD4 cells in the blood, will help you and your health care provider understand how well your HIV treatment is working to control your HIV infection. These test results will also help your health care provider decide whether he or she should make changes to your treatment.

These blood tests include regular:

- CD4 counts, and

- Viral load tests.

CD4 Count

CD4 cells, also called T-cells, play an important role in your body's ability to fight infections. Your CD4 count is the number of CD4 cells you have in your blood. When you are living with HIV, the virus attacks and lowers the number of CD4 cells in your blood. This makes it difficult for your body to fight infections.

Typically, your health care provider will check your CD4 count every 3 to 6 months. A normal range for a CD4 cell count is 500 cells to 1,600 cells per cubic millimeter of blood. A low CD4 cell count means you are at higher risk of developing opportunistic infections. These infections take advantage of your body's weakened immune system and can cause life-threatening illnesses. A higher CD4 cell count means that your HIV treatment is working and controlling the virus. As your CD4 count increases, your body is better able to fight infection. If you have a CD4 count of fewer than 200 cells per cubic millimeter of blood, you will be diagnosed as having AIDS.

Viral Load Test

Your viral load is the amount of HIV in your blood. When your viral load is high, you have more HIV in your body, and your immune system is not fighting HIV as well.

When you take a viral load test, your health care provider looks for the number of HIV virus particles in a milliliter of your blood. These particles are called "copies."

The goal of HIV treatment is to help move your viral load down to undetectable levels. In general, your viral load will be declared "undetectable" if it is under 40 to 75 copies in a sample of your blood. The exact number depends on the lab that analyzes your test.

Your health care provider will use a viral load test to determine your viral load. A viral load test will:

- Show how well your HIV treatment is controlling the virus, and

- Provide information on your health status.

You should have a viral load test every 3 to 6 months, before you start taking a new HIV medicine, and 2 to 8 weeks after starting or changing medicines.

Can I Transmit HIV If I Have an Undetectable Viral Load?

Antiretroviral therapy (ART) reduces viral load, ideally to an undetectable level. If your viral load goes down after starting ART, then the treatment is working. Having an undetectable viral load greatly lowers your chance of transmitting the virus to your sexual and drug-using partners who are HIV-negative. However, even when your viral load is undetectable, HIV can still exist in semen, vaginal and rectal fluids, breast milk, and other parts of your body, so you should continue to take steps to prevent HIV transmission. For example:

- HIV may still be found in genital fluids (semen, vaginal fluids). The viral load test only measures the amount of HIV in the blood. Although ART also lowers viral load in genital fluids, HIV can sometimes be present in genital fluids even when it is undetectable in the blood.

599

- Your viral load may go up between tests. When this happens, you may be more likely to transmit HIV to your partner(s). Your viral load may go up without you knowing it because you may not feel any different.

- Sexually transmitted diseases (STDs) increase viral load in genital fluids. This means that if you are living with HIV and also have an STD, you may be able to transmit HIV to your partner(s) even if the blood viral load is undetectable.

Researchers are studying how much you can lower your chances of transmitting HIV when your viral load is undetectable, and we should know more when these studies are complete.

If you are taking ART, follow your health care provider's advice. Visit your health care provider regularly and always take your medicine as directed. This will give you the greatest chance of having an undetectable viral load. Taking other actions, like using a condom consistently and correctly, can lower your chances of transmitting HIV or contracting an STD even more.

Chapter 56

Meeting the Cost for Medical Care

Cost of HIV Treatment

Living with HIV can bring up a lot of questions and concerns, especially about how to pay for treatment. Fortunately, resources and programs are available that may help.

Health Insurance

Understanding your health insurance options is key to maintaining good health.

Will My Health Insurance Cover My HIV Treatments?

There is no simple answer to this question. Getting health insurance to help pay for HIV care and treatment can be a challenge for some people living with HIV.

If you are already covered by a private group health insurance plan, such as insurance you have through your employer or a private individual plan, it will typically cover your HIV care, just as it covers care for other medical conditions. Most group health plans require that you pay a portion of your medical costs through:

This chapter includes text excerpted from "Cost of HIV Treatment," Centers for Disease Control and Prevention (CDC), February 8, 2016.

Regular payments (sometimes called "premiums"), which are usually subtracted from your paychecks, and/or

Co-pays, payments made at the time you receive health care services or medications.

If you are covered by a private health insurance policy, review your policy to find out what HIV care and treatment your insurance provider covers. If your policy does not cover portions of your HIV care, some government and private programs may be able to help pay for or provide these services.

What If I Don't Have Health Insurance?

A number of programs may help pay for your care and treatment if you do not have health insurance or if your health insurance doesn't cover the care you need. A social worker or your case manager can help you determine if you are eligible and apply for these programs.

These programs include:

- **Ryan White HIV/AIDS Program:** The Ryan White HIV/AIDS Program provides HIV-related services (like medical care and medications) in the United States for people who do not have enough health care coverage or financial resources to pay for care. The program fills gaps in care not met by other payers. Persons need to meet certain eligibility requirements to access this program. You can call your State HIV/AIDS Hotline and ask them to refer you to the nearest Ryan White provider, or talk to your social worker or case manager to find out more.

- **Medicaid:** The federal-state health insurance program pays for medical care for people with low incomes, older people, and people with disabilities. States manage the Medicaid program, and each state decides who is eligible and what the program covers. Medicaid is currently the biggest source of insurance coverage for people living with HIV. The Affordable Care Act (ACA) expands Medicaid so that, in participating states, more people with HIV who did not qualify in the past can get coverage.

- **Medicare:** The federal health insurance program is for people who are 65 and older or are disabled. All Medicare drug plans cover all HIV medications.

Ask for help. Working with your social worker, case manager, or patient navigator will help you get the care, treatment, and support you need.

How Will the Affordable Care Act Help Me Get Coverage for or Pay for HIV Care and Treatment?

The Affordable Care Act (ACA) is a law that was passed to help ensure that Americans have secure, stable, and affordable health insurance. The ACA created several changes that expand access to coverage for people living with HIV. Because coverage varies by state, talk to your health care provider or social worker to get information about the coverage available where you live. You can also contact the ACA helpline at 1-800-318-2596 for more information.

Can I Get Care and Treatment from a Government Community Health Center?

More than 8,000 Community Health Centers are operated by the U.S. Department of Health and Human Services, Health Resources and Services Administration (HRSA). They help more than 20 million people with limited access to health care. HRSA Community Health Centers provide HIV testing and some offer other services to people with HIV, including medical care. Fees are based on a person's ability to pay. Some patients receive care services at the center itself, while others are referred to an HIV specialist if the Community Health Center does not provide HIV care. Talk to your case manager or social worker for more information on Community Health Centers and whether you are eligible to receive HIV care and treatment from a center near you.

Paying for Medication

Paying for your HIV medication can be a challenge. Fortunately, there are government and private programs that can help pay for medication if you are eligible. Some of these programs include:

- **Ryan White AIDS Drug Assistance Program:** The Ryan White AIDS Drug Assistance Program (ADAP) provides HIV- and AIDS-related prescription drugs to uninsured and underinsured individuals living with HIV and AIDS. ADAP funds are used by states to provide medications to treat HIV, or to prevent the serious deterioration of health, including measures for the prevention and treatment of opportunistic infections. As a payer of last resort, ADAP only helps individuals who have neither public nor private insurance or cannot get all of their medication needs met through their insurance payer. The medication provided by this drug program varies by state. Call your state's HIV and AIDS hotline to ask about the ADAP program in your state or speak to your case manager or social worker.

- **Medicare Prescription Drug Coverage Plans:** Medicare Prescription Drug Coverage Plans are required to provide coverage for common medications that people living with HIV use. Talk to your case manager or social worker to learn more about these plans.

- **Private Prescription Assistance Programs:** Some major drug companies offer patient co-pay savings programs to people living with HIV. In addition, other assistance is available to help qualifying patients with no prescription coverage to obtain free medication. These programs can help you get the medicines you need at low or no cost. Ask your medical provider, case manager, or social worker for more information.

Your case manager, social worker, or patient navigator can help you determine your eligibility and help you apply for these types of assistance. They can also help identify other assistance programs available in your community.

Chapter 57

The Importance of a Healthy Diet

Healthy Diet

No matter your HIV status, healthy eating is good for your overall health. If you are living with HIV, following a healthy diet offers several benefits. Good nutrition helps:

- Provide the energy and nutrients your body needs to fight HIV and other infections,

- Maintain a healthy weight,

- Manage HIV symptoms and complications, and

- Absorb medicines and help manage potential side effects.

What Types of Foods Should Be Included as Part of a Healthy, Balanced Diet?

A balanced diet includes:

- **Proteins,** which build and maintain muscle. Good sources of protein include meats, fish, beans, nuts, and legumes.

- **Fruits and vegetables,** which provide essential vitamins and minerals, fiber, and other substances necessary for good health. These foods are filling and naturally low in fat and calories.

- **Carbohydrates,** which give you energy. Complex carbohydrates are a "time-release" source of energy and include fruits,

---

This chapter includes text excerpted from "Healthy Diet," Centers for Disease Control and Prevention (CDC), January 12, 2016.

vegetables, cereals, and grains. Simple carbohydrates, or sugars, give you quick energy and can come from white flour, honey, jams, syrups, and dried fruit.

- **Fats,** which give you extra energy. The so-called "good fats" can be found in nuts, seeds, canola and olive oils, and fish. The "bad fats," which are linked with a higher risk of heart disease, are found in butter and animal fats, like red meat.

Can My HIV or My HIV Treatments Affect My Diet and Nutrition?

Yes. People living with HIV sometimes face issues that can affect their nutrition, such as:

- Changes in your body's metabolism;

- Medicines that can upset your stomach;

- Opportunistic infections that can cause issues with eating and swallowing, like oral candidiasis and Kaposi sarcoma; and

- Foods that can affect antiretroviral therapy (ART) (like raw meats and fish).

Any of these problems can affect your body's ability to absorb the nutrients necessary to stay in good health.

Talk to your health care provider about your diet, and ask specific questions about what steps you should take to maintain good nutrition. Your health care provider may recommend that you take vitamins or supplements to ensure you are getting all the nutrients you need for a balanced diet. He or she may refer you to a nutritionist or dietitian with whom you can talk about your nutrition needs.

Chapter 58

Family Planning and HIV

What Questions Should I Ask My Health Care Provider about If I Am Thinking about Having a Baby?

You might ask your health care provider some of these questions:

- When do I wish to conceive a baby?

- Is my viral load undetectable?

- If I become pregnant, will HIV cause problems for me during pregnancy or delivery?

- What's the safest way to conceive?

- How do I avoid transmitting HIV to my partner, surrogate, or baby during conception, pregnancy, and delivery?

- Will my baby have HIV?

- If my partner is on PrEP, will we have a lower chance of transmitting HIV to our baby?

- Will my HIV treatment cause problems for my baby?

- If I become pregnant, what medical and community programs and support groups can help me and my baby?

This chapter includes text excerpted from "Family Planning," Centers for Disease Control and Prevention (CDC), January 12, 2016.

- If I don't want to become pregnant, what birth control methods are best for me?

Answers to these questions can help you make the best informed family planning decisions possible.

As a Woman Living with HIV, What If I Become Pregnant Unexpectedly?

If you have HIV and become pregnant, talk to your health care provider right away about medical care for you and your baby. You might also need to plan for your child's future in case you were to get sick.

If you were being treated for HIV before you became pregnant, your HIV treatment will not change very much from what it was before you became pregnant. You should have a pelvic examination and be tested for sexually transmitted diseases (STDs) during your pregnancy. Your health care provider will order tests and suggest medicines for you to take. Talk with your health care provider about all the pros and cons of taking medicine while you are pregnant.

As a Woman Living with HIV, How Can I Reduce the Chance of Transmitting HIV to My Baby?

If you have HIV, the most important thing you can do is to take medicines to treat HIV infection (called antiretroviral therapy or ART) the right way, every day.

If you're pregnant, talk to your health care provider about getting tested for HIV and other ways to keep you and your child from getting HIV. Women in their third trimester should be tested again if they engage in behaviors that put them at risk for HIV.

If you are HIV-negative but you have an HIV-positive partner and are considering getting pregnant, talk to your doctor about taking pre-exposure prophylaxis (PrEP) to help keep you from getting HIV. Encourage your partner to take medicines to treat HIV (ART), which greatly reduces the chance that he will transmit HIV to you.

If you have HIV, take medicines to treat HIV (ART) the right way, every day. If you are treated for HIV early in your pregnancy, your risk of transmitting HIV to your baby can be 2% or less. After delivery, you can prevent transmitting HIV to your baby by avoiding breastfeeding, since breast milk contains HIV.

Is Adoption an Option?

Adopting a baby can be an option for people with HIV who want to begin or expand their families.

The American with Disabilities Act (ADA) does not allow adoption agencies to discriminate against individuals or couples with HIV. If you are interested in adoption, contact your HIV service provider for help in getting referred to organizations or agencies.

Chapter 59

Smoking, Substance Abuse, and HIV

Smoking

Tobacco use is the leading cause of preventable illness and death in the United States, causing nearly one out of five deaths in the United States each year.

Why Is Smoking a Concern If I'm Living with HIV?

Smoking increases your risk of developing lung cancer, other cancers, heart disease, chronic obstructive pulmonary disease (COPD), asthma, and other diseases, and of dying early. For these reasons, smoking is an important health issue for everyone, but it is a greater concern for people living with HIV, who tend to smoke more than the general population.

About 1 in 5 U.S. adults smoke. Among adults living with HIV, the number of people who smoke is 2 to 3 times greater. Smoking has many negative health effects on people who are living with HIV. For example, smokers living with HIV:

This chapter contains text excerpted from the following sources: Text beginning with the heading "Why Is Smoking a Concern If I'm Living with HIV?" is excerpted from "Smoking," Centers for Disease Control and Prevention (CDC), September 10, 2015; Text under the heading "How Can Substance Use Affect My Health?" is excerpted from "Substance Use," Centers for Disease Control and Prevention (CDC), January 12, 2016.

- Are at higher risk than nonsmokers with HIV of developing lung cancer, head and neck cancers, cervical and anal cancers, and other cancers;

- Are more likely than nonsmokers with HIV to develop bacterial pneumonia, Pneumocystis jiroveci pneumonia, COPD, and heart disease;

- Are more likely than nonsmokers with HIV to develop conditions that affect the mouth, such as oral candidiasis (thrush) and oral hairy leukoplakia; and

- Have a poorer response to antiretroviral therapy (ART).

People with HIV who smoke have a greater chance of developing a life-threating illness that leads to an AIDS diagnosis. People who smoke and live with HIV also have a shorter lifespan than people living with HIV who do not smoke.

What Are the Benefits of Quitting Smoking?

Quitting smoking has major and immediate health benefits for tobacco users, including people living with HIV. These benefits include:

- Lowering your risk of lung cancer, other cancers, heart disease, chronic obstructive pulmonary disease (COPD), and stroke,

- Reducing HIV-related symptoms, and

- Having an improved quality of life.

You can learn about the benefits of quitting smoking and get tips for quitting from CDC's national tobacco education campaign—Tips From Former Smokers (Tips). The Tips campaign profiles real people—not actors—who are living with serious long-term health effects from smoking and secondhand smoke exposure. You can also view a story and tips from a person living with HIV who quit smoking.

Substance Use

Substance use refers to using legal drugs (like prescription pain medicines or alcohol) and/or illegal drugs (like cocaine, heroin, or methamphetamines). Substance abuse means that a person is using drugs or alcohol in a way that is harmful to his or her health and well-being.

How Can Substance Use Affect My Health?

Substance use, abuse, and dependence may damage your body and brain, and drug overdoses can cause death. This damage to your body and brain can negatively affect your health and well-being in many ways.

- **Physical effects:**
  - Methamphetamines can lead to brain, liver, and kidney damage, impaired blood circulation, significant weight loss, and tooth decay.
  - Drugs like cocaine and heroin can seriously damage your respiratory and circulatory systems.
  - Methamphetamines and cocaine can negatively affect your immune system, making it easier for your body to get an infection.
  - Some substances interfere with HIV medicines that are part of an overall treatment plan.

- **Other effects:**
  - The after-effects of a drug or alcohol "high" can create feelings of depression, exhaustion, pain, and/or irritability.
  - Getting high may cause you to forget to take your HIV medicines or forget to make and keep doctor and clinic appointments.
  - Using drugs can make it hard for you to maintain your house, job, relationships, and social supports—all of which are important for your well-being.
  - Using drugs can make you more prone to risky practices, such as sharing needles or not using condoms. This increases the chance that you could transmit HIV or get a sexually transmitted disease (STD) that could make your infection worse.

What Treatment or Support Programs Are Available to Help Me with a Substance Use or Dependence Problem?

Choosing to stop using drugs or alcohol is not easy, but it can be done. Quitting will improve your health, well-being, and relationships with others.

- Different types of substance use require different types of treatment. Based on your level of dependence, you may need medical treatment and/or psychological therapy to help you quit. Talk with your health care provider to explore treatment options that are specific to your type of substance use.

- Peer support and faith-based recovery groups may also help you manage substance use and dependence.

Support is available. Many organizations provide hotlines and guidance on substance abuse treatment options:

- Use the Substance Abuse and Mental Health Services Administration (SAMHSA) Substance Abuse Treatment Facility Locator to find alcohol and substance abuse treatment facilities and programs near you.

- Find treatment options for opioid abuse by specific drug or by state. Use SAMHSA's Opioid Treatment Program Directory and Buprenorphine Physician and Treatment Program Locator for information you can use.

- CDC offers more information on substance abuse and treatment.

Chapter 60

Things to Be Aware of While Traveling Abroad

Travel Abroad-Check List

- Before you go on a trip outside the United States, talk to your doctor about your destinations and planned activities.

- Take special care with food and water.

- Protect your health (and the health of others) just as you do at home.

Each year, millions of Americans travel abroad. Even though travel outside the United States can be risky for anyone, it may require special precautions for individuals living with HIV infection. For example, travel to some developing countries can increase the risk of getting an opportunistic infection. For some destinations, certain vaccines that contain live viruses may be required, and your health care provider needs to review your medical record to ensure they are safe for you.

The most important things you can do is **see your health care provider before you travel,** know the medical risks you might face, and learn how to protect yourself.

This chapter includes text excerpted from "Travel Abroad," Centers for Disease Control and Prevention (CDC), December 16, 2015.

Before You Travel

- Talk to your health care provider or an expert in travel medicine about health risks in the places you plan to visit. Ideally, this conversation should take place at least 4–6 weeks before your scheduled departure. Your health care provider can advise you on preventive medicines you may need, specific measures you need to take to stay healthy, and what to watch out for. He or she may also be able to provide you with the name(s) of health care providers or clinics that treat people with HIV infection in the region you plan to visit. Your health care provider may also:

  - recommend you pack a supply of medicine, such as antibiotics to treat travelers' diarrhea

  - recommend certain vaccinations

- Consult CDC Health Information for International Travel (commonly called the Yellow Book). The section on Immunocompromised Travelers has an extensive amount of information that may be useful for you. Make sure your health care provider knows about this source of information.

- If you are traveling to an area where insect-borne diseases (such as dengue fever, yellow fever, or malaria) are common, minimize the risk of getting bitten by mosquitoes or ticks. Remember to:

  - Pack a good supply of insect repellent that contains at least 30 percent DEET;

  - Wear lightweight long pants and shirts with long sleeves;

  - Wear a hat and inspect your scalp and body daily for ticks.

  - You doctor may also recommend:

  - Sleeping under a mosquito net to prevent mosquito bites;

  - Taking medicine to prevent getting malaria.

- Educate and prepare yourself

  - **About your destination:** Make sure you know if the countries you plan to visit have special health rules for visitors, especially visitors with HIV infection.

  - **About your insurance policies:** Review your medical insurance to see what coverage it provides when you are away from home. You may purchase supplemental traveler's insurance to cover the cost of emergency medical evacuation by air and the cost of in-country care, if these costs may are not covered by your regular insurance.

- Take proof of insurance, such as a photocopy or scan your policy and send the image to an e-mail address you can access both in the United States and abroad. Leave a copy at home and tell your friends or family where it is located.

When You Travel Abroad

- **Food and water** in developing countries may contain germs that could make you sick.
- **Do not**
  - eat raw fruit or vegetables that you do not peel yourself;
  - eat raw or undercooked seafood or meat;
  - eat unpasteurized dairy products;
  - eat anything from a street vendor;
  - drink tap water (in developing countries some hotels may purify their own water but it is safer to avoid it), drinks made with tap water, or ice made from tap water.
- **Do** eat and drink:
  - hot foods;
  - hot coffee or tea;
  - bottled water and drinks (make sure the seals are original and have not been tampered with);
  - water that you bring to a rolling boil for one full minute then cool in a covered and clean vessel;
  - fruits that you peel;
  - wine, beer and other alcoholic beverages are also safe.
- **Tuberculosis** is very common worldwide, and can be severe in people with HIV. Avoid hospitals and clinics where coughing TB patients are treated. See your doctor upon your return to discuss whether you should be tested for TB.

- **Animal wastes,** such as fecal droppings in soil or on sidewalks, can pose hazards to individuals with weakened immune systems. Physical barriers, such as shoes, can protect you from direct contact. Likewise, towels can protect you from direct contact when lying on a beach or in parks. If you are in physical contact with animals, wash your hands thoroughly afterwards with soap and water.

- **Take all your medications** on schedule, as usual.

- **Stick to your special diet,** if you are on one.

- **Take the same precautions** that you take at home to prevent transmitting HIV to others.

Part Seven

Additional Help and Information

Chapter 61

Glossary of Terms Related to Sexually Transmitted Diseases

abstinence: Not having sexual intercourse.

acquired immunodeficiency syndrome (AIDS): A disease of the immune system due to infection with HIV (human immunodeficiency virus). HIV destroys the CD4 T lymphocytes (CD4 cells) of the immune system, leaving the body vulnerable to life-threatening infections and cancers. Acquired immunodeficiency syndrome (AIDS) is the most advanced stage of HIV infection.

adherence: Taking medications exactly as prescribed. Poor adherence to an HIV treatment regimen increases the risk for developing drug-resistant HIV and virologic failure.

antiretroviral therapy (ART): The recommended treatment for HIV infection. Antiretroviral therapy (ART) involves using a combination of three or more antiretroviral (ARV) drugs from at least two different HIV drug classes to prevent HIV from replicating.

bacterial vaginosis (BV): A vaginal infection that develops when there is an increase in harmful bacteria and a decrease in good bacteria in the vagina.

This glossary contains terms excerpted from documents produced by several sources deemed reliable.

biopsy: Removal of tissue, cells, or fluid from the body for examination under a microscope. Biopsies are used to diagnose disease.

cervical cancer: A type of cancer that develops in the cervix. Cervical cancer is almost always caused by the human papillomavirus (HPV), which is spread through sexual contact.

chancroid: A sexually transmitted disease caused by the bacterium *Haemophilus ducreyi*. Chancroid causes genital ulcers (sores).

chlamydia: A common sexually transmitted disease caused by the bacterium *Chlamydia trachomatis*. Chlamydia often has mild or no symptoms, but if left untreated, it can lead to serious complications, including infertility.

coinfection: When a person has two or more infections at the same time. For example, a person infected with HIV may be coinfected with hepatitis or tuberculosis (TB) or both.

condom: A device used during sexual intercourse to block semen from coming in contact with the inside of the vagina. Condoms are used to reduce the likelihood of pregnancy and to prevent the transmission of sexually transmitted disease, including HIV. The male condom is a thin rubber cover that fits over a man's erect penis. The female condom is a polyurethane pouch that fits inside the vagina.

dental dam: A thin, rectangular sheet, usually latex rubber, used as a barrier to prevent the transmission of sexually transmitted infections during oral sex.

drug resistance: When a bacteria, virus, or other microorganism mutates (changes form) and becomes insensitive to (resistant to) a drug that was previously effective.

dysplasia: The development of precancerous changes in cells. Dysplasia can affect various parts of the body, including the cervix or prostate. The extent of dysplasia within body tissue can be mild (grade 1), moderate (grade 2), or severe (grade 3).

fallopian tubes: Tubes on each side of ovaries to the uterus.

genital warts: A sexually transmitted disease caused by the human papillomavirus (HPV). Genital warts appear as raised pink or flesh-colored bumps on the surface of the vagina, cervix, tip of the penis, or anus.

gonorrhea: A sexually transmitted disease caused by the bacterium *Neisseria gonorrhoeae*. Gonorrhea can also be transmitted from an infected mother to her child during delivery. Gonorrhea often has mild or no symptoms. However, if left untreated, gonorrhea can lead to infertility, and it can spread into the bloodstream and affect the joints, heart valves, and brain.

hepatitis B virus (HBV) infection: Infection with the hepatitis B virus (HBV). HBV can be transmitted through blood, semen, or other body fluids during sex or injection-drug use. Because HIV and HBV share the same modes of transmission, people infected with HIV are often also coinfected with HBV.

hepatitis C virus (HCV) infection: Infection with the hepatitis C virus (HCV). HCV is usually transmitted through blood and rarely through other body fluids, such as semen. HCV infection progresses more rapidly in people coinfected with HIV than in people infected with HCV alone.

herpes simplex virus 2 (HSV-2) infection: An infection caused by herpes simplex virus 2 (HSV-2) and usually associated with lesions in the genital or anal area. HSV-2 is very contagious and is transmitted by sexual contact with someone who is infected (even if lesions are not visible).

human immunodeficiency virus (HIV): The virus that causes AIDS, which is the most advanced stage of HIV infection. HIV is a retrovirus that occurs as two types HIV-1 and HIV-2. Both types are transmitted through direct contact with HIV-infected body fluids, such as blood, semen, and genital secretions, or from an HIV-infected mother to her child during pregnancy, birth, or breastfeeding (through breast milk).

human papillomavirus (HPV): The virus that causes human papillomavirus (HPV) infection, the most common sexually transmitted infection. There are two groups of HPV types that can cause genital warts and types that can cause cancer. HPV is the most frequent cause of cervical cancer.

injection drug use: A method of illicit drug use. The drugs are injected directly into the body into a vein, into a muscle, or under the skin with a needle and syringe. Blood-borne viruses, including HIV and hepatitis, can be transmitted via shared needles or other drug injection equipment.

microbicide: A drug, chemical, or other substance used to kill microorganisms. Increasingly, the term is used specifically for substances that prevent or reduce the transmission of sexually transmitted diseases, such as HIV.

molluscum contagiosum: A common, usually mild skin disease caused by the virus Molluscum contagiosum and characterized by small white, pink, or flesh-colored bumps with a dimple in the center. Molluscum contagiosum is spread by touching the affected skin of an infected person or by touching a surface with the virus on it. The bumps can easily spread to other parts of the body if someone touches or scratches a bump and then touches another part of the body.

mother-to-child transmission (MTCT): When an HIV-infected mother passes HIV to her infant during pregnancy, labor and delivery, or breastfeeding (through breast milk). Antiretroviral (ARV) drugs are given to HIV-infected women during pregnancy and to their infants after birth to reduce the risk of mother-to-child transmission (MTCT) of HIV.

occupational exposure: Contact with a potentially harmful physical, chemical, or biological agent as a result of one's work. For example, a health care professional may be exposed to HIV or another infectious agent through a needlestick injury.

opportunistic infection (OI): An infection that occurs more frequently or is more severe in people with weakened immune systems, such as people with HIV or people receiving chemotherapy, than in people with healthy immune systems.

Pap test: A procedure in which cells and secretions are collected from inside and around the cervix for examination under a microscope. Pap test also refers to the laboratory test used to detect any infected, potentially precancerous, or cancerous cells in the cervical cells obtained from a Pap test.

pelvic inflammatory disease (PID): Infection and inflammation of the female upper genital tract, including the uterus and fallopian tubes. Pelvic inflammatory disease is usually due to bacterial infection, including some sexually transmitted diseases, such as chlamydia and gonorrhea. Symptoms, if any, include pain in the lower abdomen, fever, smelly vaginal discharge, irregular bleeding, or pain during intercourse. PID can lead to serious complications, including infertility, ectopic pregnancy (a pregnancy in the fallopian tube or elsewhere outside of the womb), and chronic pelvic pain.

post-exposure prophylaxis (PEP): Short-term treatment started as soon as possible after high-risk exposure to an infectious agent, such as HIV, hepatitis B virus (HBV), or hepatitis C virus (HCV). The purpose of post-exposure prophylaxis (PEP) is to reduce the risk of infection.

An example of a high-risk exposure is exposure to an infectious agent as the result of unprotected sex.

pubic lice: Also called crab lice or crabs, pubic lice are parasitic insects found primarily in the pubic or genital area of humans.

scabies: An infestation of the skin by the human itch mite (*Sarcoptes scabiei var. hominis*). The microscopic scabies mite burrows into the upper layer of the skin where it lives and lays its eggs. The most common symptoms of scabies are intense itching and a pimple-like skin rash. The scabies mite usually is spread by direct, prolonged, skin-to-skin contact with a person who has scabies.

semen: A thick, whitish fluid that is discharged from the male penis during ejaculation. Semen contains sperms and various secretions. HIV can be transmitted through the semen of a man with HIV.

sexually transmitted disease (STD): An infectious disease that spreads from person to person during sexual contact. Sexually transmitted diseases, such as syphilis, HIV infection, and gonorrhea, are caused by bacteria, parasites, and viruses.

spermicide: A topical preparation or substance used during sexual intercourse to kill sperm. Although spermicides may prevent pregnancy, they do not protect against HIV infection or other sexually transmitted diseases. Irritation of the vagina and rectum that sometimes occurs with use of spermicides may increase the risk of sexual transmission of HIV.

sterility: The inability to get pregnant, or get someone pregnant; often caused by the effects of untreated bacterial infections such as chlamydia or gonorrhea.

syphilis: An infectious disease caused by the bacterium Treponema pallidum, which is typically transmitted through direct contact with a syphilis sore, usually during vaginal or oral sex. Syphilis can also be transmitted from an infected mother to her child during pregnancy. Syphilis sores occur mainly on the genitals, anus, and rectum, but also on the lips and mouth.

transmission: The spread of disease from one person to another.

trichomoniasis: A sexually transmitted disease caused by a parasite.

ulcer: An open lesion on the surface of the skin or a mucosal surface, caused by superficial loss of tissue, usually with inflammation.

vaccination: Giving a vaccine to stimulate a person's immune response. Vaccination can be intended either to prevent a disease (a preventive vaccine) or to treat a disease (a therapeutic vaccine).

vaginal fluid: The natural liquids produced inside a woman's vagina. In an infected person, STDs can be passed when vaginal fluids come in contact with the genital area of a woman's sex partner.

vesicle: A small, fluid-filled bubble, usually superficial, and <0.5cm

virus: A microscopic infectious agent that requires a living host cell in order to replicate. Viruses often cause disease in humans, including measles, mumps, rubella, polio, influenza, and the common cold. HIV is the virus that causes AIDS.

yeast infection: A fungal infection caused by overgrowth of the yeast Candida (usually *Candida albicans*) in moist areas of the body. Candidiasis can affect the mucous membranes of the mouth, vagina, and anus.

Chapter 62

Directory of Organizations That Provide Information about Sexually Transmitted Diseases

Government Agencies That Provide Information about STDs

Agency for Healthcare Research and Quality
540 Gaither Rd.
Ste. 2000
Rockville, MD 20850
Phone: 301-427-1104
Website: www.ahrq.gov
Email: richard.kronick@ahrq.hhs.gov

Centers for Disease Control and Prevention
1600 Clifton Rd.
Atlanta, GA 30333
Toll-Free: 800-CDC-INFO
(800-232-4636)
Phone: 404-639-3311
TTY: 888-232-6348
Website: www.cdc.gov
E-mail: cdcinfo@cdc.gov

Resources in this chapter were compiled from several sources deemed reliable; all contact information was verified and updated in April 2016.

Federal Trade Commission
600 Pennsylvania Ave. N.W.
Washington, DC 20580
Phone: 202-326-2222
Website: www.ftc.gov
E-mail: webmaster@ftc.gov

Healthfinder®
P.O. Box 1133
Washington, DC 20013-1133
Toll-Free: 800-336-4797
Phone: 301-565-4167
Fax: 301-984-4256
Website: www.healthfinder.gov
E-mail: healthfinder@nhic.org

National Cancer Institute
6116 Executive Blvd.
Ste. 300
Bethesda, MD 20892-8322
Toll-Free: 800-4-CANCER
(800-422-6237)
TTY: 800-332-8615
Website: www.cancer.gov
E-mail: cancergovstaff@mail.nih.
gov

*National Center for
Complementary and
Alternative Medicine*
P.O. Box 7923
Gaithersburg, MD 20898-7923
Toll-Free: 888-644-6226
TTY: 866-464-3615
Fax: 866-464-3616
Website: www.nccih.nih.gov
E-mail: info@nccam.nih.gov

*National Center for Health
Statistics*
3311 Toledo Rd.
Hyattsville, MD 20782
Toll-Free: 800-CDC-INFO
(800-232-4636)
Website: www.cdc.gov/nchs
E-mail: cdcinfo@cdc.gov

*National Institute of Allergy
and Infectious Diseases*
6610 Rockledge Dr.
MSC 6612
Bethesda, MD 20892-6612
Toll-Free: 866-284-4107
Phone: 301-496-5717
TDD: 800-877-8339
Fax: 301-402-3573
Website: www.niaid.nih.gov
E-mail: ocpostoffice@niaid.nih.
gov

*National Institute of Mental
Health*
6001 Executive Blvd.
Rm. 8184, MSC 9663
Bethesda, MD 20892-9663
Toll-Free: 866-615-6464
Phone: 301-443-4513
TTY: 866-415-8051
Fax: 301-443-4279
Website: www.nimh.nih.gov
E-mail: nimhinfo@nih.gov

*National Institute of
Neurological Disorders and
Stroke*
P.O. Box 5801
Bethesda, MD 20824
Toll-Free: 800-352-9424
Phone: 301-496-5751
TTY: 301-468-5981
Website: www.ninds.nih.gov
E-mail: NEXT@ninds.nih.gov

National Institute on Aging
31 Center Dr., MSC 2292
Bldg. 31, Rm. 5C27
Bethesda, MD 20892
Toll-Free: 800-222-2225
Phone: 301 496 1752
TTY: 800-222-4225
Fax: 301-496-1072
Website: www.nia.nih.gov
E-mail: niaic@nia.nih.gov

National Institutes of Health
9000 Rockville Pike
Bethesda, MD 20892
Phone: 301-496-4000
TTY: 301-402-9612
Website: www.nih.gov
E-mail: NIHinfo@od.nih.gov

*National Prevention
Information Network*
P.O. Box 6003
Rockdale, MD 20849-6003
Toll-Free: 800-458-5231
TTY: 888-232-6348
Website: www.npin.cdc.gov
E-mail: info@cdcnpin.org

*National Women's Health
Information Center*
200 Independence Ave. S.W.
Rm. 712E
Washington, DC 20201
Toll-Free: 800-994-9662
Phone: 202-690-7650
TDD: 888-220-5446
Fax: 202-205-2631
Website: www.womenshealth.
gov
E-mail: WomensHealth@hhs.gov

*Office of Minority Health
Resource Center*
P.O. Box 37337
Washington, DC 20013-7337
Toll-Free: 800-444-6472
Phone: 240-453-2882
TDD: 301-251-1432
Fax: 240-453-2883
Website: www.minorityhealth.
hhs.gov
E-mail: info@minorityhealth.
hhs.gov

*Substance Abuse and
Mental Health Services
Administration*
P.O. Box 2345
Rockville, MD 20847-2345
Toll-Free: 877-SAMHSA-7
(877-726-4727)
TTY: 800-487-4889
Fax: 240-221-4292
Website: www.samhsa.gov
E-mail: SAMHSAInfo@samhsa.
hs.gov

U.S. Department of Health and Human Services
200 Independence Ave. S.W.
Rm. 443 H
Washington, DC 20201
Toll-Free: 877-696-6775
Website: www.hhs.gov
E-mail: OCRPrivacy@hhs.gov

U.S. Food and Drug Administration
10903 New Hampshire Ave.
Silver Spring, MD 20993
Toll-Free: 888-INFO-FDA
(888-463-6332)
Website: www.fda.gov
E-mail: webmail@oc.fda.gov

U.S. National Library of Medicine
8600 Rockville Pike
Bethesda, MD 20894
Toll-Free: 888-FIND-NLM
(888-346-3656)
Phone: 301-594-5983
TDD: 800-735-2258
Fax: 301-402-1384
Website: www.nlm.nih.gov
E-mail: custserv@nlm.nih.gov

Private Agencies That Provide Information about STDs

Advocates for Youth
2000 M St. N.W., Ste. 750
Washington, DC 20036
Phone: 202-419-3420
Fax: 202-419-1448
Website: www.
advocatesforyouth.org
E-mail: anna@gcapp.org

AIDS.org
P.O. Box 69491
Los Angeles, CA 90069
Website: www.aids.org
E-mail: aidsnews@aidsnews.org

AIDS Education Global Information System
32302 Alipaz St., #267
P.O. Box 184
San Juan Capistrano, CA
92693-0184
Phone: 949-495-1952
Fax: 949-443-1755
Website: www.aegis.org
E-mail: help@aegis.org

AIDS Healthcare Foundation
6255 W. Sunset Blvd.
21st Fl.
Los Angeles, CA 90028
Phone: 323-860-5200
Website: www.aidshealth.org
E-mail: mprsupport@aidshealth.
org

American Cancer Society
250 Williams St. N.W.
Atlanta, GA 30303
Toll-Free: 800-227-2345
TTY: 800-735-2991
Website: www.cancer.org
E-mail: grants@cancer.org

American Foundation for AIDS Research
120 Wall St., 13th Fl.
New York, NY 10005-3908
Phone: 212-806-1600
Fax: 212-806-1601
Website: www.amfar.org
E-mail: information@amfar.org

American Medical Association
515 N. State St.
Chicago, IL 60654
Toll-Free: 800-621-8335
Website: www.ama-assn.org
E-mail: haley.guion@ama-assn.org

American Social Health Association
P.O. Box 13827
Research Triangle Park, NC 27709
Phone: 919-361-8400
Fax: 919-361-8425
Website: www.ashastd.org
E-mail: info@ashastd.org

American Society for Colposcopy and Cervical Pathology
152 W. Washington St.
Hagerstown, MD 21740
Toll-Free: 800-787-7227
Phone: 301-733-3640
Fax: 301-733-5775
Website: www.asccp.org
E-mail: info@asccp.org

American Society of Reproductive Medicine
1209 Montgomery Hwy
Birmingham, AL 35216-2809
Phone: 205-978-5000
Fax: 205-978-5005
Website: www.asrm.org
E-mail: asrm@asrm.org

Association of Reproductive Health Professionals
1901 L St. N.W., Ste. 300
Washington, DC 20036
Phone: 202-466-3825
Website: www.arhp.org
E-mail: ARHP@arhp.org

The Body
250 W. 57th St.
New York, NY 10107
Website: www.thebody.com

Cleveland Clinic
9500 Euclid Ave.
Cleveland, OH 44195
Toll-Free: 800-223-CARE
(800-223-2273)
Phone: 216-636-5860
TTY: 216-444-0261
Website: www.my.clevelandclinic.org
E-mail: CirjakE@ccf.org.

631

Engender Health
440 Ninth Ave.
New York, NY 10001
Phone: 212-561-8000
Website: www.engenderhealth.
org
E-mail: info@engenderhealth.org

Foundation for Women's Cancer
230 W. Monroe
Ste. 2528
Chicago, IL 60606
Toll-Free: 800-444-4441
Phone: 312-578-1439
Fax: 312-578-9769
Website: www.
foundationforwomenscancer.org
E-mail: info@
foundationforwomenscancer.org

Gay and Lesbian Medical Association
1326 18th St. N.W.
Ste. 22
Washington, DC 20036
Phone: 202-600-8037
Fax: 202-478-1500
Website: www.glma.org
E-mail: info@glma.org

Gay Men's Health Crisis
446 W. 33rd St.
New York, NY 10001-2601
Phone: 212-367-1000
Website: www.gmhc.org
E-mail: hotline@gmhc.org

Elizabeth Glaser Pediatric AIDS Foundation
1140 Connecticut Ave. N.W.
Ste. 200
Washington, DC 20036
Phone: 202-296-9165
Fax: 202-296-9185
Website: www.pedaids.org
E-mail: info@pedaids.org

Go Ask Alice!
Alfred Lerner Hall, 8th Fl.
2920 Broadway, Mail Code 2606
New York, NY 10027
Phone: 212-854-5453
Fax: 212-854-8949
Website: www.goaskalice.
columbia.edu
E-mail: alice@columbia.edu

Guttmacher Institute
125 Maiden Ln., 7th Fl.
New York, NY 10038
Toll-Free: 800-355-0244
Phone: 212-248-1111
Fax: 212-248-1951
Website: www.guttmacher.org
E-mail: media@guttmacher.org

Hepatitis B Foundation
3805 Old Easton Rd.
Doylestown, PA 18902
Phone: 215-489-4900
Fax: 215-489-4920
Website: www.hepb.org
E-mail: contact@hepb.org

*Hepatitis Foundation
International*
504 Blick Dr.
Silver Spring, MD 20904
Toll-Free: 800-891-0707
Phone: 301-622-4200
Fax: 301-622-4702
Website: www.hepfi.org
E-mail: info@
hepatitisfoundation.org

HIV InSite
4150 Clement St.
Box 111V
San Francisco, CA 94121
Fax: 415-379-5547
Website: www.hivinsite.ucsf.edu
E-mail: hivinsite@ucsf.edu

*Immunization Action
Coalition*
1573 Selby Ave.
Ste. 234
St. Paul, MN 55104
Phone: 651-647-9009
Fax: 651-647-9131
Website: www.immunize.org
E-mail: admin@immunize.org

iwantthekit.org
Toll-Free: 866-575-5504
Phone: 410-502-0764
Website: www.iwantthekit.org
E-mail: iwantthekit@jhmi.edu

Kaiser Family Foundation
2400 Sand Hill Rd.
Menlo Park, CA 94025
Phone: 650-854-9400
Fax: 650-854-4800
Website: www.kff.org
E-mail: cpalosky@kff.org

*National Coalition for LGBT
Health*
1325 Massachusetts Ave. N.W.
Ste. 705
Washington, DC 20005
Phone: 202-558-6828
Website: www.lgbthealth.net
E-mail: coalition@lgbthealth.net

*National Cervical Cancer
Coalition*
P.O. Box 13827
Research Triangle Park
NC 27709
Toll-Free: 800-685-5531
Fax: 919-361-8425
Website: www.nccc-online.org
E-mail: nccc@ashastd.org

*Nemours Foundation Center
for Children's Health Media*
1600 Rockland Rd.
Wilmington, DE 19803
Phone: 302-651-4000
Website: www.kidshealth.org
E-mail: info@kidshealth.org

Planned Parenthood
434 W. 33rd St.
New York, NY 10001
Toll-Free: 800-230-PLAN
(800-230-7526)
Phone: 212-541-7800
Fax: 212-245-1845
Website: www.
plannedparenthood.org
E-mail: info@ppnyc.org

POZ Magazine
462 Seventh Ave.
19th Fl.
New York, NY 10018-7424
Phone: 212-242-2163
Fax: 212-675-8505
Website: www.poz.com
E-mail: website@poz.com

Project Inform
273 Ninth St.
San Francisco, CA 94103
Toll-Free: 877-HELP-4-HEP
(877-435-7443)
Phone: 415-558-8669
Fax: 415-558-0684
Website: www.projectinform.org
E-mail: info@help4hep.org

Sexuality Information and Education Council of the United States
90 John St.
Ste. 402
New York, NY 10038
Phone: 212-819-9770
Fax: 212-819-9776
Website: www.siecus.org
E-mail: kromines@siecus.org

Women Alive
85 W. Burnside Ave.
Los Angeles, CA 90019
Phone: 323-292-1564
Fax: 323-292-9886
Website: www.women-alive.org
E-mail: info@women-alive.org

Index

Index